W9-BMC-360

Exercise and the Heart in Health and Disease

FUNDAMENTAL AND CLINICAL CARDIOLOGY

Series Editor

Samuel Z. Goldhaber, M.D.

Cardiovascular Division
Department of Medicine
Harvard Medical School
and Brigham and Women's Hospital
Boston, Massachusetts

Exercise and the Heart in Health and Disease

edited by

Roy J. Shephard
University of Toronto
Toronto, Ontario, Canada

Henry S. Miller, Jr.
Wake Forest University
Winston-Salem, North Carolina

Marcel Dekker, Inc.   New York • Basel • Hong Kong

Library of Congress Cataloging-in-Publication Data

Exercise and the heart in health and cardiac disease / [edited by] Roy
J. Shephard, Henry S. Miller, Jr.
     p.   cm. - (Fundamental and clinical cardiology ; v. 6)
  Includes bibliographical references and index.
  ISBN 0-8247-8633-5 (alk. paper)
  1. Exercise.   2. Exercise therapy.   3. Heart-Diseases-Exercise
therapy. I. Shephard, Roy J. II. Miller Jr., Henry S.   III. Series
    [DNLM: 1. Exercise.   2. Heart Diseases-prevention & control.
  3. Heart Diseases-rehabilitation.   W1 FU538TD v.6]
  QP301.E938   1992
  613.7'1-dc20
  DNLM/DLC
  for Library of Congress   92-4531
                                                                   CIP

This book is printed on acid-free paper.

Copyright © 1992 by MARCEL DEKKER, INC. All Rights Reserved

Neither this book nor any part may be reproduced or transmitted in any form or
by any means, electronic or mechanical, including photocopying, microfilming,
and recording, or by any information storage and retrieval system, without permission in writing from the publisher.

MARCEL DEKKER, INC.
270 Madison Avenue, New York, New York 10016

Current printing (last digit):
10 9 8 7 6 5 4 3 2 1

PRINTED IN THE UNITED STATES OF AMERICA

Series Introduction

Marcel Dekker, Inc., has focused on the development of various series of beautifully produced books in different branches of medicine. These series have facilitated the integration of rapidly advancing information for both the clinical specialist and the researcher.

In this new series, Fundamental and Clinical Cardiology, my goal as Series Editor is to assemble the talents of world-renowned authorities to discuss virtually every area of cardiovascular medicine. In the current monograph, Drs. Shephard and Miller have edited a much needed and timely book, *Exercise and the Heart in Health and Disease*. Future contributions to this series will include books on molecular biology, interventional cardiology, and clinical management of problems such as coronary artery disease and ventricular arrhythmias.

Samuel Z. Goldhaber

Preface

The last few years have seen an ever-growing interest in exercise as a means to health, particularly cardiac health, with enthusiastic participation not only by clinically healthy individuals of all ages, but also by patients with various types of cardiac disorders. Patients have even completed marathon runs after both myocardial infarction and cardiac transplant operations.

Surprisingly, the scientific evidence supporting adoption of an active lifestyle remains relatively incomplete. Secondary rehabilitation (the promotion of exercise for the clinically healthy middle-aged adult who undoubtedly has some occult atherosclerotic lesions of the coronary vessels) is based not on direct experiment, but rather on a number of epidemiological studies, the majority of which have demonstrated a low incidence of myocardial infarction in populations presumed to be physically active. Tertiary rehabilitation (the cardiac rehabilitation programs offered after myocardial infarction) has been tested by prospective experiments in which patients have been randomly assigned to either exercise or control groups, but again, individual studies of 300–700 patients have not been large enough to demonstrate a statistically significant improvement of prognosis in the exercised group. Recourse has been made to a pooling of data (the somewhat dubious approach of metanalysis) to show a relatively uniform 20–30 percent decrease of mortality in exercised patients.

Most authorities would now accept that exercise is beneficial at all ages, not only for the clinically healthy person, but for the majority of patients who have various cardiac disorders. However, to date, exercise has been accepted as a generic phenomenon, ignoring such fundamental factors as the frequency, duration, intensity and type of physical activity and environmental factors. If a little exercise is good, is more better? Does it matter whether the exercise is aerobic or anaerobic? Can strength work be substituted for a rhythmic workout? Is safety equal for the regular exerciser and for the occasional weekend athlete? How should the prescription be modified to accommodate the young, the middle-aged, the elderly, and those with established cardiac disease? What benefits may be anticipated from exercise? Are these all yielded by the same pattern of exercise?

These are some of the questions to which we have sought answers from a worldwide panel of experts.

Roy J. Shephard
Henry S. Miller, Jr.

Contents

Contributors

Gary J. Balady, M.D. Associate Professor of Medicine, Section of Cardiology, Boston University School of Medicine, and Director, Cardiovascular Exercise Center and Cardiac Rehabilitation, The University Hospital, Boston, Massachusetts

David S. Braden, M.D. Pediatric Cardiologist, Department of Pediatrics, Portsmouth Naval Hospital, Portsmouth, Virginia

Carl Foster, Ph.D. Director, Cardiac Rehabilitation and Exercise Testing, Cardiovascular Disease Section, University of Wisconsin Medical School, Sinai Samaritan Medical Center, Milwaukee, Wisconsin

Roger M. Glaser, Ph.D., FACSM Director, Institute for Rehabilitation Research and Medicine, and Professor, Department of Physiology and Biophysics, Wright State University School of Medicine, Dayton, Ohio

Jack Goodman, B.P.H.E., M.Sc., Ph.D. Assistant Professor, School of Physical and Health Education, University of Toronto, Toronto, Ontario, Canada

Terence Kavanagh, M.D.   Associate Professor, Department of Rehabilitation Medicine, and Medical Director, Toronto Rehabilitation Centre, University of Toronto, Toronto, Ontario, Canada

Arthur S. Leon, M.S., M.D.   Henry L. Taylor Professor of Exercise Science and Health Enhancement, Division of Kinesiology, College of Education; Division of Epidemiology, School of Public Health; and Section of Cardiology, Department of Medicine, the Medical School at the University of Minnesota, Minneapolis, Minnesota

Henry S. Miller, Jr., M.D.   Professor of Internal Medicine/ Cardiology, and Medical Director, Cardiac Rehabilitation Program, Section of Cardiology, Department of Medicine, Bowman Gray School of Medicine, Wake Forest University, Winston-Salem, North Carolina

Deborah Morley, Ph.D.   Research Assistant Professor, Section of Cardiology, Department of Medicine, Temple University School of Medicine, Philadelphia, Pennsylvania

Ralph S. Paffenbarger, Jr., M.D.   Professor of Epidemiology, Division of Epidemiology, Department of Health Research and Policy, Stanford University School of Medicine, Stanford, California

Roy J. Shephard, M.D., Ph.D., D.P.E.   Professor of Applied Physiology, Department of Preventive Medicine and Biostatistics, School of Physical and Health Education, University of Toronto, Toronto, Ontario, Canada

L. Kent Smith, M.D., M.P.H.   Director, Drug Research and Cardiac Rehabilitation, Arizona Heart Institute, Phoenix, Arizona

William B. Strong, M.D.   Professor and Chief of Pediatric Cardiology, Department of Pediatrics, Medical College of Georgia, and Director, Georgia Prevention Institute, Augusta, Georgia

Hoshedar P. Tamboli, M.B.B.S.   Cardiovascular Disease Section, Department of Medicine, University of Wisconsin Medical School, Sinai Samaritan Medical Center, Milwaukee, Wisconsin

Nanette Kass Wenger, M.D.   Professor of Medicine (Cardiology), Department of Medicine, Emory University School of Medicine, Atlanta, Georgia

Linda D. Zwiren, Ed.D., FACSM Professor, Department of Health and Physical Education, and Department of Biology, Hofstra University, Hempstead, New York

Exercise and the Heart in Health and Disease

1

Physiological, Biochemical, and Psychological Responses to Exercise

Roy J. Shephard

University of Toronto
Toronto, Ontario, Canada

INTRODUCTION

In this first chapter, we shall explore in general terms the various factors determining physiological, biochemical, and psychological responses to exercise at all ages, in both health and disease. The term *exercise* will first be defined. Acute responses to exercise will then be distinguished from the more chronic reactions of training, and we shall examine the influence of intensity, duration, and frequency of activity on the training response. We will consider also variations in training response with the type of exercise that is adopted and with environmental differences, and we shall then briefly summarize the postulated medical and psychological health benefits of a regular exercise regimen. A final section will discuss the strengths and weaknesses of current evidence concerning these postulated benefits.

DEFINITIONS OF EXERCISE, PHYSICAL FITNESS, AND SPORT EXERCISE

Exercise implies, strictly speaking, the voluntary performance of one or more bouts of physical activity with the deliberate intention of improving some aspect of health (22).

Physical Fitness

An increase of physical fitness is the normal consequence of regularly repeated bouts of exercise. Nevertheless, a fair part of the variance in most physiological indices of fitness is attributable to a combination of social and genetic inheritance rather than the patterns of habitual exercise that the individual has adopted in recent months (100,122, 123,154).

Sport

Sport may be considered as a particular variant of exercise, where the primary motive for participation is found in such factors as the excitement of competition, the thrills of rapid body movement, or an increase of opportunities for social contacts (91) rather than an improvement of health.

Physical Activity

Physical activity encompasses all forms of movement, whether undertaken voluntarily (exercise and sport) or unavoidably (the performance of occupational and domestic chores). In the past, a substantial part of the total daily physical activity of most adults was attributable to occupational and domestic responsibilities, but with current trends to mechanization and automation in developed societies, humans must turn increasingly to their leisure time if they are to engage in sufficient physical activity either to develop or to sustain their physical condition (106).

ACUTE AND CHRONIC RESPONSES TO EXERCISE

Acute Responses

Duration

The duration of an acute bout of exercise can vary from less than 10 s (as in a 50-m dash), to an athletic event lasting 24 h or more (for example, a 100-km run). The responses of the body show a corresponding gradation. Although the average intensity of effort is usually higher during a brief event, the disturbance of normal physiological, biochemical, and psychological functions is more profound and more long-lasting with a sustained, 24-h bout of physical activity (Table 1).

Very Brief Exercise. Physiological reactions to a very brief (5–10 s) and exhausting bout of physical activity are limited largely to a depletion of

Table 1   Factors Limiting Exercise in Relation to the Duration of Activity

0–10 s	10–60 s	1–60 min	60–120 min	2–5 h	>5 h
← Motivation, release of inhibition, arousal →					
Anerobic power	Anerobic capacity	$\dot{V}O_{2\,max}$	Fluid and mineral loss	Glycogen stores	Fat mobilization
Reaction time	Strength	Strength	Heat elimination	Fluid and mineral loss	Fat stores
Strength	Skill		$\dot{V}O_{2\,max}$	Heat elimination	Food intake
Skill				Fat mobilization	Protein reserves
Flexibility				$\dot{V}O_{2\,max}$	Bone and joint strength

Source: From Ref. 156, used with permission.

anaerobic energy reserves (adenosine triphosphate and creatine phosphate) within the active muscles. These "phosphagen stores" are rapidly replenished after cessation of exercise, the half-time of the recuperative process averaging 22 s (34).

Brief Exercise.   If the exercise bout continues for somewhat longer (1–2 min), there is then a substantial accumulation of lactic acid in the active tissues. The intramuscular concentration of lactate may rise as high as 30 mM/L at exhaustion (68). The blood lactate also rises over the course of brief exhausting exercise, typically to a limiting value of 10–12 mM/L (154,156), and there is an associated feeling of muscle weakness, with vigorous hyperventilation.

Endurance Exercise.   If the period of all-out physical activity is further extended to that of an endurance event (a total of 5–10 min), the exerciser usually develops a plateau of oxygen intake (the peak oxygen intake for the task, 10–12 times the resting oxygen consumption in a young adult who is engaged in a "large muscle" exercise such as running on a treadmill or pedaling a cycle ergometer [154]).

Associated with this aerobic response, there is a large increase of cardiac output (from the resting value of 5–6 L/min to a maximum of 25–30 L/min in a young man) and an even greater augmentation of respiratory minute volume (156). If the intensity of effort is such that the rate of accumulation of lactate in the bloodstream exceeds its rate of clearance (the so-called anaerobic threshold, around 70% of maximal oxygen intake [189]), then the ventilation becomes disproportionate to oxygen consumption.

There are also increments of blood catecholamine levels (187) (larger for exciting sports than for equivalent intensities of laboratory exercise on a cycle ergometer [15]).

Sustained Aerobic Exercise.   If the exercise is continued yet longer (20–30 min), there are changes in the blood levels of many hormones. For instance, there is an increased output of cortisol (an index of stress), growth hormone (probably to facilitate fat mobilization [165,168]), and the hormones concerned with mineral and fluid balance (157,158).

The local temperature within the active tissues rises by 1–2°C over the first 5 min of exercise, whereas the core temperature of the body tends to stabilize at a level 1–4°C above the resting value over 15–30 min of vigorous physical activity (6). Sweating is induced with a lag of a few minutes relative to the onset of exercise. Under adverse conditions, a vigorous bout of physical activity can stimulate a flow of up to 2 L of sweat/h (1); the corresponding tendency to depletion of fluid and mineral reserves (156) is partially offset by the liberation of "bound" water, as glycogen is metabolized.

Prolonged Exercise.   Muscle glycogen stores vary with the extent of training that has been undertaken and with the recent diet of the individual (78a). In the average adult, carbohydrate reserves can be exhausted by about 100 min of exercise at 75% of maximum oxygen intake (the typical intensity adopted in prolonged bouts of an aerobic pursuit such as cross-country skiing, [141]).

Exercise bouts of 1 h and longer also tend to cause a secretion of β-endorphins, with a corresponding elevation of mood (65,132).

If the exercise bout is both prolonged and intense, it may cause a leakage of key proteins from the active skeletal muscles (and to a lesser extent from the myocardium). Such leakage is readily detected as increases in the serum concentrations of creatine kinase and lactate dehydrogenase. This response needs to be distinguished carefully from the increased serum enzyme levels that accompany myocardial infarction, for instance by a study of isozyme patterns, or the use of more specific markers of cardiac damage such as an increased blood level of cardiac troponin (29).

Psychological Reactions.   The immediate psychological response to a bout of vigorous exercise is generally an increase of arousal (102,200). If the exerciser initially feels bored or depressed, then exercise may relieve such sensations, and indeed many individuals make the comment that they exercise to "feel better" (158). On the other hand, if a person is initially anxious or overaroused, then the acute effect of a bout of activity may be to increase such anxiety.

Whether exercise serves to increase or to decrease an individual's anxiety depends very much upon its ambience. If relaxation is an important goal, then a walk in the country may be a much more effective remedy than a vigorous game of squash with the employer (161). Those interested in the psychological benefits of exercise are increasingly commending moderate rather than all-out effort.

Because of immediate arousal, if vigorous exercise is taken too close to the time of retiring at night, it may cause a loss of sleep (188). On the other hand, if moderate exercise is taken earlier in the evening, it appears to facilitate sleep, enhancing the important slow-wave component of the electroencephalogram (36).

Chronic Responses

Effects of Training

If a subject repeats a given bout of exercise on a regular basis, as in a normal training regimen, the body undergoes a progressive adaptation to the particular pattern of stress that has been imposed. Among functional consequences are: (a) the ability to undertake that particular form of activity is increased (that is, a higher peak rate of working becomes possible), (b) the disturbance of body function associated with a given intensity and duration of that form of physical activity is progressively reduced, and (c) the rate of recovery following a given bout of exercise is speeded (153).

Specificity of Training

The adaptation of body function tends to be relatively specific to the type of training that has been practiced. For example, there is little cross-transfer between cardiorespiratory and muscular types of training (indeed, very vigorous cardio-respiratory training may impede muscular development). Likewise, endurance training of the arm muscles has little beneficial effect upon performance when the subject is using the legs (99), although some 50% of the training effects developed by regular leg exercise can be transferred to the subsequent performance of work by the arms (27).

Habituation and Learning

The earliest adaptations to repeated bouts of exercise are cerebral in type, arising largely in the prefrontal cortex (51). Over the first few days, the body in essence becomes "habituated" to a particular exercise situation, so that performance of what is becoming a familiar task induces less arousal (151).

There is a parallel decrease in such physiological markers of arousal as the increment of heart rate and the rise of blood pressure observed at a given intensity of effort.

Learning of the task also makes it more automatic. Control is transferred from the motor cortex to the cerebellum, and there is a mechanically more efficient performance, with a corresponding decrease in the loading of the cardiorespiratory system.

Functional Adjustments

The next group of training responses are functional in type—for instance, the total blood volume and the tone of the peripheral veins are both increased by habitual physical activity, so that the stroke volume is better sustained during vigorous effort, and the peak cardiac output is augmented (77).

At the same time, the distribution of the available blood flow becomes more effective from the viewpoint of performing physical work, so that the maximum arteriovenous oxygen difference is increased (83). In a trained individual, the circulation to the inactive tissues shows a greater than normal reduction during the exercise bout, whereas there is an increase of flow to the active tissues (and to the skin in a hot climate) (135,136,171,172). In consequence, the maximum arteriovenous oxygen difference is larger than in an untrained person (83,171,172).

The muscles also appear stronger after training. This reflects an increased synchronization of neural firing, the mobilization of an increased fraction of the total motoneuron pool, and possibly a greater relaxation of antagonists (45). There are quite rapid increases of enzyme concentrations in the active muscles as training continues. However, the precise balance of change between aerobic and anaerobic enzyme systems is somewhat specific to the type of exercise that has been pursued (56,76).

Structural Changes

If the training is both protracted and vigorous, there are eventual structural adaptations. If the emphasis has been upon endurance training, there may be a progressive hypertrophy of the left ventricular wall (28,73,94,137); this reduces unit work per sarcomere in the ventricular wall (63), facilitating maintenance of the cardiac stroke volume at high work rates (178) and thus the development of a large maximum cardiac output. There may also be some increases in the dimensions of either the coronary arteries or the collateral blood supply (75,86,182), with an increase in the ventricular fibrillation threshold (112).

Likewise, a strengthening of the respiratory muscles allows the subject to develop and sustain a larger maximum voluntary ventilation (130).

If the emphasis of the training regimen has been upon isometric and isotonic muscle-building exercises, there will be an increase of muscle bulk in those body parts that have been active (45). In consequence, a given task can be performed at a smaller fraction of maximum muscle force, with a smaller rise of blood pressure, and less danger for the cardiovascular system.

A further consequence of repeated, prolonged, moderate bouts of activity will be a progressive replacement of fat by lean tissue (163,170), sometimes without any net change of body mass. The flexibility of the exercised joints is increased, tendons and articular cartilages are strengthened (103), and the density of weight-bearing bones is increased (25,176,193).

In general, hormonal reactions to a given intensity of exercise are reduced after training. For instance, there is a lesser secretion of catecholamines at any given rate of working (187). A given bout of exercise is usually perceived as less stressful (19), and depending upon initial reactions, there may be an increase or a decrease in the secretion of cortisol (165).

At any given intensity of effort, the tendency to tissue damage is also reduced with training, and in consequence there is a lesser release of enzymes such as creative kinase (CK) and lactic dehydrogenase (LDH) into the circulation (5).

Psychological Responses

Psychological responses to a training program vary very much with the initial status of the individual. If the exerciser initially had a well-balanced personality, then little change of mood state is likely despite repeated bouts of exercise. However, in those individuals who are initially anxious or depressed (for instance, as a consequence of a recent myocardial infarction), restoration of a more normal mood state is apparently helped by regular participation in an endurance training program (87). Perhaps because of the mood changes induced by a secretion of endorphins, there is some evidence that people can become addicted to prolonged bouts of aerobic exercise (140).

Time Course

The time course of the various physiological, biochemical, and psychological adaptations to the onset or cessation of habitual exercise varies with the health of the individual, the pattern of the chosen training regimen (a progressively increasing load, or a fixed intensity program), and the precise intensity of training that has been adopted.

Much of the advantage of physical condition normally enjoyed by an endurance athlete is lost as a consequence of 2–3 weeks of enforced bedrest (144,179). Conversely, most of the physical condition that has been lost over several weeks of bedrest can be regained over a few weeks of renewed training (144) (Fig 1). Hickson and associates (72)

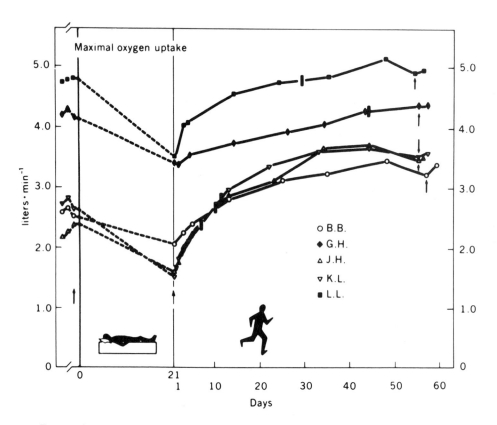

Figure 1   Decrease of maximal oxygen intake over 21 days of bedrest and time course of recovery with resumption of training. Data for three sedentary and two active young men. (From Saltin, B., Blomqvist, B., Mitchell, J. H., Johnson, R. L., Wildenthal, K., and Chapman, C. B., Response to submaximal and maximal exercise after bed rest and training. *Circulation, 38* (Suppl. 7): 1–68, used with permission.)

suggested that the half-time of response for one specific component of physical fitness (the maximum oxygen intake) was as little as 10 days, given exposure of the subjects to a constant training stimulus. However, critics of this work have pointed out that the normal training plan involves a progressive increase of both intensity and duration of effort (85).

Given a progressive training plan, healthy 65-year-old subjects are still able to make quite large gains in their maximal oxygen intake over as little as 7 weeks of training (169). On the other hand, a person who has sustained a myocardial infarction finds difficulty in exercising hard during the first few months following the clinical incident. In such patients (Fig. 2), the early training responses involve the peripheral rather than the central circulation (121), although after some 12 months of exercise at progressively higher intensities, some increase of cardiac stroke volume is eventually seen (61,121). The increase of maximal oxygen intake in "postcoronary" patients can continue slowly over several years, provided that they are following a progressive exercise program (155).

Not all elements of the body's response change in parallel. For instance, Saltin (142) drew attention to a discrepancy between the concentrations of tissue enzymes (which usually change rapidly, over 7–10 days of training or detraining [71]) and the increments of maximal oxy-

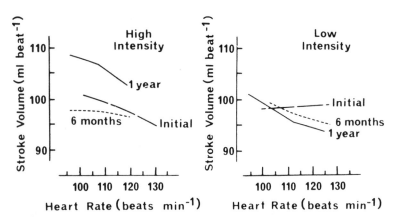

Figure 2 Influence of progressive endurance training on cardiac stroke volume. Data obtained on postcoronary patients following high-intensity or low-intensity exercise program for 6 and 12 months (From Ref. 121; used with permission.)

gen intake (which may continue over the course of many weeks, if not months). In Saltin's view, the difference of time course is good evidence that the increase of maximal oxygen intake reflects central changes (particularly an increase of maximal cardiac output) rather than peripheral adaptations (an increased extraction of oxygen, associated with an enhanced local activity of enzymes in the active tissues). Smith and O'Donnell (175) also suggested that changes in anaerobic threshold developed faster than gains of maximal oxygen intake, which in turn was modified more rapidly than the heart rate response to submaximum exercise. In contrast, Rogers et al. (131) noted an improvement of submaximal responses before gains in maximal oxygen intake. Possibly, such differences reflect differences in the type or intensity of training.

The time course of the psychological changes is known less precisely than that for the physiological and biochemical responses to training, since the tests of mood state which are currently available do not lend themselves to frequent repetition. However, we have observed substantial improvements of affect in postcoronary patients over the course of a year of progressive training (187).

Effects of Intensity, Frequency, and Duration of Exercise

The response to a training program is influenced by the intensity, frequency, and duration of the prescribed effort relative to the initial fitness of the individual. Other potential variables are the age of the individual, fiber composition (those with a high proportion of slow-twitch fibers are more susceptible to endurance training [139]), and other interindividual constitutional differences yet to be clarified.

Intensity

Need to Define Threshold. Whether the intent has been to develop the cardiorespiratory performance or to enhance the muscular strength of an individual, much of the literature on training has been built around the concept that a critical threshold intensity of exercise must be reached in order to initiate a training response.

Definition of an appropriate intensity of exercise training has physiological, biochemical, and psychological implications. It has been regarded as important by both the busy executive (who wishes to minimize personal investment of both time and effort in exercise) and by the international athlete (who wishes to maximize the training response, without causing "staleness" or the tissue damage associated with "overtraining").

It has further been assumed that as a person becomes older, or is adversely affected by some chronic disease process, the margin between an effective and a dangerously intensive exercise program becomes narrower, with a corresponding need for greater sophistication in the prescription of exercise.

Need for Overloading. In physiological terms, some overloading of the body systems must occur if there is to be a training response. For instance, if exercise is performed in an upright posture, cardiac stroke volume is not maximized until at least 50% of maximal oxygen intake is developed (8,40,171,172), (Table 2). The accompanying rise of systolic blood pressure (which offers an afterload to the ventricular muscle) is proportional to both the intensity of effort and its duration.

There have been occasional suggestions that prolonged and intensive cardiovascular effort may cause both cardiac fatigue and pulmonary edema even in a healthy young adult, but in general, a small excess of preloading or afterloading is not critical. On the other hand, an excessive rise of systolic pressure in a patient with coronary atherosclerosis can provoke myocardial ischemia, ventricular fibrillation, and even cardiac failure (120,155). Likewise, heavy preloading can provoke decompensation in a patient with a tendency to congestive heart failure. In skeletal muscle, also, it is necessary to develop an increase of tension for hypertrophy to occur (185), but an excessive loading can give rise to microscopic or gross muscular damage.

At the cellular level, the hypertrophy of skeletal and cardiac muscle is dependent upon changes in both membrane permeability and the rate of protein transcription. Booth and Watson (18) found that in

Table 2 Cardiovascular Responses to Arm (A) and to Leg (L) Exercise

Oxygen consumption ($L\ min^{-1}$ STPD)	Stroke volume (ml)		Heart rate (beats min^{-1})		Cardiac output ($L\ min^{-1}$)		Arteriovenous oxygen difference (ml/L)	
	A	L	A	L	A	L	A	L
1.5	96	125	132	96	12.3	13.2	123	120
2.0	101	131	155	117	14.9	15.9	133	127
2.5	108	138	174	142	18.5	18.5	139	135
Maximum (2.79, A; 3.70, L)	103	138	178	179	18.3	24.7	144	150

Source: From Ref. 172, used with permission.
Note that in both forms of activity, the stroke volume of the heart shows a small increase to more than 50% of the task-specific peak oxygen intake.

rats muscle protein synthesis was decresed over the first 30 min of exercise, but by 7 h there was an increase in the net rate of protein formation. Potential triggers to the increased protein synthesis include an increased intracellular concentration of amino acids brought about by a tension-induced degradation of protein, an increased influx of amino acids via the stretched sarcolemma of the loaded muscle, and an impact of decreasing intracellular adenosine triphosphate (ATP) and pH levels upon Ca^{2+}-mediated stimulation of ribonucleic acid (RNA) transcription (18). Plainly, there is scope for overintensive exercise to induce both local hypoxia and excessive changes of membrane permeability, with a leakage of vital cellular constituents into the extracellular space, and the development of frank microtraumas (10,29).

From a psychological perspective, a moderate overload is again desirable. The subject must in essence regard the intensity of effort as appropriate to personal training goals. Recruits will sometimes drop out of exercise classes, either because they are perceived as lacking sufficient challenge, or because the required program seems beyond the capacity of the participant.

Cardiovascular Threshold. The concept of a cardiovascular training threshold is commonly attributed to Karvonen et al. (82). The Helsinki-based investigators studied the training responses of a single population of young adults (male medical students). In some of the students, the required speed of running was such as to yield an average heart rate of 135 beats/min at the end of exercise sessions. In this group, no training occurred. A second group of students were exercised more vigorously, reaching a final heart rate in the range 160–180 beats/min. In the case of the more vigorously exercised individuals, the training response was such that it was found necessary to increase the treadmill speed by 25–30% over a 4-week period in order to maintain a consistent exercise heart rate.

Subsequent authors have sought to apply the findings of Karvonen et al. (82) to subjects of all ages, regardless of their initial physical condition. Some investigators have interpreted the cardiorespiratory training threshold as lying at 60% of the difference between resting and maximum heart rates (a figure of 145 beats/min in a young adult), others have suggested that Karvonen and associates demonstrated a threshold at 60% of maximum oxygen intake (a heart rate of about 135 beats/min in a young adult), and a few authors have even spoken of the cardiovascular threshold as lying at 60% of maximum heart rate (a figure of about 117 beats/min). In fact, the Finnish studies did not define any precise and universally generalizable threshold, although it was shown that if the stimulus was a relatively brief period of treadmill exercise, a cardiovascular training response occurred at a heart rate of 170 beats/min, but not at 135 beats/min.

If there is indeed a precise intensity threshold for cardiorespiratory training, its location is probably modified by both the initial fitness of the individual and by the duration of the activity. Certainly, there are circumstances where training can occur at exercise heart rates of less than 160–180 beats/min. Thus Bouchard et al. (20) apparently produced some cardiovascular training by having their subjects perform cycle ergometer exercise at a heart rate of 130 beats/min for no more than 10 min per day. Likewise, Durnin et al. (38) reported substantial improvement in the endurance fitness of young soldiers who were required to march 10–30 km/day at heart rates which are unlikely to have exceeded 120 beats/min.

Oja (118) maintained that physiological responses to walking matched those obtained with a jogging regimen. One possible factor contributing to the effectiveness of walking programs for the middle aged and elderly is that fast walking is enough to carry most such individuals to 70% or more of their maximal oxygen intake (128). A further consideration is that a sedentary lifestyle has increased responsiveness to training. Restriction of recent activity is a particular feature of patients who have recently been hospitalized for myocardial infarction, and among such individuals there may be an initial training response to exercise heart rates as low as 110 beats/min (84).

In a series of treadmill experiments where young and healthy male subjects were randomly allocated to laboratory-controlled training regimens differing in intensity, frequency, and duration (150), a multiple regression analysis demonstrated that the most important determinant of the individual's adaptive response was the intensity of effort relative to their initial fitness (Fig. 3).

Subsequent experiments, mainly with university-age males, have not clarified the determinants of the cardiorespiratory training response greatly. Reports have claimed an effect of intensity (42), of intensity but not initial fitness (52), of both fitness and intensity (149), with the latter variable becoming insignificant after equating the total amount of work performed (148), of intensity despite equation of initial fitness and total amount of work performed (190), and of intensity and duration (32).

Wenger and Bell (191) further claimed that the impact of a training program continued to increase with intensity of exercise up to loads demanding 90–100% of maximal oxygen intake.

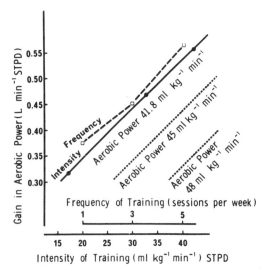

Figure 3 Factors influencing the training response of young men. The response to any given intensity of training varies inversely as the initial aerobic power of the group. If intensity and initial fitness are held constant, there is also a difference of response between one, three, and five training sessions per week (From Ref. 150; used with permission.)

The issues of initial physical condition and of training intensity are particularly critical when comparing the training response of young and elderly subjects. If the assessment of initial physical condition is based upon absolute figures rather than age-related standards, reactions may be compared (inappropriately) between a sedentary young adult and an extremely fit senior citizen. Likewise, if the intensity of training prescribed for a 65-year-old subject is equated with that of a young adult in terms of the absolute oxygen consumption developed during the required exercise program (145), then the stimulus applied to the older person is much greater, and in consequence they may be judged as having a better training response than a younger individual. However, if the comparison is based upon programs demanding an equivalent fraction of the individual's maximal oxygen intake, then the training response is seen to depend much less strongly upon the age of the participant (161a).

Current wisdom holds that an optimal intensity of training for cardiorespiratory (endurance) training lies at or just below a work rate where lactate begins to accumulate (the so-called anaerobic threshold). This amounts to 60–70% of personal maximal oxygen intake in most sedentary individuals, but may reach 75–80% of aerobic power in endurance competitors (2). An appropriate intensity of effort can be set for each individual in terms of a prescribed distance and pace (84,85). Alternatively, the subject may be instructed to count the pulse rate immediately following exercise (17), or to seek an intensity of exercise that initiates sweating (92) and is perceived as moderate while allowing a continuation of normal conversation (16,19,24).

Much higher intensities of training are tolerated with programs of brief interval training (for instance, 10- to 30-s bouts of activity, followed by 10- to 30-s recovery periods). By suitably adjusting the length of exercise and recovery phases, it is possible to use interval training as a means of enhancing the function of systems responsible for anaerobic power, anaerobic capacity, or aerobic power (7,39). For instance, training at intensities above the lactate threshold seems necessary in order to increase the lactate threshold (67). One possible method of training the anaerobic energy systems is to increase the effective body mass during exercise sessions; for example, by wearing a 9- to 10-kg vest while training (138). Brief interval training leads to an increase of both glycogen stores and alkaline reserve in the active limbs, with increased local concentrations of ATP, myoglobin, and possibly of glycolytic enzymes (156). More prolonged bouts of interval training (1-min bouts of exercise, followed by 1-min recovery periods) are particularly effective in enhancing the performance of patients when endurance activity would otherwise be halted by anginal pain (86a).

Muscle-Training Threshold.   The required intensity of effort has an influence upon the patterns of muscle fiber recruitment and thus the localization of training responses within the skeletal muscles. Moderate effort recruits predominantly the slow-twitch fibers, leading over the course of some weeks to a selective enhancement of their function, with an increased tolerance of fatiguing muscular activity. In particular, there is a training-induced increase in the size, the number, and the complexity of mitochondria within the active fibers, with a corresponding increase in the local activity of aerobic enzymes (76) (Fig 4). One effect is to encourage the metabolism of fat rather than glycogen during prolonged bouts of activity (157) (Fig 5). The cross-sectional area of the individual muscle fibers increases relatively little with this pattern of training.

More intensive resistance and isometric programs lead to a selective recruitment of fast-twitch (Type II) fibers, with hypertrophy (183) and sometimes a splitting of the individual Type II fibers (57). However, investigators have yet to substantiate a true hyperplasia, with the

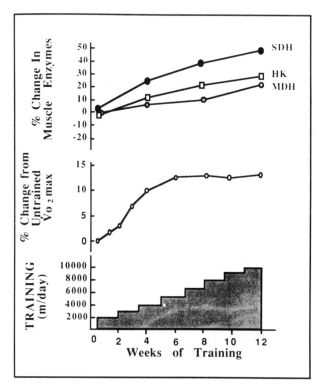

Figure 4 Changes in muscle enzyme activities and maximal oxygen intake in response to 12 weeks of swim-training. SDH, HK, and MDH signify succinate dehydrogenase, hexokinase, and malate dehydrogenase, respectively. (From Wilmore, J. H., and Costill, D. L., *Training for Sport and Activity*. 3rd Ed. W. C. Brown, Dubuque, Iowa (1988); used with permission.)

formation of new muscle fibers (180). Because of the increased amount of contractile protein within individual fibers, hypertrophy may lead to some diminution in the volume density of the muscle mitochondria (101). The acute cellular response to functional overload is a slowing of protein synthesis within the muscle sarcoplasm, but within 24 h supranormal rates of protein formation are observed. If the overload is too great, the muscles may become sore; there is then a disruption of connective tissue elements and an increase in the hydroxyproline/ creatine ratio for the tissue (184), while the mitochondria may also show evidence of damage, particularly a swelling and destruction of their cristae (5,10,44).

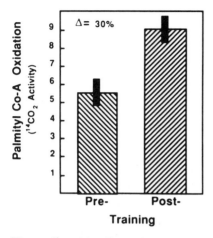

Figure 5 The effect of 8 weeks of endurance training upon the ability of skeletal muscle to oxidize fats. (From Wilmore, J. H., and Costill, D. L., *Training for Sport and Physical Activity*. 3rd Ed. W. C. Brown, Dubuque, Iowa; used with permission.)

Muscle training is usually associated with some change in the relative proportions of Type IIa (fast oxidative glycolytic) and Type IIb (fast glycolytic) fibers. Moreover, there is increasing evidence that high-intensity intermittent training may convert Type I (slow-twitch) fibers into type II (35,78,173,181).

The appropriate intensity of effort for muscle-building exercises is usually established in terms of the fraction of maximum voluntary force that must be exerted. For example, muscle endurance is developed by frequently repeated sets of contractions at a relatively low intensity such as 60% of maximum voluntary force, whereas strength is enhanced by high-intensity contractions with only a limited number of repetitions (4,59,64). However, during isometric effort there also appears to be an interaction between the intensity and the duration of contraction. Thus, Hettinger (70) observed a training response to maximum contractions which were held for 1–2 s, but if the intensity of effort was reduced to 67% of maximum force, then the minimal duration of contraction for a training response was 4–6 s; with a further prolongation of the contraction, a training response was observed at forces as low as 40–50% of maximum voluntary effort.

Psychological Threshold.   There is little objective information on an appropriate intensity of training from the viewpoint of inducing psychological gains. However, if the training program is to be perceived by the individual as achievable and yet effective, the optimum intensity is probably similar to that discussed in connection with physiological and biochemical gains. Most subjects perceive effort at the anaerobic threshold as moderately demanding.

Frequency.

Relation to Recovery Processes. The optimal frequency of a training program has physiological, biochemical, and psychological connotations which can be related to the anticipated time course of both acute exercise responses and the speed of recovery processes following an initial bout of exercise.

The on-transient has been discussed above. The likely speed of recovery varies with the type, intensity, and duration of activity that has been undertaken. Muscle phosphagen stores can be replenished extremely rapidly (34), allowing a second burst of activity which draws upon such stores within a few seconds of the first. Forms of interval training designed to train anaerobic power may thus allow recovery periods as short as 10–60 s (196).

If activity continues for sufficient time that lactate accumulates in the working muscles, local concentrations are substantially reduced over the first 15–30 min of recovery. Thus, if a local accumulation of lactic acid has been the main factor limiting an initial training session, a further bout of activity is possible on the same day. Such patterns of training tend to maximize anaerobic capacity.

On the other hand, the main concerns may be to allow a sufficient recovery period to permit an increase of protein synthesis and a restoration of glycogen reserves, together with the repair of any exercise-induced microtraumas. The person prescribing exercise must then recognize that glycogen stores peak as late as 2 days after a prolonged bout of exercise (143), while abnormal blood enzyme concentrations also persist for several days after a very strenuous bout of exercise (29). Thus, prolonged bouts of high-intensity exercise should either be limited to alternate days, or at most arranged as alternating "light" and "heavy" days of training.

Empirical Data. Some empirical data sets have demonstrated an increase of training response as the frequency of sessions is increased from one to five sessions per week (125,150,169), but other studies have not found this (11). One variable is probably the extent of overtraining that occurs in individual exercise sessions. There may also be some interindividual variation; thus Linden et al. (97) found that some subjects could maintain their physical condition by as little as two bouts of exercise per week, but others needed daily training. Moreover, it has been suggested that the effectiveness of an increase in the frequency of sessions is strongly related to a consequent increase in the total amount of exercise that is taken (74). Plainly, many of the processes involved in training, whether the increase of protein synthesis in the muscle sarcoplasm or the metabolism of excess body fat, must be related in a semiquantitative fashion to the number of times that a given stress is presented and/or the total quantity of work that is performed.

Psychological Considerations. The main psychological argument against recommending a low frequency of exercise (such as one or two sessions per week) is that the prescription is then easily forgotten by the patient. The intensity of individual bouts must also be increased in order to obtain the same response, with a danger that the participant will become excessively fatigued. In contrast, if sessions are incorporated into a daily routine (for instance, a regular walk to the bus or the subway station), they become much more automatic. Habit is an important determinant of both general and specific exercise behavior (53) (Fig 6).

At the opposite extreme, if the frequency of exercise sessions is perceived as excessively time consuming, then the subject may complain of staleness, fatigue, or boredom, and there is again a strong likelihood that the prescribed program will be abandoned. Psychological problems are particularly likely if the patient has pursued the activity to the point of excluding normal social contacts, if a further investment of time and effort does not appear to be yielding commensurate gains of physical condition, or if muscle soreness, pain, and injuries have resulted from excessively vigorous exercise.

The ideal program is thus sufficiently frequent to become habitual, but leaves the participant ample opportunity for other pursuits, and produces no more than a pleasant sensation of tiredness on the following day.

Duration. As with the frequency of repetitions, the duration of the individual exercise bout influences the impact of a given intensity of exercise upon training responses. However, because of the acute adaptive reactions which develop over a single, sustained bout of physical activity, two moderate-length bursts of exercise may induce a larger training response than a single bout of equivalent total duration.

This generalization is particularly true of neurological and psychological adaptations—for instance, the progressive decrease of exercise heart rate with habituation to a given form of physical activity

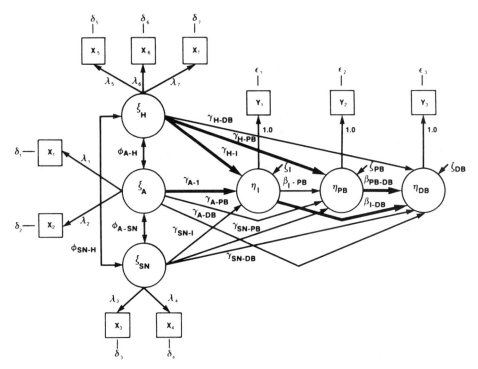

Figure 6 An empirical model illustrating the factors influencing exercise behavior. The technique of path analysis has been used to examine relationships between habit (H), attitude (A), subjective norms (SN), behavioral intention (I), proximal behavior (PB), and distal behavior (DB). The strongest correlations are indicated by heavy arrows. Thus, attitudes influence intention and distal behavior, while habits have a strong influence upon intention and proximal behavior. (From Godin, G., Valois, P., Shephard, R. J., and Desharnais, R., Prediction of leisure-time exercise behavior: A path analysis (Lisrel V) model. *J. Behav. Med.*, **10**: 145–158 (1987); used with permission.)

depends more upon the number of times the activity has been attempted than upon the duration of individual sessions.

If a primary intent of the prescribed program is to consume an excess of body fat, there is a roughly stoichimetric relationship between fat loss and the added energy cost of the exercise plus any subsequent postexercise stimulation of metabolism. However, prolonged bouts of exercise tend to induce a progressive increase in the metabolic response to a given rate of external working (23). Moreover, because more fat and less carbohydrate is metabolized during low-intensity effort, prolonged slow walking may be a more effective method of inducing fat loss than an apparently equivalent energy expenditure that is developed by short bursts of more intensive activity. Optimization of the blood lipid profile requires the covering of a total walking or jogging distance of at least 18–20 km/week (89,194) (Fig 7), again a measure of the quantity of exercise that is undertaken rather than frequency or duration of individual bouts.

On the other hand, some of the physiological reactions to over-load, for instance, the rise of blood pressure with sustained rhythmic or isometric exercise (96), are proportional to the duration of the activity. A short bout of vigorous activity may provide a very valuable training stimulus to both the cardiovascular system and the skeletal

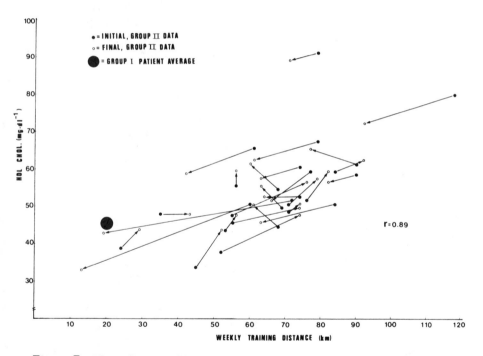

Figure 7 The influence of weekly jogging distance on serum levels of HDL-cholesterol. Data for postcoronary patients. Each line joins observations on a single subject over a period of 1 year. During this period, some subjects increased and some decreased their weekly jogging distance, generally with a corresponding change in HDL-cholesterol concentrations. The large circle indicates average values for patients content with a more modest exercise prescription (From Ref. 89; used with permission.)

muscles, but if the effort is more prolonged, it may give rise to acute manifestations of myocardial ischemia or strain of the skeletal muscles. Biochemical (29), humoral (93), and immunological (90) evidence of overstrain is associated particularly with very prolonged bouts of exercise, whereas the development of gross musculoskeletal injuries can also be correlated with attempts to cover more than a specific jogging distance per week (127). For the average middle-aged person, a useful ceiling of effort is probably a weekly fast walking or jogging distance of about 50 km; that is, 10 km/day, 5 days/week.

Empirical data show that while the duration of activity has some influence upon the magnitude of the training response, the impact of this variable is less than that of intensity (32,150). Nevertheless, prolonged moderate activity such as brisk walking may be a more practical form of training than shorter periods of more intensive effort, both for a person who wishes to exercise while en route to a workplace that lacks shower facilities, and for an older individual who might be endangered by a more intensive bout of physical effort.

Effects of Type of Exercise

Endurance Training. Assuming that intensity, duration, and frequency of exercise are controlled, does it matter what type of endurance training is undertaken? In terms of one criterion of physiological response (the increment of maximal oxygen intake), Beaudet (13) found no difference in reactions to swimming, running, and cycling programs. Likewise, Milburn and Butts (105) reported that in terms of gains of oxygen transport, aerobic dance was just as effective as a jogging program.

Nevertheless, some specificity of the training response can be identified with respect to task learning, habituation, and local circulatory adaptations. Other important issues are the volume of muscle that is activated, the effects of adopting different postures while exercising, and subjective preferences.

Task Learning. As a specific task is repeated, the various component movements become more automatic in type; control is progressively transferred from the motor cortex to the cerebellum. At the same time, the required movements are performed with an ever greater mechanical efficiency, and in consequence the oxygen cost of working at a specific speed is decreased (150). Such task learning affects the heart rate response and the perception of effort for a given task, but except in exceptional circumstances there is little transfer of the skills that are acquired from one task to another.

Habituation.   Habituation is a form of negative conditioning that is peculiar to a given investigator and the conditions of a particular experiment (51). Initially, the anxiety provoked by the investigator and the laboratory setting may cause a substantial cardiac response for about one subject in four. As the required exercise task is repeated and it becomes perceived as less threatening, the heart rate, blood pressure, and ventilatory reactions all diminish. This type of adaptation depends upon the integrity of the prefrontal cortex (51).

Much of the adjustment of habituation occurs over the first two or three exposures to the unfamiliar situation. While a part of the process is highly task specific, there may also be a partial transfer of adaptations to similar tasks, particularly if the investigator and the general laboratory setting remain unchanged.

Local Circulatory Adaptations.   If training is undertaken by a relatively small group of muscles, for instance, when using an arm ergometer, a pulley system (60), or a swim-bench (49), the circulatory adaptations that occur seem mostly local in type. The subject is able to develop a larger than initial peak oxygen intake while using the arms, but little of this gain in performance can be transferred to forms of exercise that use the legs (27,99,133). During maximal leg effort, such specificity of training seems more marked for the cycle ergometer than for the treadmill (probably because cycling is heavily dependent on quadriceps strength). However, during submaximal effort, the converse seems to be true, adaptations to the treadmill being more specific than those for a cycle ergometer (43); this may possibly reflect the perceived safety of the two types of exercise.

The precise mechanisms responsible for any local improvement of performance with endurance training are still being debated. Conceivably, a local strengthening of the muscles allows them to contract at a smaller fraction of their maximal voluntary force (153), facilitating a better perfusion of the working limbs; however, in general, endurance training does not induce a major hypertrophy of skeletal muscle.

Alternatively, there may be a local increase of muscle capillarization (30,147,177), with an increased activity of aerobic enzymes. Both of these changes would facilitate the local extraction of oxygen by the active muscles (30); however, the intramuscular extraction of oxygen is fairly complete even prior to training (142), and it is hard to envisage how the muscular arteriovenous oxygen difference could undergo any major increase as a result of endurance training. A third hypothesis is that training may induce a greater neural traffic between local chemoreceptors in the exercised limb and cardiovascular centers in the brain stem; this might cause a local vasodilatation and thus facilitate development of a larger peak oxygen intake.

If large muscle groups are involved in the training process, the condition of the central circulation is usually improved, and the enhanced function is then generalizable to other types of exercise (Fig 8). While there may ultimately be some cardiac hypertrophy, the immediate effects are attributable to an increased central blood volume (greater preloading), an increase of myocardial contractility, and a decrease of arterial blood pressure at a given work-rate (decreased afterloading). Thus Wilmore et al. (195) found a transfer of training from cycling or jogging to treadmill performance, and White (192) found the trampoline as effective a method of improving cardiorespiratory function as cycling or treadmill exercise. However, Daub et al. (31) suggested that ice hockey training (a more intermittent and "anaerobic" form of activity) had no influence upon the maximal oxygen intake that could be developed during such activities as skating and cycling, and Wilmore et al. (195) found no gains of treadmill performance after 20 weeks of participation in a tennis program.

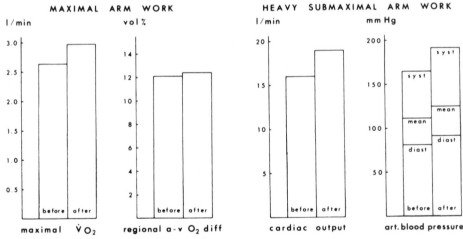

Figure 8 Data obtained during bouts of rhythmic arm exercise, performed before and after a period of leg training on a cycle ergometer. Note that some of the training response is transferable from the legs to the arms. (From Clausen, J. P., in *Limiting Factors of Physical Performance* (J. Keul, ed.). Thieme, Stuttgart (1973); used with permission.)

It may finally be asked how far cardiovascular training interferes with muscular training, or vice versa. While it is possible to develop both cardiovascular and muscular function simultaneously, an excess of endurance training does appear to hamper the development of muscular strength (37), particularly in parts of the body that are not actively involved in the aerobic performance.

Volume of Active Muscle. The volume of active muscle influences the extent of training, the resultant rise of systemic blood pressure, and the extent of any fatigue that develops.

In general, effective central, cardiovascular training requires the involvement of a substantial muscle mass. Indeed, the usual recommendation in an endurance prescription is to involve as much of the body musculature as possible. Appropriate activities to suggest include walking, jogging, running, swimming, cycling, and particularly cross-country skiing (85). However, attempts to increase the effectiveness of leg exercise by the carrying of hand-held weights have achieved only limited success (9,26). Negative features of arm-loading include greater impact stress when jogging, greater discomfort, and a larger rise of systemic blood pressure (particularly in hypertensive patients [58]).

If a similar level of oxygen consumption is developed using a smaller muscle mass, for example, the arms rather than the legs, then the increment of heart rate and blood pressure is relatively greater, with a corresponding increase of cardiac work rate and associated risks of myocardial ischemia (113). A high-intensity circuit training program that involves extensive arm work can be very stressful, with a large secretion of epinephrine and norepinephrine (121a). In general, the rise of blood pressure during muscular effort is proportional to the fraction of maximum voluntary force that is exerted (33,96), although if the active muscles are extremely small (for example, the fingers), then their impact upon systemic blood pressure is smaller (54). A further variable is fiber type; other factors being equal, the rise of systemic blood pressure during exercise is related to the proportion of fast-twitch fibers that is activated (47).

A lower peak heart rate is generally attained with arm than with leg exercise (167a,171,172); this reflects a limitation of effort by peripheral muscular fatigue rather than cardiovascular performance. The rating of perceived exertion is approximately proportional to heart rate, but the muscular component of the sensation is greater with small muscle than with large muscle effort.

The main practical justification for the deliberate training of small muscles arises if a person must undertake either dynamic or isometric exercise at work using that particular group of muscles. If weakness has developed through a period away from work (particularly immobilization or bedrest due to an injury or a heart attack), a patient may be helped by a specific training program before a return to normal or modified employment.

Posture. Most forms of human endurance exercise are performed in the standing or the sitting position. This tends to involve a large fraction of the body musculature, but has the disadvantage that the preloading of the heart is reduced, at least until function of the muscle pump has overcome gravitation pooling in the capacity vessels of the lower half of the body. A somewhat larger cardiovascular response to training might be anticipated with the one form of exercise that is easily performed from a lying position—moderate intensity swimming; in this situation, a combination of the horizontal posture and a cooling of the superficial veins by the water increase the central blood volume, and thus ventricular preloading.

Support of the body mass by immersion in water (95,160) or by sitting on a chair (104) can be particularly helpful to the frail elderly who wish to obtain some exercise despite degenerative changes in their knee joints or the lower part of the spine.

Certain postures where all or part of the body mass must be supported by prolonged isometric contraction place an additional strain upon the circulation, particularly if the subject performs the Valsalva maneuver in an attempt to increase muscular force. A rise of both systemic blood pressure and heart rate increase the cardiac work rate, and there is a corresponding increase in the risk of myocardial ischemia. An extended bout of "push-ups," for example, may be inadvisable for an older person with established cardiovascular disease.

Posture may finally be important in terms of sustaining bone mass. Some authors, at least, have argued that the prevention of osteoporosis is dependent on weight-bearing activity. If so, swimming would be a less desirable exercise prescription than rapid walking, particularly for an older person; however, the mass needed to stimulate bone growth is still vigorously debated, and one recent report noted unusual development of the playing arm in tennis players (124).

Subjective Preferences. If the physiological responses to two possible prescriptions are roughly comparable, much of the choice between alternative forms of physical activity must be based upon subjective preferences. Account must be taken of the individual's motives for exercising, available skills, and available resources.

Many otherwise excellent exercise programs are relatively ineffective because of a low level of patient compliance. Among possible techniques to improve exercise participation rates, one obvious approach is to tailor the physical activity prescription to satisfy subjective preferences. If the prime motivation of the individual is the enhancement of personal health, the meeting of an ascetic challenge, or stress-relaxation (91), a solitary activity such as jogging or rapid distance walking is probably an appropriate suggestion, but if the search is for competition, a vigorous team or individual competitive sport should be suggested. If the desire is for increased social contacts, a gymnastic or dance program may prove to be the optimum recommendation. Much depends on the need of the individual for supervision and encouragement; those with an external "locus of control" have a greater requirement for such encouragement. Bassey et al. (12) found only limited gains when an unsupervised aerobics program was made available to factory workers. Kavanagh and Shephard (88) also commented that the physiological gains realized in a home exercise program were smaller than those achieved during a standard rehabilitation center-based cardiac program.

One important factor discouraging exercise participation is that the class member fails to reach a level of performance where the activity becomes enjoyable. It is thus helpful to recommend types of activities which are well suited to the patient's body build, and where the individual has already developed some skills.

A further significant factor leading to defections from an exercise program is the existence of real and perceived barriers to participation. Account should thus be taken of equipment already available to the patient, financial resources available to purchase other items that are essential for a particular pursuit, and the opportunity costs involved in attendance at the particular place where a given activity must be pursued.

Finally, account must be taken of the negative impact of any injuries sustained by the patient or by other members of the group. Some types of programs seem more likely to cause injury than others—for example, skipping is reputed to be worse than jogging (121a). Aerobic dance also has a bad reputation, probably owing as much to program design as to improper footwear or the use of rather hard floor surfaces (48). Within a given class of activity, the risk of injury often seems associated with an excessive intensity of exercise, and even more with an excessive volume of activity per week (126).

Muscular Training. As with endurance activity, there is some communality of the training response between different types of muscle-strengthening regimens. For example, Gettman et al. (50) found similar increments of lean mass in response to isotonic or isokinetic circuit training.

In the case of strength training, there also seems some specificity of increments in force with respect to the velocity of contraction (62,81,134) and the joint angle tested; those who undertake training using explosive movements or a rapid speed of contraction develop an increase of power during rapid movements, whereas those trained with slower movement patterns demonstrate increases of strength mainly during slower contractions. Presumably, this reflects differences of muscle fiber recruitment during the two types of training. Isometric training seems particularly liable to induce gains of strength only at the specific joint angle where exercise has occurred (70). This is partly a question of very specific muscle development and partly an example of test learning, which can give a misleading impression of gains of strength in longitudinal experiments.

Effects of Environment

General Considerations. A training program in essence subjects the body to a physical and sometimes a mental stress. If exercise is performed in an adverse environment, this heightens the intensity of stress for any given level of physical activity; the training response may be increased in consequence, but at the same time there is a danger that the individual may pass the optimal or "eu-stress" level to which adaptation is possible. Certainly, the risks of an exercise prescription are increased in extreme environments, and the subject's motivation may also be reduced. The issue of danger is particularly important when recommending physical activity programs for patients who have only a small safety margin between an effective and an excessive prescription. A recommendation that would be safe under temperate conditions may become quite dangerous if it is attempted in the face of excessive heat or cold.

Given that our understanding of the training process itself is far from complete, it is not surprising that details of the interactions between training and environment remain somewhat sketchy.

Hot Environments. Certain parallels may be drawn between the processes of heat acclimatization and cardiovascular training. In both instances, there is a dynamic loading of the circulation (although in the heat this is due to an increase of skin blood flow rather than any increase of muscle flow). If exposure is prolonged, the deep body temperature rises in both situations, and there is a resultant stimulation of sweating with a progressive depletion of blood volume (156). Moreover, as the individual becomes accustomed to either heat or exercise, there is an expansion of blood volume (66), allowing cardiac output to be better sustained. With any given exposure to a heat or exercise load, the rise of body temperature also tends to be smaller, and sweating occurs earlier and in greater quantities (109,156).

It is thus logical that repeated exposure to one form of stress should be seen as helping adaptation to the other (79). Some cross-acclimatization has indeed been reported between the two stressors, although for maximum adaptation, a hot environment and vigorous exercise must be presented simultaneously (199).

There are many dangers linked with overexertion in the heat, ranging from the minor hazards of skin rashes and infections to the major risks of heat exhaustion, heat collapse, hyperthermia, and heat stroke (156). Those who are most vulnerable seem to be groups of individuals with a low maximum cardiac output—the unfit, the elderly, and particularly those with cardiac disease. Partly because of the increase in resting cardiac output, and partly because of the disturbances of mineral balance induced by prolonged sweating, spells of hot weather usually give rise to an increased cardiac mortality among such individuals (41).

In industries where hard physical work is required, experience has shown that as heat stress becomes excessive, the incidence of accidents rises (186). A similar trend to an increased risk of physical injury might be anticipated if voluntary exercise is performed in the heat. Heat and physical activity seem likely to contribute jointly to an increased level of psychological arousal, and thus a greater perception of exertion at any given fraction of an individual's maximal oxygen intake (19). Perhaps in part for this reason, people tend to take less voluntary physical activity in hot climates. Finally, a heat-induced depletion of fluid and mineral reserves can give rise to a variety of long-term pathologies, including a feeling of neurasthenia and an irritability that interferes with effective participation in team activities (198).

The primary means of avoiding exercise-induced heat problems is to change the locale or to moderate the intensity of deliberate physical activity when the wet bulb globe thermometer reading or other index of effective temperature exceeds the safe limits proposed by groups such as the American College of Sports Medicine (2) (Table 3). In gen-

Table 3 Position Statement of American College of Sports Medicine on Prevention of Heat Injuries During Distance Running

---

Based on research findings and current rules governing distance running competition, it is the position of the American College of Sports Medicine that:

1. Distance races (> 16 km or 10 miles) should *not* be conducted when the wet bulb temperature—globe temperature* exceeds 28°C (82.4°F). (1,2)
2. During periods of the year, when the daylight dry bulb temperature often exceeds 27°C (80°F), distance races should be conducted before 9:00 A.M. or after 4:00 P.M. (2,7,8,9)
3. It is the responsibility of the race sponsors to provide fluids which contain small amounts of sugar (less than 2.5 g glucose per 100 ml of water) and electrolytes (less than 10 mEq sodium and 5 mEq potassium per liter of solution.) (5,6)
4. Runners should be encouraged to frequently ingest fluids during competition and to consume 400–500 ml (13–17 oz.) of fluid 10–15 minutes before competition. (5,6,9)
5. Rules prohibiting the administration of fluids during the first 10 kilometers (6.2 miles) of a marathon race should be amended to permit fluid ingestion at frequent intervals along the race course. In light of the high sweat rates and body temperatures during distance running in the heat, race sponsors should provide "water stations" at 3–4 kilometer (2–2.5 mile) intervals for all races of 16 kilometers (10 miles) or more. (4,8,9)
6. Runners should be instructed in how to recognize the early warning symptoms that precede heat injury. Recognition of symptoms, cessation of running, and proper treatment can prevent heat injury. Early warning symptoms include the following: piloerection on chest and upper arms, chilling, throbbing pressure in the head, unsteadiness, nausea, and dry skin. (2,9)
7. Race sponsors should make prior arrangements with medical personnel for the care of cases of heat injury. Responsible and informed personnel should supervise each "feeding station." Organizational personnel should reserve the right to stop runners who exhibit clear signs of heat stroke or heat exhaustion.

It is the position of the American College of Sports Medicine that policies established by local, national, and international sponsors of distance running events should adhere to these guidelines. Failure to adhere to these guidelines may jeopardize the health of competitors through heat injury.

---

*Adapted from Minard, D. *Prevention of heat casualties in Marine Corps Recruits. Milit. Med.* 126: 261, 1961. WB-GT = 0.7 (WBT) + 0.2 (GT) + 0.1 (DBT)
Source: *Medicine & Science in Sports,* 7(1): vii (1975)

eral, appropriately cool conditions can be found by the use of a swimming pool or an air-conditioned gymnasium, or by shifting the timing of exercise sessions to the cooler temperatures of late evening and early morning. However, it is important to recognize that heat stress is not confined to tropical regions; when a radiant heat load of perhaps 100 W is imposed by exposure to bright sunshine (110), vigorous exercise can cause serious heat stress over half an hour or less, even if environmental temperatures are only moderately warm. Thus, it is important that sports physicians monitor the core temperatures of those undertaking prolonged bouts of exercise even in supposedly temperate climates.

It is possible to change from land-based activities such as jogging to water-based activities such as swimming and aquabics if unfavorable temperatures persist. Finally, patients with known cardiac disease should be counseled to moderate the intensity of their prescribed exercise and/or to seek further medical advice if they notice an increase of abnormal heart rhythms or an earlier onset of exercise-induced anginal pain as a consequence of warm conditions.

Cold Conditions. Cold exposure causes a constriction of peripheral veins. Central blood volume is thus increased, and this leads to a small immediate increase of the individual's maximal oxygen intake (21). However, there have been disparate reports of possible interactions between exercise training and cold acclimatization, and the current consensus suggests that there is little relationship between the two variables (146,160).

Fat subjects might be thought less vulnerable to cold stress than thinner individuals, but in fact much of the insulation of the body is based upon an active neurally-mediated reduction of blood flow to the limb muscles rather than a passive protection from subcutaneous fat depots. A determination of skinfold thicknesses thus provides only a limited measure of a person's cold tolerance (174). The ability to sustain shivering and to engage in prolonged and vigorous physical activity are also important protective measures, and both depend upon the extent of the individual's glycogen reserves (80). Because unfit individuals have smaller initial reserves of glycogen and are less able to sustain vigorous physical activity over a long period, they are the usual victims of hypothermia in climbing accidents (129).

In the context of exercise prescription, there has been considerable interest in the possibility that a given intensity of exercise may metabolize a larger quantity of fat if the activity is performed in a cold environment (114–117), (Fig. 9). The reasons for the phenomenon are not fully understood; increases of energy expenditure due to the wear-

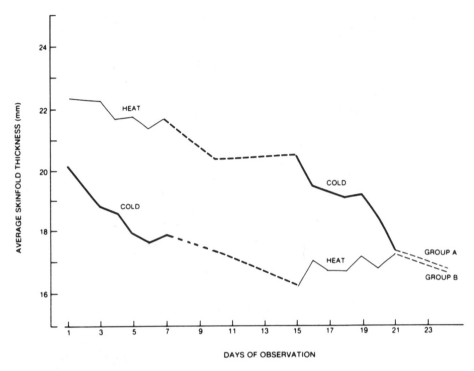

Figure 9 A comparison of the fat loss induced by a week of exercise in cold and warm environments. Crossover experiments involving two groups of young men (From Ref. 117; used with permission.)

ing of heavy clothing and boots are largely offset by a reductin of peripheral body temperatures, and thus a lower rate of basal metabolism in the cold. Possibly, catecholamine secretion is increased by the low temperatures, leading to an increase of "futile" metabolic cycles, either in brown fat or elsewhere; if so, each bout of exercise might provoke a prolonged increase of metabolic rate greater than would be observed in a temperate climate. The mobilization of depot fat also seems to cause a ketosis, with a potential loss of energy from the body as partially metabolized ketone bodies are excreted (114,115). The cold-induced fat loss apparently occurs more readily in the obese than in thinner individuals (115), and (possibly because of a need to conserve the body reserves of fat for pregnancy and lactation), the cold-induced stimulation of fat metabolism is less obvious in female than in male subjects (108).

Intensely cold conditions can be dangerous from the viewpoint of provoking both local and general problems. Patients with a poor peripheral circulation are particularly vulnerable to frostbite; the risk of damage depends on the severity of the wind-chill factor, and is exacerbated by any local disturbance of the cutaneous air-film (as might occur, for example, with the rapid body movements of downhill skiing or speed skating). A cold-induced peripheral vascular constriction raises the systemic blood pressure, thus increasing the workload upon the heart; the resultant risk of myocardial ischemia is further augmented by an associated secretion of catecholamines.

When a critical respiratory minute volume is exceeded (usually 30–40 L/min), the patient starts to breathe through the mouth as well as the nose (111); this disturbance of normal mechanisms for warming, filtering, and humidifying inspired air within the nasal passages can provoke bronchospasm, often with an associated reflex narrowing of the coronary vessels (Bezold-Jarisch reflex) and an increased risk of myocardial ischemia.

Older individuals with brittle bones and a deteriorating sense of balance are particularly vulnerable to falls under icy conditions. The older segment of the population also has an increased vulnerability to hypothermia (14,55); problems from a decline of core temperature are particularly likely to arise if prolonged bouts of exercise are performed in clothing that either lacks adequate insulation, or has lost its insulation due to soaking by rain, mist, or sweat. In the older person, the problem is further compounded by an inability to make good the heat loss by an increased rate of body heat production.

The psychological effect of moderate cold exposure is generally to encourage brisk patterns of movement. However, when the weather is extremely cold, there is a tendency to remain indoors and to allow fitness to deteriorate. There are at least two possible options in terms of maintaining physical condition during the winter months. One is to seek an indoor exercise facility. Such establishments are increasingly available in larger cities throughout the world, although some of the users of indoor tracks and gymnasia complain of drying of the throat and exercise-induced bronchospasm during the winter season because the inspired air in such buildings often has a very low water content. If a change from outdoor to indoor pursuits is indeed proposed at the onset of winter, it is important to consider whether a differing group of muscles will be stressed by the indoor activities; unless a change in the mode of exercise is accompanied by an appropriate immediate moderation of the intensity and duration of activity, overuse injuries may develop.

A second possibility, particularly for the younger adult, is to continue to exercise out-of-doors during the winter months, making an appropriate change in the type of activity that is undertaken. For instance, cross-country skiing can be quite pleasant at ambient temperatures as low as -10 to $-15°C$, given a sunny day and appropriate clothing. Indeed, the change of pursuit necessitated by winter can provide the useful psychological ingredient of variety to an exercise prescription. If the activity is to be pursued out-of-doors, it is very important to match the amount of clothing that is worn to variations in the intensity of the pursuit. Failure to take this precaution may cause a soaking of the protective garments with sweat, and the resultant loss of insulation will then allow a rapid cooling of the body when a rest pause is taken.

High Altitudes.   At the time of the Mexico City Olympics there was considerable interest in the possibility of enhancing training responses by the sustained exposure of athletes to high altitudes (152). The physiological effects of exposure to high altitudes include an increase of hemoglobin concentrations (which develops progressively over several weeks), a decrease of cerebrospinal fluid bicarbonate levels over the first 12 h of exposure, slower adjustments of acid/base balance that normalize both blood and tissue pH over the course of the first week, and a decrease of blood volume (which can persist for several weeks).

As in "blood-doping," the altitude-induced increase of hemoglobin concentration has the potential to enhance endurance performance, provided that the individual's myocardial contractility is adequate to sustain the stroke volume in the face of some increase in blood viscosity. However, any increase of endurance is short lived, since the hemoglobin concentration reverts to normal within 2–3 weeks of a return to sea-level conditions (156). The altitude-induced decrease of cerebrospinal fluid and serum bicarbonate concentrations has a negative impact upon anaerobic performance, while the decrease of blood volume also reduces the ability to undertake sustained bouts of endurance exercise during the first few weeks at high altitudes.

From the viewpoint of the safety of a vigorous exercise prescription, there are a number of hazards specific to high altitude, particularly if the person concerned is unacclimatized to the new environment. Particular dangers include acute mountain sickness and pulmonary edema. There is also some evidence that the risk of heart attacks is increased by exposure to high altitude, particularly in patients with a preexisting myocardial ischemia.

High Ambient Pressures.   Recreational diving is rapidly becoming a popular form of exercise. Some of the risks of the diving-induced increase of ambient pressure and subsequent decompression are relatively independent of the pattern of exercise that is being undertaken. However, the danger of exhaustion of gas supplies while underwater is proportional to both the intensity of effort and the period of submersion. Likewise, the risks of nitrogen narcosis, oxygen poisoning, and decompression sickness all increase as the period underwater is extended, and problems from an excessive work of breathing are particularly likely if intensive activity is attempted at substantial depths (156).

However, the main danger of underwater activity for the person with cardiac disease is the immediate cardiovascular shock that is encountered on first entering the water. A reflex constriction of the cutaneous vessels caused by immersion of the face (the diving reflex) and an augmented secretion of catecholamines increase the workload of the heart, and arrhythmias may be seen at this stage. Body temperature drops progressively throughout most types of underwater activity, and this may further augment the secretion of catecholamines, with a risk of cardiac arrest. Another possible cause of cardiovascular problems is an adverse reaction to myocardial oxygen lack in the later stages of a breath-hold dive; this type of response is particularly likely to occur in a person with a poor coronary vascular supply. Finally, the development of pressure differentials between the peripheral veins and the interior of the thoracic cavity (a "pulmonary squeeze") can considerably increase the preloading of the heart, with potential adverse effects upon the person with a poor myocardial contractility. The tone of the peripheral veins progressively decreases while the individual is lying submerged, and the blood pressure may fall abruptly as the upright posture is resumed on climbing from the water; a hypotensive episode, with loss of consciousness, is particularly likely in a person who is unfit, or is receiving hypotensive medication for the treatment of hypertension.

Other risks of the underwater environment include drowning secondary to a disturbance of cardiac rhythm and a resultant loss of consciousness, and physical injury associated with a hypotensive episode on emerging from the water.

Air Pollution.   Catastrophic episodes of air pollution in London, England, during 1952 and 1956 (123a) demonstrated that those most vulnerable to the adverse health effects of air contaminants were the very young and the frail elderly. A fatal outcome was particularly linked to advanced age and the presence of chronic cardiac or respiratory disease.

Exercise increases exposure of the individual to air pollutants from several perspectives. First, there is often a two- to threefold gradient in the peak concentrations of air contaminants from ambient air to the more protected environment of a home with closed windows. Second, both particulate and gas-phase contaminants generally reach the body via the respiratory tract. Thus, an exercise-induced increase of respiratory minute volume tends to induce *at least* a proportionate increase in exposure to the toxic material. Finally, if the intensity of exercise is sufficient to induce mouth breathing (usually initiated at a respiratory minute volume of 30–40 L/min [111]), the pulmonary exposure to air contaminants is increased about tenfold because the normal scrubbing and filtration mechanisms of the nose are bypassed; the proportion of soluble vapors absorbed in the trachea and larger bronchi is also less if the speed of transit of the inspirate is increased.

There are two broad categories of air pollution: reducing smog (an accumulation of the combustion products of fossil fuels) and oxidant smog (the end result of an accumulation of automobile exhaust in bright sunlight). Reducing smog (SO_2, SO_3, and soot particles) was apparently responsible for the 5000 fatalities which occurred during the London smog episodes of 1952 and 1956, but at normally encountered urban concentrations the oxides of sulfur do little except to provoke a mild bronchospasm, with an increase of respiratory rate. This can exacerbate any inherent tendency of the individual to exercise-induced bronchospasm. There may also be a temporary paralysis of the tracheal ciliae, and this leaves the respiratory tract more vulnerable to infecting microorganisms.

Oxidant smog includes carbon monoxide, ozone, and various oxides of nitrogen; all of these substances are derived from automobile exhaust, which undergoes complex chemical changes in the upper atmosphere in the presence of sunlight. Although the concentrations of oxidant pollutants are influenced by traffic density, atmospheric stability and the number of hours of recent sunshine are other critical variables influencing the accumulation of oxidant contaminants. If the exposure to an oxidant smog is brief, the dose of carbon monoxide that is received varies with the individual's respiratory minute volume and pulmonary blood flow (and hence with the intensity of exercise) (Table 4). However, after several hours of exposure to a high concentration of carbon monoxide, an equilibrium is reached that is independent of the intensity of effort (158). Carbon monoxide exposure can impair both oxygen transport and psychomotor function, but from the health point

Table 4 Influence of Atmospheric Partial Pressure of Carbon Monoxide, Duration of Exposure, and Intensity of Exercise on Blood Carboxyhemoglobin Levels (%)

Partial pressure of carbon monoxide (Pa)	Duration of exposure, intensity of work, and COH̄b%								
	15 min			60 min			480 min		
	S	M	H	S	M	H	S	M	H
0.5	0.5	0.5	0.6	0.6	0.6	0.7	0.9	0.9	0.9
1.0	0.6	0.6	0.7	0.7	0.9	1.1	1.5	1.7	1.7
2.5	0.7	0.8	1.0	1.1	1.7	2.2	3.3	4.1	4.2
5.0	0.8	1.2	1.6	1.7	3.0	4.1	6.4	8.0	8.3
20.0	1.8	3.5	5.2	5.4	11.0	15.5	24.5	31.7	32.9

Predictions based upon model of Coburn et al., *J. Clin. Invest.* 44: 1899–1910, 1965, and calculations of World Health Organization (Health Aspects Related to Indoor Air Quailty, WHO Regional Office for Europe Copenhagen, 1979), for sedentary subjects (S), subjects undertaking moderate activity (M), and subjects undertaking heavy work (H) sufficient to induce a respiratory minute volume of 30 L min^{-1} and a pulmonary diffusing capacity of 60 ml min^{-1} Torr^{-1}.
Source: Shephard, R. J., *Carbon Monoxide: The Silent Killer.* Springfield, Illinois, Charles C Thomas; used with permission.

of view, the most important consequence is an exacerbation of the effects of preexisting cardiovascular disease. The time to onset of angina is reduced during an exercise bout, and the risk of cardiac arrest is also increased. Carbon monoxide induces a tissue hypoxia, and the toxic effects of exposure to this gas are thus exacerbated at high altitudes. Ozone is a respiratory irritant. At the concentrations sometimes encountered in urban air, it causes bronchospasm, with rapid shallow breathing and a decrease of maximal oxygen intake (46). For the reasons noted above, the threshold concentration for measurable effects drops from about 0.75 ppm at rest to about 0.1 ppm during vigorous exercise. There has been less formal study of the nitrogen oxides, although they are known to cause pulmonary edema if concentrations are high. Such a response becomes more likely during intensive exercise, partly because the toxic gas is drawn more deeply into the lungs, partly because more gas in inhaled, and partly because prolonged intensive exercise itself gives some tendency to the development of pulmonary edema.

Psychological Stress. The level of psychological stress encountered during exercise varies enormously from one situation to another. Moreover, it is important to consider the psychological environment, since this influences not only performance, but also the cardiovascular risks of physical activity (155).

In some instances, the pressures of time, perceived hostility, and other stressors may be brought from the home or the office to the gymnasium or exercise site. A person who is conscious of such pressures may need to moderate the intensity of an exercise prescription if abnormalities of cardiac rhythm are not to develop, since the emotional disturbance can increase heart rate, blood pressure, and catecholamine secretion in response to a given exercise load. Moreover, a change in the type of exercise may be helpful for such individuals—as an example, a peaceful walk in the countryside may do more to relieve occupational or domestic pressures than a challenging game of squash that the patient is determined to win.

Excitement and competition inherent to the chosen form of physical activity may be a significant additional source of stress. Thus, Blimkie et al. (15) observed that catecholamine levels were much higher when young men were playing a game of hockey than when they were undertaking an equivalent intensity of exercise on a cycle ergometer (Fig. 10). Cardiovascular problems are particularly likely if the intensity of competition is severe or seems beyond the capacity of the participant. Whereas a patient with a relaxed, "Type B" personality may accept defeat graciously, those with "Type A," hostile and competitive behavioral traits often remain determined to win even when

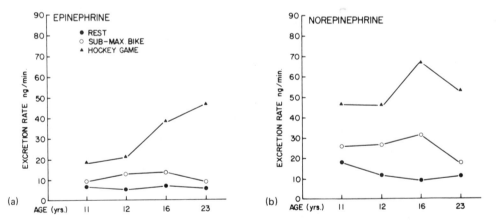

Figure 10 Urinary excretion of epinephrine and norepinephrine in males aged 11, 12, 16, and 23 years. Samples collected at rest, immediately after a game of ice hockey, and immediately after submaximal cycle ergometer exercise of comparable metabolic intensity (From Ref. 15; used with permission.)

they are conscious of physical exhaustion. Politicians participating in "fun runs" seem especially vulnerable to exceeding the prudent limits imposed by their physical capacities. Often, they are reluctant to admit to any physical limitations while under the spotlight of the television cameras.

Any unfamiliar situation can be a further source of psychological stress. About one-quarter of patients are very anxious on the first occasion that they are tested in an exercise laboratory. The increase of heart rate, blood pressure, and ventilation induced by such anxiety not only tends to invalidate the test results, but it also reduces the margin of safety for any procedure that is being carried out. Ideally, patients should be habituated to the general environment of the test laboratory by one or more preliminary visits (151). Care should also be taken to explain all intended procedures in a calm and reassuring manner, allowing the patient to experiment with unfamiliar devices before beginning a definitive test. The claim is sometimes made that the physiological effects of psychological stress are seen mainly at low intensities of effort. Given that most laboratories proceed from a low to higher intensities of exercise, using a progressive test protocol, some familiarization is undoubtedly possible as the required form of physical activity develops. Moreover, the effect of a 10 beats/min anxiety-induced increase of heart rate is relatively larger (in percentage terms) at rest than during maximal exercise. However, in our experience the psychological impact of a first progressive exercise test upon a nervous subject does not abate as maximal effort is approached. Indeed, impending exhaustion may increase the level of anxiety and thus absolute increases of heart rate and blood pressure.

POSTULATED HEALTH BENEFITS OF REGULAR EXERCISE

The acute health benefits of a regular exercise program include an improvement of overall lifestyle, gains of perceived health, and an improved mood state. Chronic health benefits have also been postulated, including a decreased risk of ischemic heart disease and hypertension; the control of obesity, maturity-onset diabetes, and cholecystitis; a strengthening of ligaments, cartilage, and bone structure; and a reduced incidence of certain forms of malignant disease. For reasons to be discussed in the following section, it is difficult to obtain conclusive experimental proof of the postulated chronic benefits of regular exercise.

Improvement of Lifestyle

Participation in a regular program of physical activity may encourage other favorable changes of lifestyle, such as a more careful consideration of diet or the cessation of smoking (164). The majority of reports to date have been cross-sectional in type, and it is then difficult to decide which variable is cause and which effect. Indeed, several favorable aspects of lifestyle may have a common basis in a high socioeconomic status or other independent determinants.

An uncontrolled longitudinal experiment seemed to suggest that the involvement of Masters' athletes in long-distance running had encouraged a much higher percentage of successful cigarette withdrawals than would have been likely in the general population (106a). However, further study of Masters' competitors (88a,88b) established that the cigarette withdrawal often antedated competitive involvement; both the interest in competitive exercise and smoking cessation were more properly attributable to an overall interest in a healthy lifestyle. On the other hand, controlled trials of exercise programs that have also included substantial amounts of deliberate health education (14a,166) have had a favorable impact upon cigarette and alcohol consumption, obesity, and overall health knowledge.

If regular physical exercise does indeed have a specific effect upon other facet of lifestyle, one might anticipate maximal benefit from those forms of physical activity that the individual perceives as being health related. The demands of the exercise prescription should be realistic, so that participation improves self-image and feelings of self-efficacy. The patient will then find motivation to begin and to sustain a fight against other adverse and addictive forms of behavior such as smoking, over consumption of alcohol, and overeating.

Various other interactions between exercise and lifestyle may be suggested. The vigorous breathing of endurance exercise brings to light the dyspnea which is caused by smoking, encouraging evaluation of a cigarette addiction. An alcoholic may be helped by a pattern of exercise that optimizes arousal and thus counters the depression underlying the alcohol addiction. The compulsive eater may be acutely dissuaded from unnecessary eating if the blood sugar is raised temporarily by a brief bout of intensive exercise; however, more prolonged sessions of moderate exercise are needed to establish a good long-term balance between food intake and energy consumption.

Perceived Health

The World Health Organization (197) has stressed the importance of a positive approach to health. Physicians should seek not merely the absence of disease, but an optimization of human potential, with complete social, psychological, and mental well-being. Most people will agree that the main reason why they exercise is to "feel better"; in essence, this comment reflects an improvement of perceived health. An individual operates along a continuum stretching from optimal health to overt disease (69), and one important effect of involvement in a regular program of physical activity is a displacement of the individual toward the optimal health end of this continuum. Such a change is probably the main factor responsible for the reduction of demand for medical and hospital services (161) seen over the first few months of involvement in a physical activity program.

The type of activity most likely to maximize such wellness is relatively specific to a given individual. In some, the sensation of optimal health may be due to the added arousal induced by a few minutes of vigorous exercise, but in other people the key factor may be the stress-relaxation associated with a much longer period of more gentle activity. Some individuals may respond positively to an enhancement of their body image and the feelings of self-efficacy that are associated with a trim body figure or well-toned muscles, whereas others may sense the lessening of fatigue during daily tasks as endurance fitness is increased. A few may describe the euphoria which has been linked to an increased output of β-endorphins in very prolonged bouts of vigorous exercise.

STRENGTHS AND WEAKNESSES OF CURRENT EVIDENCE

A general principle of medical science is that, where possible, an important hypothesis should be tested by means of well-controlled experiments using randomly allocated subjects. However, there are substantial obstacles when attempting to apply this type of approach to an evaluation of the long-term benefits of physical exercise.

There is some possibility of conducting experiments where light electrical stimulation is applied to the muscles of sleeping patients, but with this one exception, humans are well aware when they have engaged in an exercise training program. Reactions are thus colored by their atitudes, positive or negative, toward voluntary physical activity. Moreover, when arranging an exercise class for high-risk individuals, it is commonly thought desirable to assure a close medical supervision of participants, and such regular contact with a medical team in itself provides emotional support, advice on lifestyle, and a closer monitoring of clinical condition than that which occurs in any control group. If subjects are randomly assigned between treatment and control groups, further problems arise; there is usually a selective loss of patients from the treatment group (those of low socioeconomic status, with a poor lifestyle and an above-average severity of disease), while those who are assigned to the control group are equally liable to a selective contamination with an interest in physical activity (those most vulnerable to contamination are patients of high socioeconomic status and those who are health conscious). When investigating issues like the prevention of ischemic heart disease, it is finally necessary to recruit and to retain large samples (around 5000 cases). Even if several major university centers agree to cooperate in the necessary research, such numbers are difficult to obtain and almost impossible to retain.

Investigators have thus attempted to accumulate sufficient evidence by a pooling of results from all large trials of adequate quality (the technique of meta-analysis [119,128a,164a]); Unfortunately, the policies at individual centers vary with respect to diagnostic criteria, date of entry into the trial, exercise program, ancillary treatment, duration of observation, and diagnostic endpoints. While the requisite 5000 patients can be accumulated in short order by a meta-analytic approach (Table 5), and differences between experimental and control groups may reach conventional levels of statistical significance (p <0.05), it remains uncertain exactly what exercise hypothesis has been proven by the manipulation of such disparate data.

The alternative approach commonly adopted by the exercise scientist is to attempt to draw inferences from epidemiological data, comparing the health experience of groups supposedly varying in their levels of physical activity. The criteria suggested by the eminent statistician Bradford Hill can then be applied to examine whether any observed associations between exercise and health are casual or causal.

Strength of the Association

The strength of the association between regular exercise participation and disease prevention is relatively weak—For example, there seems to be a 25-50% reduction in the risk of fatal myocardial infarction among

Table 5 To Illustrate the Potential for Pooling of Data from Controlled Trials of Exercise in Postcoronary Rehabilitation

Author[a]	Sample size	Entry	Follow-up	Treatment
Kentala (1972)	298 (165)[b]	6–8 wk	1 yr	Individually supervised, 2–3/wk
Kallio (1981)	375 (74F, 301M)	Hospital discharge (2 wk)	3 yr	Exercise + health education
[c]Kallio et al. (1988)	375 (74 F, 301 M)	Hospital discharge (2 wk)	10 yr (3 yr prog.)	Exercise + health education
[c]Hamalainen et al. (1988)	456	Hospital discharge (2 wk)	6 yr (3/12 program)	Exercise + health education (controls received community-based program)
Palatsi (1976)	380	2–3/12	29 months (1 yr program)	Daily home program (nonrandomized allocation)

[a] See (164a) for details of references.
[b] Numbers suitable for long-term follow-up.
[c] Coronary deaths, assuming 4-year follow-up of all subjects.
Source: From Ref. 164a; used with permission.

active subjects relative to those who are inactive, compared with the nine- to 10-fold increase in the risk of bronchial carcinoma which is observed when a non-smoker is compared to a heavy smoker.

Consistency of the Association

The consistency of the association between an active lifestyle and the prevention of disease is generally good, but there are occasional anomalies. For instance, athletes may be quite active and yet remain vulnerable to a particular disease because a particular body build associated with an increased risk of the disorder is also a criterion for success in the sport under examination. Likewise, laborers who undertake hard physical work in a particular industry may fail to show the anticipated protection from their daily stint of exercise because a low socioeconomic status encourages other bad health habits such as smoking.

An Appropriate Lag Period

While some of the favorable responses to exercise occur almost immediately, others only become apparent after a long lag period during which exercise participation has been consistently sustained. Analysis is complicated by persistent uncertainties regarding the length of the lag period for various diseases, and relatively few epidemiological studies have accumulated convincing data on long-term activity patterns. Nevertheless, the available information seems consistent with anticipated lag periods for the development of protection.

Biological Gradient

The studies of Paffenbarger (119b) provided some evidence of a biological gradient linking the magnitude of weekly leisure energy expenditures with the extent of protection against fatal ischemic heart disease, although the relationship was nonlinear, and at the highest energy expenditures, risk was again increased.

Likewise, in terms of the prevention of osteoporosis and the strengthening of bone, moderate weight-bearing exercise seems beneficial, but overvigorous exercise augments the risks of osteoporosis and stress fractures.

Plausibility

If an association is causal, it should seem plausible from a theoretical standpoint. There are plainly many plausible mechanisms whereby exercise could reduce the impact of various disease processes. Some are relatively independent of the intensity of the exercise program; for example, the incidental advice on personal lifestyle, companionship, mutual support, and joie de vivre that are almost inevitably gained through membership in an exercise class. Some benefits (such as the metabolizing of excess fat and cholesterol and the lowering of resting blood sugar) require the weekly expenditure of substantial additional amounts of energy, although in terms of metabolizing excess fat, a low intensity of activity may be more effective than shorter bouts of very vigorous exercise. Some benefits require regular moderate endurance activity; for instance, the lowering of exercise heart rate, blood pressure, and cardiac work-rate, an increase of plasma volume and total hemoglobin, and an increased secretion of fat-mobilizing hormones (growth hormone and cortisol). However, a few of the possible benefits require intensive bursts of activity; among these items are habituation to the sensations of all-out effort and a decreased secretion of catecholamines during maximal exertion.

Specificity

In many of the disease conditions for which regular physical activity is advocated (for example, ischemic heart disease, maturity-onset diabetes, osteoporosis, and intestinal tumors) there is a long latent period before clinical symptoms become apparent. Moreover, there are many situational factors that influence whether or not the disease process has clinical manifestations.

For example, a given degree of coronary narrowing may cause a myocardial infarction, but it may also remain as a silent myocardial ischemia. Likewise, a given severity of osteoporosis may lead to a fracture, but it may only be discovered on a routine radiograph. There may thus appear to be a lack of specificity in the relationship between physical inactivity and disease. However, the relationship becomes more specific if, for instance, the prevalence of myocardial ischemia or of reduced bone density is correlated with habitual patterns of physical activity.

A further factor leading to a lack of specificity is the multifactorial nature of many diseases—for instance, some patients are vulnerable to ischemic heart disease despite a lifetime of vigorous physical activity because they have a severe congenital disorder of lipid metabolism.

Coherence

Ideally, all observable facts should be explained if the relationship is causal. It could be argued that the exercise hypothesis fails to satisfy this criterion. For instance, in the study of London bus workers, the incidence of angina was higher in the active group (the "conductors") than in the sedentary group (the drivers [107]). Possibly, the added physical demands of work brought subclinical disease to light at an earlier stage among the conductors.

Likewise, in some instances, vigorous exercise increases rather than decreases the immediate risk of a heart attack (155).

Experimental Verification

The ultimate test of any hypothesis is experimental verification. Some of the obstacles to a controlled experiment testing the exercise hypothesis have been noted above. Observations on experimental animals have not been very satisfactory. The restricted diet and cramped living quarters of the average laboratory animal are not typical of normal life, and it is surprisingly difficult to persuade most species to undertake regular vigorous exercise while they are confined to a laboratory.

Further, there are no good animal models for such chronic disease conditions as atherosclerosis. Arterial lesions can only be produced by the constraints of providing a very high fat diet to rigorously caged animals. Finally, the long lag period which preceeds the appearance of clinical disease makes any experiments that are attempted very costly to conduct.

Analogous Mechanisms

Epidemiologists hope to find analogous mechanisms as evidence to support a causal hypothesis. For example, it is hypothesized that if smoking exposes the lungs to carcinomatous tars, then it should be possible to induce carcinomatous changes by painting the skin of mice with the tars formed during the combustion of cigarettes.

There is little analogous evidence concerning the beneficial effects of physical activity. The recurrence of fatal myocardial infarction is reduced by the regular administration of β-blocking drugs (155), pointing to an analogy with the exercise-induced reduction of catecholamine output. Likewise, if blood cholesterol levels are reduced by a regular daily dose of cholestyramine, there is some reduction in the incidence of fatal heart attacks among patients with a high risk of cardiovascular disease (98), supporting the benefit of an analogous exercise-induced amelioration of the blood lipid profile.

SUMMARY

In summary, there is much evidence suggesting the benefit of increased physical activity in the secondary and the tertiary prevention of a variety of chronic disorders. However, for various technical reasons, it is difficult to mount conclusive double-blind experiments.

Not all of Bradford Hill's criteria of a causal linkage between regular exercise and good health are fully satisfied. Nevertheless, in most conditions where exercise is commonly proposed, the benefits of enhanced physical activity seem to outweigh any disadvantages. An increase of physical exercise can thus be commended not only in terms of the probable control of disease, but also (and more importantly) in terms of an enhancement of the quality of life.

REFERENCES

1. Adams, W.C., Fox, R.H., Fry, A.J., and MacDonald, I. C., *J. Appl. Physiol., 38*:1030–1037 (1975).
2. American College of Sports Medicine, *Med. Sci. Sports,* 7:vii–viii (1975).
3. American College of Sports Medicine, *Guidelines for Graded Exercise Testing and Prescription.* 3rd Ed. Lea & Febiger, Philadelphia (1986).
4. Anderson, T., and Kerney, J.T., *Res. Quart., 53*: 1–7 (1982).
5. Armstrong, R.B., *Sports Med., 3*: 370–381 (1986).
6. Asmussen, E., and Bøje O., *Acta Physiol. Scand., 10*: 1–22 (1945).
7. Åstrand, I., Åstrand, P.O., Christensen, E.H., and Hedman, R., *Acta Physiol. Scand., 48*: 448–453 (1960).
8. Åstrand, P.O., Cuddy, T.E., Saltin, B., and Stenberg, J., *J. Appl. Physiol., 19*: 268–274 (1964).
9. Auble, T.E., Schwartz, L., and Robertson, J., *Phys. Sportsmed.,* 15(6):133–140 (1987).
10. Banister, E.W., in *Frontiers of Fitness* (R.J. Shephard, ed.). Charles C Thomas, Springfield, Illinois, pp. 5–36 (1971).
11. Bartels, R., Billings, C.E., Fox, E.L., Mathews, D.K., O'Brien, R., Tauz, D., and Webb, W., Abstracts, AAHPER Convention, p. 13 (cited by Pollock, 1973) (1968).
12. Bassey, E.J., Patrick, J.M., Irving, J.M., Blecher, A., and Fentem, P.H., *Eur. J. Appl. Physiol., 52*: 120–125 (1983).
13. Beaudet, S.M. *Ergonomics,* 27:955–957 (1984).
14. Besdine, R.W. and Harris, T.B., in *Principles of Geriatric Medicine* (R. Andres, E.L. Bierman, and W.R. Hazzard, eds.). McGraw-Hill, New York, pp. 209–217 (1985).
14a. Blair, S.N., Piserchia, P.V., Wilbur, C.S., and Crowder, J.H. *JAMA 255:* 921–926 (1986).
15. Blimkie, C.J., Cunningham, D.A., and Leung, F.Y. in *Frontiers of Activity and Child Health* (H. Lavallée and R.J. Shephard, eds.). Editions du Pélican, Quebec City, pp. 313–321 (1977).
16. Birk, T.J., and Birk, C.A., *Sports Med., 4*: 1–8 (1987).
17. Boone, T., and Edwards, C.A., *Ann. Sports Med., 4*: 29–31 (1988).
18. Booth, F.W. and Watson, P.A., *Fed. Proc., 44*: 2293–2300 (1985).
19. Borg, G., in *Frontiers of Fitness* (R.J. Shephard, ed.). Charles C Thomas, Springfield, Illinois, pp. 280–294 (1971).
20. Bouchard, C., Hollmann, W., Venrath, H., Herkenrath, G., and Schlussel, H., *Sportarzt u Sportmedizin, 7*: 348–357 (1966).
21. Bryan, C., *Can. Med. Assoc. J., 96*: 804 (1967).
21a. Buyze, M.T., Foster, C., Pollock, M.L., Sennett, S.M., Hare, J., and Sol, N., *Phys. Sportsmed.,* 14(11): 65–69 (1986).
22. Caspersen, C.J., Powell, K.E., and Christenson, G.M., *Publ. Health Rep., 100*: 126–131 (1985).
23. Chad, K.E., and Wenger, H.A., *Can. J. Sport Sci., 13*: 204–207 (1989).
24. Chow, R.J., and Wilmore, J.H., *J. Cardiac Rehab., 4*: 382–387 (1984).

25. Chow, R.K., Harrison, J.E., Sturtridge, W., Josse, R., Murray, T.M., Bayley, A., Dornan, J., and Hammond, T., *Clin. Invest. Med.* *10*(2): 59–63 (1987).
26. Claremont, A.D., and Hall, S.J., *Med. Sci. Sports Exerc.*, *20*: 167–171 (1988).
27. Clausen, J.P., *Physiol. Rev.*, *57*:779–815 (1977).
28. Cox, M.L., Bennett, J.B., and Dudley, G.A., *J. Appl. Physiol.*, *61*: 926–931 (1986).
29. Cummins, P., Young, A., Auckland, M.L., Michie, C.A., Stone, P.C.W., and Shepstone, B.J., *Eur. J. Clin. Invest.*, *17*: 317–324 (1987).
30. Daub, W.D., Green, H.J., Houston, M.E., Thomson, J.A., Fraser, I.G., and Ranney, D.A., *Can. J. Physiol.*, *60*: 628–633 (1982).
31. Daub, W.D., Green, H.J., Houston, M.E., Thomson, J.A., Fraser, I.G., and Ranney, D.A., *Med. Sci. Sports Exerc.*, *15*: 290–294 (1983).
32. Davies, C.T.M., and Knibbs, A.V., *Int. Z. Angew. Physiol.*, *29*: 299–305 (1971).
33. Davies, C.T.M., and Starkie, D.W., *Eur. J. Appl. Physiol.*, *53*: 359–363 (1985).
34. di Prampero, P.E. in *Frontiers of Fitness* (R.J. Shephard, ed.). Charles C Thomas, Springfield, Illinois, pp. 155–173 (1971).
35. Donselaar, Y., Eerbeek, O., Kernell, D., and Verhey, B.A. *J. Physiol. (Lond.)*, *382*: 237–254 (1987).
36. Driver, H.S., Meintjes, A.F., Rogers, G.C., and Shapiro, C. M., *Acta Physiol. Scand*, *133*(Suppl. 574): 8–13 (1988).
37. Dudley, G.A., and Fleck, S.J., Strength training and endurance training. *Sports Med.*, *4*: 79–85 (1987).
38. Durnin, J.V.G.A., Brockway, J.M., and Whitcher, H.W., *J. Appl. Physiol.*, *15*: 161–165 (1960).
39. Edwards, R.H.T., Ekelund, L.G., Harris, R.C., Hesser, C.M., Hultman, E., Melcher, A., and Wigertz, O., *J. Physiol. (Lond.)*, *234*: 481–497 (1973).
40. Ekblöm, B., and Hermansen, L., *J. Appl. Physiol.*, *25*: 619–625 (1968).
41. Ellis, F.P., *Environ. Res.*, *5*: 1–4 (1972).
42. Faria, I.E., *Res. Quart.* *41*: 44–50 (1970).
43. Fernhall, B., and Kohrt, W., *Med. Sci. Sports Exerc.*, *17*: 225 (1985).
44. Friden, J. *Int. J. Sports Med.*, *5*: 57–66 (1984).
45. Fried, T., and Shephard, R.J., *Can. Med. Assoc. J.*, *103*: 260–266 (1970).
46. Folinsbee, L., Shephard, R.J., and Silverman, F., *J. Appl. Physiol.*, *42*: 531–536 (1977).
47. Frisk-Holmberg, M., Essén, B., Fredrickson, M., Ström, G., and Wibell, L., *Acta Med. Scand.*, *213*: 21–26 (1983).
48. Garrick, J.G., Gillien, D.M., and Whiteside, P., *Am. J. Sports Med.*, *14*: 67–72 (1986).
49. Gergley, T., McArdle, W., DeJesus, P., Toner, M., Jacobwitz, S., and Spina, R., *Med. Sci. Sports Exerc.*, *16*: 125 (1984).
50. Gettman, L.R., Culter, L.A. and Strathman, T.A., *J. Sports Med. Phys. Fitness*, *20*: 265–274 (1980).
51. Glaser, E.M., *The Physiological Basis of Habituation.* Oxford University Press, London, pp. 1–102 (1966).

52. Gledhill, N., and Eynon, R.B., in *Training: Scientific Basis and Application* (A.W. Taylor, ed.). Charles C Thomas, Springfield, Illinois, (1972).
53. Godin, G., and Shephard, R.J., *Sports Med.* 10: 103–121, (1990).
54. Going, S.B., Ball, T.E. and Massey, B.M., *Med. Sci. Sports Exerc.*, 15: 163 (Abstr.) (1983).
55. Goldman, A., Exton-Smith, A.N., G. Francis, et al., *J.R. Coll. Phys. (Lond.)*, 11: 291–306 (1977).
56. Gollnick, P.D., and Hermansen, L., *Exerc. Sport Sci. Rev.*, 1: 1–43 (1973).
57. Gonyea, W., Ericson, G.C., and Bonde-Peterson, F., *Acta Physiol. Scand.*, 99: 105–109 (1977).
58. Graves, J.E., Pollock, M.L., Montain, S.J., Jackson, A.S., and O'Keefe, J.M., *Med. Sci. Sports Exerc.*, 19: 260–265 (1987).
59. Grimby, G., *Sports Med.*, 2: 309–315 (1985).
60. Grogan, J.W., and Kelly, J.M., *Med. Sci. Sports Exerc.*, 17: 268–269 (1985).
61. Hagberg, J.M., Ehsani, A.A., and Holloszy, J.O., *Circulation*, 67: 1194–1199 (1983).
62. Hakkinen, K., and Komi, P.V., *Eur. J. Appl. Physiol.*, 55: 147–155 (1986).
63. Hamrell, B.B., and Hultgren, P.B., *Fed. Proc.*, 45: 2591–2596 (1986).
64. Hansen, J.W., *Int. Z. Angew. Physiol.*, 23: 367–370 (1967).
65. Harber, V.J., and Sutton, J.O. *Sports Med.*, 1: 154–171 (1984).
66. Harrison, M.H., *Sports Med.*, 3: 214–223 (1986).
67. Heinritze, J., Weltman, A., Schurrer, R.L., and Barlow, K., *Eur. J. Appl. Physiol.*, 54: 84–88 (1985).
68. Hermansen, L., in *Muscle Metabolism During Exercise* (B. Pernow and B. Saltin, eds.). Plenum Press, New York, pp. 401–408 (1971).
69. Herzlich, C. *Health and Illness*. Academic Press, New York (1973).
70. Hettinger, T., *Physiology of Strength*. Charles C Thomas, Springfield, Illinois (1961).
71. Hickson, R.C., and Rosenkoetter, M.A., *Am. J. Physiol.*, 241: C140–C144 (1981).
72. Hickson, R.C., Hagberg, J.M., Ehsani, A.A., and Holloszy, J. O., *Med. Sci. Spt. Exerc.*, 13: 17–20 (1981).
73. Hickson, R.C., Kanakis, C., Davis, J.R., Moore, A.M., and Rich, S., *J. Appl. Physiol.*, 53: 225–229 (1982).
74. Hill, J.S., Wearing, G.A., and Eynon, R.B., *Med. Sci. Sports*, 3: k (1971).
75. Ho, K.W., Roy, R.R., Taylor, J.F., Heusner, W.W., and Van Huss, W.D., *Med. Sci. Sports Exerc.*, 15: 472–477 (1983).
76. Holloszy, J.O., and Booth, F.W., *Ann. Rev. Physiol.*, 38: 273–291 (1976).
77. Holmgren, A., *Can. Med. Assoc. J.*, 96: 697–702 (1967).
78. Howald, H., *Int. J. Sports Med.*, 3: 1–12 (1982).
78a. Hultman, E. Muscle glycogen stores and prolonged exercise. in *Frontiers of Fitness*. R.J. Shephard, ed. Springfield, Illinois: Charles C. Thomas, 1971.
79. Inbar, O., Gutin, B., Dotan, R., and Bar-Or, O., *Med. Sci. Sports*, 10: 62 (1978).
80. Jacobs, I., Romet, T.T. and Kerrigan-Brown, D., *Eur. J. Appl. Physiol.*, 54: 35–39 (1985).
81. Kanehisa, H., and Miyashita, M. *Eur. J. Appl. Physiol.*, 52: 104–106 (1983).

82. Karvonen, M.J., Kentala, E., and Mustala, O., *Ann. Med. Exp. Fenn., 35*: 307–315 (1957).
83. Katz, A., Sharp, R.L., Armstrong, L.E., and King, D.S., *Can. J. Appl. Spt. Sci., 9*: 11–15 (1984).
84. Kavanagh, T., *Heart Attack? Counter Attack!* Van Nostrand, Toronto (1976).
85. Kavanagh, T. *The Healthy Heart Programme.* Van Nostrand, Toronto (1980).
86. Kavanagh, T. *Phys. Sportsmed., 17*(1): 96–114 (1988).
86a. Kavanagh, T. and Shephard, R.J. Conditioning of post-coronary patients: comparison of continous and interval training. *Arch. Phys. Med. Rehab. 56*: 72–76, (1975),
87. Kavanagh, T., Shephard, R.J., Tuck, J.A., and Qureshi, S., *Ann. N.Y. Acad. Sci., 301*: 1029–1038 (1977).
88. Kavanagh, T., and Shephard, R.J., *Arch. Phys. Med. Rehab., 61*(3): 114–118 (1980).
88a. Kavanagh, T. and Shephard, R.J., *Physician Sports Medicine 18*(6): 94–103 (1990).
88b. Kavanagh, T. Lindley, L.J., Shephard, R.J., and Campbell, R. *Ann. Sport Med. 4*: 55–64 (1988).
89. Kavanagh, T., Shephard, R.J., Lindley, L.J., and Pieper, M., *Arteriosclerosis, 3*: 249–259 (1983).
90. Keast, D., Cameron, K., and Morton, A.R., *Sports Med., 5*: 248–267 (1988).
91. Kenyon, G.S., *Res. Quart., 39*: 566–574 (1968).
92. Kohl, H.W., Blair, S.N., Paffenbarger, R.S., Macera, C.A., and Kronenfeld, J.J., *Am. J. Epidemiol., 127*: 1228–1239 (1988).
93. Kuipers, H., and Keizer, H.A., *Sports Med., 6*: 79–92 (1988).
94. Landry, F., Bouchard, C., and Dumesnil, J., *J.A.M.A., 254*: 77–80 (1985).
95. Lawrence, G., *Aqua-Fitness for Women.* Personal Library Publishers, Toronto, (1981).
96. Lind, A.R., and McNicol, G.W., *Can. Med. Assoc. J., 96*: 706–712 (1967).
97. Linden, R.J., Mary, D.A.S.G., and Winter, C., *J. Physiol. (Lond.), 357*: 100P (1984).
98. Lipid Research Clinics, *J.A.M.A., 251*: 351–364; 365–374 (1984).
99. Loftin, M., Boileau, R.A., Massey, B.H., and Lohman, T.G., *Med. Sci. Sports Exerc., 20*: 136–141 (1988).
100. Lortie, G., Bouchard, C., LeBlanc, C., Tremblay, A., Simoneau, J.A., Thériault, G., and Savoie, J.-P., *Hum. Biol., 54*: 801–812 (1982).
101. MacDougall, J.D., Sale, D.G., Moroz, J.R., Elder, G.C.B., Sutton, J.R., and Howald, H., *Med. Sci. Sports, 11*: 164–166 (1979).
102. Martens, R., *Exerc. Sports Sci. Rev., 2*: 155–188 (1974).
103. Matsuda, J.J., and Vailas, A.C., *Med. Sci. Sports Exerc., 16*: 120 (1984).
104. McNamara, P.S., Otto, R.M., and Smith, T.K., *Med. Sci. Sports Exerc., 17*: 266 (Abstr.) (1985).
105. Milburn, S., and Butts, N.K., *Med. Sci. Sports Exerc., 15*: 510–513 (1983).
106. Montoye, H.J., *Physical Activity and Health: An Epidemiological Study of an*

Entire Community. Prentice Hall, Englewood Cliffs, New Jersey (1975).
106a. Morgan, W.P., Gildiner, M. and Wright, G.R. *CAHPER J* 42: 36–43 (1976).
107. Morris, J.N., and Crawford, M.D., *Lancet*, 2: 1053–1057, 1111–1120 (1958).
108. Murray, S.J., Shephard, R.J., Greaves, S., Allen, C., and Radomski, M., *Eur. J. Appl. Physiol.*, 55: 610–618 (1986).
109. Nadel, J., *Problems with Temperature Regulation During Exercise.* Academic Press, New York (1977).
110. Nielsen, B., Kassow, K., and Aschengreen, F.E., *Eur. J. Appl. Physiol.*, 58: 189–196 (1988).
111. Niinimaa, V., Cole, P., Mintz, S., and Shephard, R.J., *Resp. Physiol.*, 43: 69–75 (1979).
112. Noakes, T.D., Higginson, L., and Opie, L.H., *Circulation*, 67: 24–30 (1983).
113. Noble, B.J., Kraemer, W.J., Clark, M.J., and Culver, B.W., *Med. Sci. Sports Exerc.*, 16: 146 (1984).
114. O'Hara, W.J., Allen, C., and Shephard, R.J., *Eur. J. Appl. Physiol.*, 37: 205–218 (1977).
115. O'Hara, W.J., Allen, C., and Shephard, R.J., *Can. Med. Assoc. J.*, 117: 773–779 (1977).
116. O'Hara, W.J., Allen, C., and Shephard, R.J., *Can. J. Physiol.*, 55: 1235–1241 (1978).
117. O'Hara, W.J., Allen, C., Shephard, R.J., and Allen, G., *J. Appl. Physiol.*, 46: 872–877 (1979).
118. Oja, P., *Finn. Spts. Exerc. Med.*, 2: 62–71 (1983).
119. Oja, P., Vuori, I., Nieminen, R., Kukkonen-Harjula, K., and Niittymaki, S., *Med. Sci. Sports Exerc.*, 17: 270 (1985).
119a. Oldridge, N.B., Guyatt, G.H., Fischer, M.E., and Rimm, A.A. *JAMA* 260: 945–50 (1988).
119b. Paffenbarger, R.S. *Med. Sci. Sports Exerc.* 20: 426–438 1988.
120. Parker, J.O., DiGiorgi, S., and West, R.O., *Am. J. Cardiol.*, 17: 470–483 (1966).
121. Paterson, D.H., Shephard, R.J., Cunningham, D., Jones, N.L., and Andrew, G., *J. Appl. Physiol.*, 47: 482–489 (1979).
121a. Pels, A.E., Pollock, M.I., Dohmeier, T.E., Lemberger, K.A., and Dehrlein, B.F. *Med. Sci. Sports Exerc.* 19: 66–70 (1987).
122. Pérussue, L., Lortie, G., LeBlanc, C., Tremblay, A., Thériault, G., and Bouchard, C., *Ann. Hum. Biol.*, 14: 425–434 (1987).
123. Pérusse, L., LeBlanc, C., and Bouchard, C., *Can. J. Sport Sci.*, 13: 8–14 (1988).
123a. Phair, J.J., Carey, G.C.R., and Shephard, R.J. Measuring human reactions to air pollution. *Monograph 4.* Washington: Franklin Institute, (1958).
124. Pirnay, F., Bodeux, M., Crielaard, J.M., and Franchimont, P. *Int. J. Sports Med.*, 8: 331–335 (1987).
125. Pollock, M. *Exerc. Sport Sci. Rev.* 1: 155–188 (1973).

126. Pollock, M.L., *Phys. Sportsmed.*, 6(6): 50–64 (1979).
127. Pollock, M.L., Miller, H.S., Linnerud, A.C., and Cooper, K. H., *Arch. Phys. Med. Rehab.*, 56: 141–145 (1975).
128. Porcari, J., McCarron, R. , Kline, G., Freedson, P.F., Ward, A., Ross, J.A., and Rippe, J.M., *Phys. Sportsmed.*, 15(2): 119–129 (1987).
128a. Powell, K.E., Thompson, P.D., Caspersen, C.J., and Kendrick, J.S., *Ann. Rev. Publ. Hlth.* 8: 253–287 (1987).
129. Pugh, L.G.C.E., in *Environmental Effects on Work Performance* (G.R. Cumming, D. Snidal, and A.W. Taylor, eds.). Canadian Association of Sport Sciences, Ottawa (1972).
130. Robinson, E.P., and Kjellgaard, J.M., *J. Appl. Physiol.*, 52: 1400–1406 (1982).
131. Rogers, M.A., Yamamoto, C., Hagberg, J.M., Martin, W.H., Ehsani, A.A., and Holloszy, J.O., *Med. Sci. Sports Exerc.*, 20: 260–264 (1988).
132. Rosch, P.J., in *Psychosomatic Cardiovascular Disorders—When and How to Treat* (P. Kielholz, W. Siegenthaler, P. Taggart, and A. Zanxhetti, eds.). Huber, Bern (1981).
133. Rösler, K., Hoppeler, H., Conley, K.E., Claassen, H., Gehr, P., and Howald, H., *Eur. J. Appl. Physiol.*, 54: 355–362 (1985).
134. Rösler, K., Conley, K.E., Howald, H., Gerber, C., and Hoppeler, H., *J. Appl. Physiol.*, 61: 30–36 (1986).
135. Rowell, L.B., *Physiol. Rev.*, 54: 75–159 (1974).
136. Rowell, L.B., in *Handbook of Physiology*. Vol. 27. American Physiological Society, Washington, D.C., pp. 967–1023 (1985).
137. Rubal, B.J., Al Muhailani, A.R., and Rosentswieg, J., *Med. Sci. Sports Exerc.*, 19: 423–429 (1987).
138. Rusko, H., and Bosco, C., *Eur. J. Appl. Physiol.*, 56: 412–418 (1987).
139. Rusko, H., and Rahkila, P., *J. Sports Sci.*, 1: 185–194 (1983).
140. Sachs, M.L., in *The Exercising Adult* (R.C. Cantu, ed.). Heath, Lexington, Massachusetts, pp. 19–27 (1982).
141. Saltin, B., in *Textbook of Work Physiology*. McGraw-Hill, New York, p. 466 (1970).
142. Saltin, B., in *Limiting Factors of Physical Performance* (J. Keul, ed.). Thieme, Stuttgart (1973).
143. Saltin, B., and Hermansen, L., in *Nutrition and Physical Activity* (G. Blix, ed.). Almqvist and Wiksell, Uppsala, p. 32 (1967).
144. Saltin, B., Blomqvist, G., Mitchell, J.H., Johnson, R.L., Wildenthal, K., and Chapman, C.B., *Am. Heart Assoc. Monogr.*, 23: 1–68 (1968).
145. Saltin, B., Hartley, L.H., Kilbom, Å., and Åstrand, I., *Scand. J. Clin. Lab. Invest.*, 24: 323–334 (1969).
146. Schwartz, E., Glick, Z., and Magazanik, A., *Aviat. Space Environ. Med.*, 48: 254–260 (1977).
147. Sexton, W.L., Korthuis, R.J., and Laughlin, M.H., *Am. J. Physiol.*, 254: H274–H278 (1988).
148. Sharkey, B.J., *Med. Sci. Sports*, 2: 197–202 (1970).
149. Sharkey, B.J., and Holleman, J.P., *Res. Quart.*, 38: 698–704 (1967).

150. Shephard, R.J., *Int. Z. Angew. Physiol.*, *26*: 272–278 (1968).
151. Shephard, R.J., *Int. Z. Angew. Physiol.*, *28*: 38–48 (1969).
152. Shephard, R.J., *Br. J. Sports Med.*, *8*: 38–45 (1974).
153. Shephard, R.J., *Endurance Fitness*. 2nd Ed. University of Toronto Press, Toronto (1977).
154. Shephard, R.J., *Human Physiological Work Capacity*. Cambridge University Press, London (1978).
155. Shephard, R.J., *Ischemic Heart Disease and Exercise*. Croom Helm, London (1981).
156. Shephard, R.J., *Physiology and Biochemistry of Exercise*. Praeger Publishing, New York (1982).
157. Shephard, R.J., *Biochemistry of Exercise*. Charles C Thomas, Springfield, Illinois (1983).
158. Shephard, R.J., *Canad. Med. Assoc. J.*, *128*: 525–530 (1983).
159. Shephard, R.J., *Sports Med.*, *2*: 59–71 (1985).
160. Shephard, R.J., *CAHPER J.*, *50*(6): 2–5, 20 (1985).
161. Shephard, R.J., *Economic Benefits of Enhanced Fitness*. Human Kinetics, Champaign, Illinois (1986).
161a. Shephard, R.J., *Physical Activity and Ageing*. 2nd Ed. Croon Helm Publishing, London.
162. Shephard, R.J., in *Olympic Book of Sports Medicine* (A. Dirix, H.G. Knuttgen, and K. Tittel, Eds.). Blackwell Scientific, Oxford. (1988).
163. Shephard, R.J. *The Determination of Body Composition in Biological Anthropology*. Cambridge University Press, London (1989).
164. Shephard, R.J. *Br. J. Sports Med. 23*: 11–22.
164a. Shephard, R.J., *Can. J. Sport Sci. 14*: 74–84 (1989).
165. Shephard, R.J., and Sidney, K.H., *Exerc. Sport Sci. Rev.*, *3*: 1–30 (1975).
166. Shephard, R.J., Corey, P., and Cox, M., *Can. J. Publ. Health*, *73*: 183–187 (1982).
167. Shephard, R.J., Kavanagh, T., and Klavora, P., *J. Cardiac Rehab.*, *5*: 480–484 (1985).
167a. Shephard, R.J., Bouhlel, E., Vandewalle, H., and Monod, H. *J. Appl. Physiol. 64*: 1472–1479 (1988).
168. Sidney, K.H., and Shephard, R.J., *Can. J. Appl. Spt. Sci.*, *2*: 189–194 (1978).
169. Sidney, K.H., and Shephard, R.J., *Med. Sci. Sports Exerc.*, *10*: 125–131 (1978).
170. Sidney, K.H., Shephard, R.J., and Harrison, J., *Am. J. Clin. Nutr.*, *30*: 326–333 (1977).
171. Simmons, R., and Shephard, R.J., *Int. Z. Angew. Physiol.*, *30*: 73–84 (1971).
172. Simmons, R., and Shephard, R.J., *Int. Z. Angew. Physiol.*, *29*: 159–172 (1971).
173. Simoneau, J.A., Lortie, G., Boulay, M.R., Marcotte, M., Thibault, M.C., and Bouchard, C., *Eur. J. Appl. Physiol.*, *54*: 250–253 (1985).
174. Sloan, E.R.G., and Keatinge, W.R., *J. Appl. Physiol.*, *16*: 167–169 (1973).

175. Smith, D.A., and O'Donnell, T.V., *Clin. Sci.*, *67*: 229–236 (1984).
176. Stillman, R.J., Lohman, T.G., Slaughter, M.H., and Massey, B. H., *Med. Sci. Sports Exerc.*, *18*: 576–580 (1986).
177. Tamaki, N., *Eur. J. Appl. Physiol.*, *56*: 127–131 (1987).
178. Tanaka, K., Yoshimura, T., Sumida, S., Mitszono, R., Tanaka, S., Konishi, Y., Watanabe, H., Yamada, T., and Maeda, K., *Eur. J. Appl. Physiol.*, *55*: 356–361 (1986).
179. Taylor, H.L., Henschel, A., Brozek, J., and Keys, A., *J. Appl. Physiol.*, *2*: 223–239 (1949).
180. Taylor, N.A.S., and Wilkinson, J.G., *Sports Med.*, *3*: 190–200 (1986).
181. Tesch, P., Karlsson, J., and Sjödin, B., in *Exercise and Sport Biology* (P.V. Komi, ed.). Human Kinetics, Champaign, Illinois (1982).
182. Thomas, D.P., *Med. Sci. Sports Exerc.*, *17*: 546–553 (1985).
183. Thorstensson, A., *Acta Physiol. Scand.*, *443* (Suppl.): 1–45 (1976).
184. Turto, H., Lindy, S., and Haline, J., *Am. J. Physiol.*, *226*: 63–65 (1974).
185. Vandenburgh, H.H., *Med. Sci. Sports Exerc.*, *19*: S142 (1987).
186. Vernon, H.M., Bedford, T., and Karner, C.F., *Rep. Industr. Fatigue Res. Bd. (Lond.)*, *39*: His Majesty's Stationery Office, London.
187. Von Euler, U.S., *Med. Sci. Sport*, *6*: 165–173 (1974).
188. Vuori, I., Urponen, H., Hasan, J., and Partinen, M., *Acta Physiol. Scand.*, *133* (Suppl. 574): 3–7 (1988).
189. Wasserman, K., Whipp, B.J., Koyal, S.N., and Beaver, W.L., *J. Appl. Physiol.*, *35*: 236–243 (1973).
190. Wenger, H.A., and MacNab, R.B.J., in *Application of Science and Medicine to Sport* (A.W. Taylor, ed.). Charles C Thomas, Springfield, Illinois (1972).
191. Wenger, H.A., and Bell, G.J., *Sports Med.*, *3*: 346–356 (1986).
192. White, J.R., *Med. Sci. Sports*, *12*: 103 (1980).
193. Williams, J.A., Wagner, J., Wasnich, R., and Heilbrun, L., *Med. Sci. Sports Exerc.*, *16*: 223–227 (1984).
194. Williams, P.T., Wood, P.D., Haskell, W.L., and Vranizan, K. *J. A.M.A.*, *247*: 2672–2679 (1982).
195. Wilmore, J.H., Davis, J.A., O'Brien, R.S., Vodak, P.A., Walder, G.R., and Amsterdam, E.A., *Med. Sci. Sports*, *12*: 1–8 (1980).
196. Wilt, F., in *Exercise Physiology* (H. Falls, ed.). Academic Press, New York (1968).
197. World Health Organisation, *Report of 29th General Assembly*. World Health Organisation, Geneva. (1975).
198. Wyndham, C.H., and Strydom, N.B., in *Zentrale Themem der Sportmedizin* (W.R. Hollman, ed.). Springer Verlag, Berlin (1972).
199. Wyndham, C.H., Strydom, N.B., Benade, A.J.S., and Van Rensbury, A.J., *J. Appl. Physiol.*, *35*: 454–458 (1973).
200. Yerkes, R.M., and Dodson, J.D., *J. Comp. Neurol. Psychol.*, *18*: 459–482, 1908 (1908).

2

Assessment of Exercise Capacity and Principles of Exercise Prescription

Jack Goodman

University of Toronto
Toronto, Ontario, Canada

INTRODUCTION

The general assessment of fitness should encorporate four basic components, including aerobic power ($\dot{V}O_{2\,max}$), muscular strength and endurance, flexibility, and body composition. Depending on the precision desired, there are a number of methods to assess each of these components, with both specificity and reproducibility dependent upon the sophistication of the instrumentation used. This chapter will provide an overview of methods to assess these components, and outline strategies for improving cardiorespiratory fitness.

ASSESSMENT OF CARDIOVASCULAR FITNESS

Basic Principles

An increase in oxygen consumption ($\dot{V}O_2$) is brought about by an increase in cardiac output and peripheral extraction of oxygen. Cardiac output is augmented by increases in both heart rate (HR) and stroke volume, the latter through two mechanisms: increases in end-diastolic volume (EDV) via the Frank-Starling relationship, and reduction in end-diastolic volume (ESV) via an augmented contractile state. The increase in EDV may occur predominantly during submaximal exercise below the ventilatory threshold (VT) (20), whereas changes in ESV occur at all intensities of exercise. Increased extraction of oxygen ($a\bar{v}O_2$ difference) is achieved by maximizing the arterial content of O_2 (CaO_2) and subsequent extraction at the muscle level. Factors determining maximal CaO_2 include the arterial oxygen pressure $PaiO_2$ (affected by pulmonary diffusion), and the hemoglobin concentration. Complete extraction, represented by the lowest possible mixed venous oxygen content ($C\bar{v}O_2$), is dependent on capillary density (affecting tissue diffusion capacity), aerobic enzyme function, and fiber type. The functional limit to oxygen consumption can therefore be expressed by the Fick equation for O_2, where:

$$\dot{V}O_2 = (\text{cardiac output}) \times (a\bar{v}O_2 \text{ difference})$$

Maximal values of each component will provide a physiological limit to $\dot{V}O_{2\,max}$, depicted during graded exercise as a plateau of oxygen consumption despite increasing work rates; this in turn defines a functional limit or capacity. The linear relationship which exists between work rate and $\dot{V}O_2$ provides the basis for submaximal predictive tests of aerobic power (see Fig. 1). Since heart rate and work output are linearly related, use of a submaximal work rate and heart rate

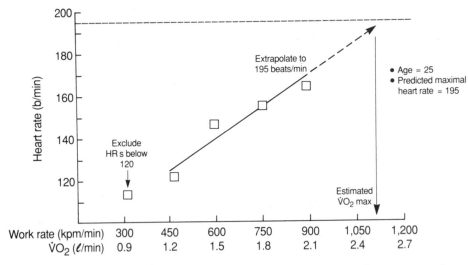

Figure 1 Pattern of $\dot{V}O_2$ during progressive exercise on a cycle ergometer. A linear increase in $\dot{V}O_2$ is observed during graded, submaximal exercise. The linear relationship allows extrapolation from submaximal levels of exercise to an age-predicted heart rate and corresponding O_2 consumption.

can provide an indirect assessment of maximal oxygen consumption, providing the mechanical efficiency of effort remains constant.

Techniques for measuring ventilatory gas exchange can noninvasively determine the functional limit of the cardiovascular system, using the basic equation.

$$\dot{V}O_2 = (\dot{V}_I \cdot F_{IO_2}) - (\dot{V}_E \cdot F_{EO_2})$$

where V_I and V_E are the inspiratory and the expiratory minute volumes, respectively, and F_{IO_2} and F_{EO_2} are the corresponding fractional concentrations of oxygen.

Various calculations and assumptions are required for a true measure of $\dot{V}O_2$, and these are described below. Direct gas-exchange measurements using rapid-response O_2 and CO_2 analyzers (see below) can provide measures of $\dot{V}O_{2\,max}$, VT, and other common gas-exchange parameters which are useful in the clinical assessment of cardiopulmonary impairment or general fitness (Table 1). Clinical exercise testing in some facilities now includes measurement of $\dot{V}O_{2\,max}$ and other gas-exchange variables, since $\dot{V}O_{2\,max}$ and the VT may provide more objective information on prognosis and functional status in certain cardiac disease states versus traditional measures such as left ventricular ejection fraction alone (55). When facilities for these determinations are unavailable, $\dot{V}O_{2\,max}$ can be estimated by various methods.

Submaximal (Predictive) versus Maximal Exercise Testing

Prediction of maximal aerobic power ($\dot{V}O_{2\,max}$) remains the most common method to assess functional capacity, particularly during clinical exercise testing. Advantages over maximal, direct measures of $VO_{2\,max}$ include: a) short test duration, b) greater safety, c) low cost, d) less equipment required, e) less expertise required, and f) group testing may be possible (15,52). Predictive tests are based upon the linear relationship between heart rate and O_2 consumption, and require the establishment of a steady-state heart rate at a given work rate. However, the error of predictive tests can range from 10 to 15%, thus for greatest accuracy, direct measures of maximal O_2 consumption are recommended. Such evaluation provides data which describe the cardiopulmonary response to exercise, and can be used to differentiate pulmonary from cardiovascular limitations in a range of diseases (54).

Supine versus Erect Exercise

Supine clinical exercise tests are slowly being supplanted with upright protocols in North America; however, European testing is still dom-

Table 1 Common Gas-Exchange Measurements, Definitions, and Normal Ranges

Measurement	Definition	Normal Range
$\dot{V}O_{2\,max}$	Upper limit for O_2 consumption obtained despite increase in work rate. Functional limit of cardiovascular system.	Male: 4.2–.0032 (age) L/min (SD ±0.4); 60–0.55 (age) ml/kg/min (SD ±7.5)[a] Female: 2.6–0.014 (age) L/min (SD ±0.4); 48–0.37 (age) ml/kg/min (SD ±7.0)[a]
$\dot{V}O_2$ slope ($\Delta\dot{V}O_2/\Delta WR$)	Aerobic contribution to exercise; low slope implies greater anaerobic contribution to work.	8.6–12 ml/min/W
O_2 pulse ($\dot{V}O_2/HR$)	Proportional to $a\overline{v}O_2$ dif. when SV is constant. Varies with age, sex, height, haemoglobin; higher in endurance trained. Can reflect changes in SV at maximum exercise if $a\overline{v}O_2$ is constant.	10–14 (males) 7–10 (female)
Ventilatory threshold (VT)	Noninvasive index of the nonlinear increase in blood lactate. Disproportionate increase in $\dot{V}E$ vs $\dot{V}O_2$, or other criteria (see text)	Absolute (% $\dot{V}O_2$ max): 45–65% Relative (ml/kg/min): >25 ml/kg/min
$\dot{V}E/MVV$ (dyspnea index)	Index providing analysis of balance between demand and capacity of ventilatory system.	65–80%
HR_{max}	Maximal heart rate obtained during maximal-effort exercise test. Age dependent.	$HR_{max} = 210 - 0.65$ age $= 220 -$ age
RER_{max} ($\dot{V}CO_2/\dot{V}O_2$)	Indicates substrate utilization (1 = complete carbohydrate metabolism). Rest = 0.75–0.85.	Values > 1.10–1.15 indicate maximal effort reached (when used in conjunction with other criteria—see text).
VD/VT	Physiological dead space/tidal volume ratio. Indicates matching of ventilation to perfusion. Falls with exercise, high in obstructive lung disease.	25–40% at rest; 5–20 during exercise.

Abbreviations: HR = heart rate; MVV = maximum voluntary ventilation; RER = respiratory gas exchange ratio; $\dot{V}O_2$ = oxygen consumption; $\dot{V}CO_2$ = carbon dioxide production; VD = dead space; $\dot{V}E$ = ventilation; VT = tidal volume.

[a] From Ref. 31; used with permission.

inated by supine cycle ergometry. Supine testing offers the advantage in detection of myocardial ischemia, with a greater likelihood of ST-segment abnormalities being observed (17). In this position, left ventricular (LV) end-diastolic volume is maximal, thereby increasing LV wall stress (and thus myocardial oxygen demand), with little change in stroke volume observed throughout exercise. Measures of $\dot{V}O_{2\,max}$ are typically 12–18% less during supine exercise testing, and therefore results must be interpreted carefully relative to data obtained from upright protocols.

Choice of Ergometer and Protocol

Measures of $\dot{V}O_{2\,max}$ vary depending on the type of ergometer used for testing. Treadmill testing yields a "true" $\dot{V}O_{2\,max}$ when subjects are properly motivated, and is therefore used as a gold standard for the assessment of functional capacity. Supine cycle ergometry will yield a $\dot{V}O_{2\,max}$ 12–18% less than treadmill testing, whereas upright cycle ergometry produces values 90–96% of those obtained during maximal treadmill testing (38). Arm cranking yields a peak $\dot{V}O_2$ 30–35% less than treadmill running. These discrepancies are due in part to the muscle mass involved, and can be directly related to the cardiac output seen in each case. The choice of ergometer depends on various factors, each device having advantages and disadvantages over its rivals (Table 2). The most common ergometers for exercise testing include the step-bench, treadmill, and cycle ergometer; these are briefly described below. For clinical exercise testing, cycle ergometers are more popular in Europe, whereas in the United States, treadmills are the common modality (15). Step-bench ergometers have gained popularity for sub-maximal testing; however, they are not well suited for maximal exercise testing, and largely remain an option for screening healthy individuals prior to the prescription of exercise.

Whether using the cycle or treadmill ergometer, the optimal test duration for eliciting a true $\dot{V}O_{2\,max}$ is 8–10 min (15,54), with a 1- to 2-minute low-load warm-up period preceding the exercise stress.

Three commonly used protocols used in testing $\dot{V}O_{2\,max}$ are: (a) Intermittent incremental loading, where successive work rates are separated by a short rest period; (b) Continuous step incremental loading, where increasing work rates are applied continuously with individual stages lasting from 1–3 min; this method usually involves achieving a "steady-state" heart rate and/or $\dot{V}O_2$; (c) Continuous incremental loading, or Ramp loading.

Table 2 Comparison of Testing Ergometers–Advantages and Disadvantages

Ergometer	Advantages	Disadvantages
Step-bench	Low cost	Maximal testing not possible
	Low maintenance	
		Ancillary measures difficult
	No calibration	
	Habituation easy	
		Limited by anthropometric factors
Treadmill	Yields a plateau in $\dot{V}O_2$	Costly
		Noisy
	Effort is not self-paced	Ancillary measures difficult
	Common activity (walking)	
		Hazardous (running)
		Habituation difficult
Cycle ergometer	Ancillary measures easy	Pedaling frequency affects loading
	Habituation easy	
	Reproducible work rates	Limited by muscle strength
		Requires regular calibration (mechanically braked)
	High mechanical efficiency	
	Easily calibrated	
		Plateau in VO_2 not usually obtained in sedentary subjects
	Occupies little space	

Source: Modified from Ref. 38; used with permission.

Step-Bench Ergometer

This method is simple, inexpensive, requires little habituation, and offers low maintenance; however, it is not widely accepted for maximal testing (38). Resistance is provided by body mass, frequency of stepping, and height of the step(s). Because the mechanical efficiency of stepping is relatively low and has a small range (15–19%), stepping frequency (footplants) should not exceed 150 footplants/min. Oxygen consumption can be determined (38):

$$\dot{V}O_2\,(L/min) = [(0.0179)\,(F)\,(f)\,(H) + (0.134\,BSA)],$$

where F, f, H, and BSA are force (kg), step frequency (footplants/min), step height (cm), and body surface area, respectively.

The Canadian Standard Test of Fitness (9) uses a Master-type two-step configuration; although designed as a motivational tool, scores can yield a submaximal prediction of $\dot{V}O_{2\,max}$ (28). The test can be used in either a field or laboratory setting for simple approximate quantification of aerobic power. Cadence is controlled by music, progressing in speed every 3 min until 70% of predicted heart rate is obtained, with normative scores available for comparison.

Cycle Ergometers

Both mechanically and electrically braked cycle ergometers are widely used for clinical and laboratory exercise testing. Stable monitoring of blood pressure, facility of ECG recording, sampling for blood, easy habituation, and cost make this type of ergometer popular. Furthermore, work and power output can be easily measured and reproduced. Because leg fatigue often limits performance on this modality, $\dot{V}O_{2\,max}$ is often 8–10% lower than treadmill scores (38,46). Pedaling frequencies used for testing range from 50 (Åstrand-Ryhming test) to 90 rpm for well-trained cyclists. Oxygen consumption, reported in L/min, is calculated as follows (38):

$$\dot{V}O_2\,(L/min) = [(0.0125)\,(R)\,(C)\,(f)\,(p{:}f) + (0.134\,BSA)]$$

where R, C, f, p:f, and BSA are resistance (newtons), circumference (cm), pedaling frequency (rpm), gear ratio, and body surface area, respectively.

Åstrand (3) described a nomogram for estimating $\dot{V}O_{2\,max}$ based upon the linear relationship between $\dot{V}O_2$ and heart rate, with provision to correct for the age-related decline in heart rate (if subjects are >30 years, or if maximal heart rate is known). Essentially, the slope of this relationship dictates fitness, with a lower HR/$\dot{V}O_2$ slope indicating better fitness. A nomogram providing an estimation of $\dot{V}O_{2\,max}$ has

been constructed (Fig. 2), and is based upon the heart rate achieved at
a single work rate performed for 6 min, sufficient to elicit a heart rate
between 125 and 170 beats/min. Because data used to derive this prediction were obtained from young subjects (<30 years), correction factors were provided for use in older subjects, adjusting for the age-
dependent decline in maximal heart rate.

A modified YMCA protocol (48) uses the Åstrand and Ryhming
nomogram (Fig. 2) and incremental work rates until subjects reach 70%
of the age-predicted heart rate. An initial work rate of 25 W is used for
females and males >35 years of age, with males <35 years beginning
at 50 W. In each case, work rate is increased by the initial amount
every 2 min, until 60–70% of the age-predicted heart rate is obtained.
After this point, work rate is increased by 25 W and exercise continues
for 2 additional minutes. $\dot{V}O_{2\,max}$ (L/min) is estimated by using the
Åstrand nomogram and the equations provided below (48):

males: $\dot{V}O_{2\,max} = 0.348\,(X) - 0.035\,(age,\ years) + 3.011$
females: $\dot{V}O_{2\,max} = 0.302\,(X) - 0.019\,(age,\ years) + 1.593$

where X is the $\dot{V}O_{2\,max}$ obtained from the Åstrand nomogram.

Figure 2 The Åstrand nomogram for determination of maximal oxygen consumption during submaximal cycle ergometry or step testing. Heart rates at a
given work rate correspond to an estimated $\dot{V}O_{2\,max}$. A line is connected from
the work rate scale to the observed pulse rate at that work rate, providing a
predicted maximal oxygen uptake. Two examples are provided here (dashed
lines), with work rates of 100 and 200 W achieved during a cycle ergometer
test. A correction factor for age should be applied if subjects are >30 years
old, using the following equation: Corrected $\dot{V}O_2 = 1.189 - 0.0086\,(age,\ yrs)$,
or by using the table below if either age or maximal heart rate is known:

Age	Factor	HR_{max}	Factor
15	1.1	210	1.12
25	1.0	200	1.00
35	0.87	190	0.93
40	0.83	180	0.83
45	0.78	170	0.75
50	0.75	160	0.69
55	0.71	150	0.64
60	0.68		
65	0.65		

(From Ref. 3; used with permission.)

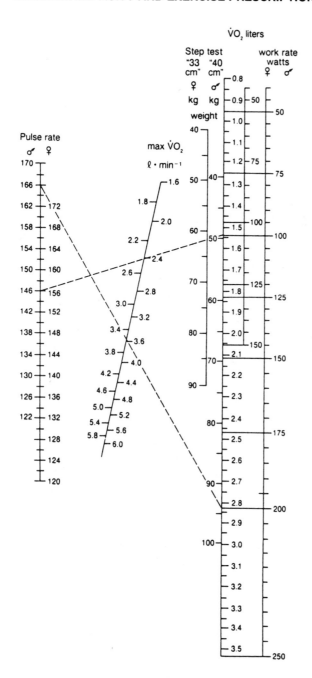

Another submaximal protocol (2) uses an extrapolation technique, where $\dot{V}O_2$ is estimated at several submaximal work rates, and a line of best-fit is extrapolated to an age-predicted maximal heart rate. Load selection varies according to the activity level and body mass of the individual (Table 3), with step increments in work rate (e.g., every 3 min). The initial work rate should elicit a minimum heart rate of 120–125 beats/min, since stroke volume contributes less to increases in cardiac output and hence $\dot{V}O_2$ above this level. At least three work rates are performed. Maximal work rate and $\dot{V}O_{2\,max}$ are gauged by extrapolation to the estimated maximal heart rate (see Fig. 1).

Treadmill Testing

A number of the available clinical protocols are summarized in Figure 3. These predict functional capacity in terms of either metabolic equivalents (METS), or $\dot{V}O_2$. All use step increments in work rate, and are therefore not advised for determination of the VT, but they are generally used during ECG stress testing. The Bruce protocol (8) increases grade and speed every 3 min. Although basically a walking protocol, running may be required in well-trained individuals who reach the final stages; however, the test is usually completed rapidly and is widely used in clinical settings. The Balke and Ware (4) protocol was first designed to test military personnel, and offers smaller increments of work rate (2% in first minute, 1% each minute thereafter), at a set speed of 5.3 km/h. The disadvantage of this protocol is the length of time required to complete the testing of most subjects. A modified version uses greater increments in grade (5% every 3 min). The Ellestad protocol (14) begins at 2.7 km/h, increasing to 9.7 km/h; the grade begins at 10% and finishes at 15% by 11 min. The Naughton protocol

Table 3 Cycle Ergometry Protocols and Load Selection: American College of Sports Medicine Protocol

Protocol	Test stage (min)			
	1 (1–2)	2 (3–4)	3 (5–6)	4 (7–8)
A	25	50	75	100
B	25	50	100	150
C	50	100	150	200

A: Body mass <73 kg; inactive or active; 74–90 kg, inactive.
B: Body mass 74–90 kg, active; >91 kg, not active.
C: Body mass >91 kg, active.
Source: Modified from Ref. 2; used with permission.

(35) uses a constant speed (3.2 km/h and 5.3 km/h), with 2.5–3.5% grade increments every 3 min. Each work rate corresponds to an increase of 3.5 ml O_2/kg/min.

Small but rapid increments in work rate are preferred for maximal exercise testing when direct measurement of $\dot{V}O_{2\,max}$ and the VT are desired. Weiner and Lourie (56) describe a widely used protocol in which subjects choose a comfortable running speed, with grade increasing 2% every 2 min. Recommended running speeds are 11.3 km/h for females, 12.1 km/h for female runners, 12.9 km/h for males, and 13.7 km/h for male runners (52).

Direct Measurement of Maximal Oxygen Consumption

The use of on-line computer-driven metabolic carts have made measurement of $\dot{V}O_{2\,max}$ simple and expeditious. With proper adherence to calibration procedures and careful maintenance, the test-retest reliabil-

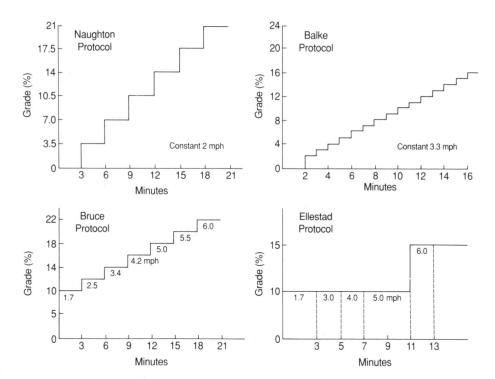

Figure 3 Treadmill protocols are compared graphically, depicting differences in loading schedules during exercise (From Ref. 2; used with permission.)

ity is 0.95% with a coefficient of variation of 2.4% (31). Equipment commonly used involves semiautomatic, or fully automated systems, incorporating either mixing chamber systems for time-average sampling of expired gases, or those that provide breath-by-breath analysis. Breath-by-breath measurement systems are costly, and are not advised unless particularly advanced measures of pulmonary/respiratory function are required for research or clinical assessment.

Methods used to calculate $\dot{V}O_2$ vary; however, in general, equations transform data to standard temperature and pressure, dry gas (STPD), account for discrepancies of volume between inspired and expired gas samples, and assume there is no use of nitrogen as a substrate (Haldane transformation). Thus, the simplified equation to determine $\dot{V}O_2$ is:

$$\dot{V}O_2 = VE \times [0.265 \times (1.0 - F_{EO_2} - F_{ECO_2}) - F_{EO_2}].$$

A flow meter is required to measure $\dot{V}E$. The expired volume of ventilation ($\dot{V}E$) is converted from ambient temperature and pressure saturated (ATPS) to STPD conditions, for use in this equation. This correction allows standard comparisons of data despite varying environmental conditions. Ventilation and tidal volumes obtained under ATPS conditions are typically reported under BTPS conditions. As mentioned above, various gas-exchange data can then be determined, and in conjunction with heart rate data, can provide important information relating to cardiopulmonary status (Table 1) and potential factors limiting exercise performance. Metabolic carts are now capable of generating graphic reports, illustrating the HR and $\dot{V}O_2$ response to exercise, and identifying the VT in normal or pathological conditions (Fig. 4). Use of the VT and $\dot{V}O_{2\,max}$ has gained popularity in the clinical evaluation of cardiovascular disease states (55).

Instrumentation—Component Design and Configuration

Various commercially designed systems are available for the measurement of gas-exchange variables during exercise; the "best" system for any particular facility depends largely on the information required, the computer support desired, and financial resources available.

Configurations Used for Gas-Collection

Timed-Average Gas Collection Technique. Prior to the advent of rapid-response CO_2 and O_2 analyzers, one-way breathing valves and meteorological balloons (or Douglas bags) were used to collect samples for chemical analysis. With this approach, samples are collected over a fixed period of time, with volume and gas samples carefully (and

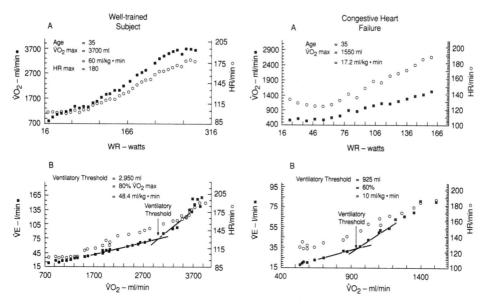

Figure 4 Ventilatory gas-exchange data obtained during graded exercise to maximum in well-trained subjects, and patients with congestive heart failure. Data are averaged over 30 s, obtained from breath-by-breath sampling. In each example, Graph A illustrates the heart rate/$\dot{V}O_2$ response; Graph B illustrates identification of the ventilatory threshold from $\dot{V}E$ and $\dot{V}O_2$ data. Highly deconditioned subjects or those with pathological conditions limiting cardiovascular function exhibit a lower $\dot{V}O_{2\,max}$, and ventilatory threshold. (Courtesy of J. Goodman, P. Liu, The Toronto Hospital, Toronto, Canada.)

laboriously) measured. Drawbacks of this technique include the necessity of a steady-state (plateaued $\dot{V}O_2$) exercise intensity (requiring 2–4 min per exercise stage), and the cumbersome nature of the equipment.
Mixing Chamber Technique. This method (Fig. 5) uses a rigid (Plexiglas) or nonrigid (bag) mixing chamber of 5–8 L volume to collect air from a one-way breathing valve placed in the mouth. Expired gas is then pumped into the gas analyzers. Volume determination is performed by either a pneumotachograph or turbine system (see below). Data are averaged over 15- or 30-s intervals. Steady-state protocols are not required using this method, and most manufacturers claim linearity of response to ventilations of greater than 300 L/min. However, end-tidal gas sampling is not possible with this method.
Breath-by-Breath Technique. Breath-by-breath (B × B) measurement of oxygen consumption and CO_2 production requires rapid response

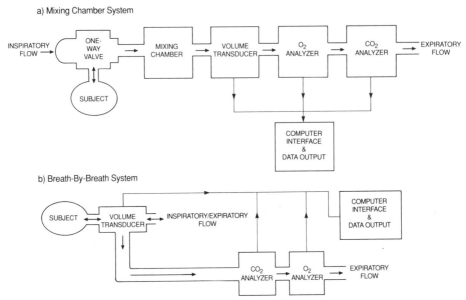

Figure 5 Schematic representation of the mixing chamber (a) and breath-by-breath (b) systems of collecting expired gases and subsequent determination of $\dot{V}E$, $\dot{V}CO_2$, and $\dot{V}CO_2$.

(80–100 ms) and stable (± 0.1–0.2%) O_2 and CO_2 analyzers, which are now common equipment on commercially available metabolic carts, even if these have been designed as mixing chamber systems. Gas is collected from a low dead space one-way valve at a high flow rate (e.g., 5 ml/s); it is then delivered to the rapid response analyzers for continuous sampling (see Fig. 5). The gas-transit and analysis times must be calibrated and temporally aligned with the gas sample (CO_2 or O_2) and integrated with the expiratory and expiratory times; $\dot{V}O_2$ and $\dot{V}CO_2$ are finally determined using appropriate algorithms. Various commercial B × B models are available; however, the costs are somewhat prohibitive—typically priced in excess of $60,000 U.S. It remains debatable whether or not clinical test settings require such instrumentation. Furthermore, there is concern about reporting a transient B × B sample as an authentic value for either $\dot{V}O_{2\,max}$ or $\dot{V}E_{max}$, and it is recommended that all *maximal* values should be reported from 15- to 30-s *averaged* data. While B × B systems are the choice method of the future, these systems are *not* without their current problems, and unless there is a particular need for such data, mixing chamber systems may offer more reliable data at significant capital savings.

Gas Analyzers

Commonly, CO_2 analyzers utilize an infrared system; the energy absorbed from a sample gas mixture is electronically compared to a reference standard, the difference being proportional to the partial pressure of the CO_2 sample. Common types of O_2 analyzers currently used include those that use zirconium oxide sensors, super-heated (700–750°C), and sensitive to PO_2 differences between the inside and outside of a gas-reference chamber. Like the CO_2 system described above, the difference is represented as an electrical voltage difference. Other systems utilize gold/silver anode sensors (polarographic). In these systems, the electrical current across an oxygen-permeable membrane is proportional to the partial pressure of O_2 (55).

Ventilation Monitors

Various devices are currently available, ranging from the gold-standard Tissot spirometer to sophisticated electronic modules. Anemometers have been used to measure ventilation; these are continuously heated, and exploit the proportional relationship between flow rate and heat loss across an electrical circuit. Such devices are of questionable reliability and stability, but they have the advantage of being independent of ambient pressure, water vapor, and ambient temperature (55).

Pneumotachographs utilize a fine wire screen which offers a laminar flow resistance and measures the pressure differential across the screen. Most are heated to eliminate water vapor and to establish standard temperature conditions. These devices are usually most stable and require little maintenance or calibration, providing the wire screen remains clear of water, saliva, or protein buildup.

The vane-turbine system is probably the most commonly used flow-sensing device in commercially available systems. Most designs use a low-mass vane which is highly sensitive to flow direction and speed. The speed of rotation of the turbine is electronically proportional to flow rate; rotation interrupts a series of light-emitting diodes, yielding a flow signal identifying inspiratory and expiratory cycles. Linearity is excellent to flows >300 L/min, and although the turbine is quite fragile, maintenance is not required.

Quality Control

Accurate and reproducible measures of gas exchange require daily and test-by-test calibration. Ventilation devices should be calibrated daily against a known volume, introduced at various flow rates, using an accurate volume syringe (1–3 L is usually required). Gas analyzers require more frequent calibration, using zero (nitrogen) and span gases (similar to the expired concentrations observed during exercise—e.g., 4% CO_2 and 16% O_2). These gases should be 100% pure, and verified using Scholander or Lloyd-Haldane analysis. When using systems that "autocalibrate," careful attention must be given to correction factors and gas-transit times, which should fall within the manufacturer's recommended limits. Failure to satisfy these conditions may result in poor temporal alignment of gas and ventilatory signals. Finally, calibration of both analyzers should be performed before each test.

Combined Cardiopulmonary Exercise Testing

Concurrent radionuclide angiography (RNA) and gas-exchange measurements provide comprehensive information on cardiopulmonary status (19,20). In our protocol, upright cycle ergometry with graded exercise (15-Watt increments every minute) is performed in conjunction with first-pass RNA measurements at peak exercise. Determination of the VT and $\dot{V}O_{2\,max}$ is possible, in combination with other variables (Table 1). Following a rest period, gated RNA is performed at rest, during submaximal (below the VT), and near peak exercise.

Criteria Used to Establish Attainment of $\dot{V}O_{2\,max}$

A number of gas-exchange variables and ancillary data provide evidence of the attainment of a true maximal effort. Failure to increase O_2 consumption despite an increase in work rate represents the functional limit of the cardiorespiratory system; further work can be performed anaerobically, but a test rarely proceeds more than 60–90 s beyond this point. Taylor et al. (50) first described acceptable criteria for a plateau of O_2 consumption during an interrupted progressive treadmill test less than a 2.1 ml/kg min rise (150 ml/min) in O_2 consumption with an increase in work rate (2.5% grade at 11.3 km/h). Other criteria include the attainment of an age-predicted heart rate (see below), a respiratory gas exchange ratio > 1.10, and blood lactate > 10 mmol/L (47).

In well-trained subjects, a plateau in $\dot{V}O_2$ can be achieved in a high percentage of cases ($> 80\%$); however, Taylor et al. (50) reported that only 75% of their subjects reached a plateau. Others have reported various success rates, ranging from 7 to 80%, depending on the exercise mode and protocol used for testing; however, use of the treadmill offers a greater likelihood of attaining a plateau.

Classification of Aerobic Power

Maximal aerobic power is dependent on sex, age, genotype, and level of habitual activity, and can be acutely altered by drugs, anemia, ambient PO_2, and other factors (15,46). Table 4 provides general classification of $\dot{V}O_{2\,max}$ for healthy individuals. Subjective means of classifying functional status in patients with heart failure, such as the New York Heart Association levels 1–4, are now being replaced by more objective measures according to $\dot{V}O_{2\,max}$ and the VT (see Table 5) (55). Other gas-exchange variables which add information to cardiopulmonary status are presented in Table 1. World-class endurance athletes have values for $\dot{V}O_{2\,max}$ in excess of 70–80 ml/kg/min, and some paraplegic athletes are capable of reaching 60 ml/kg/min. Correspondingly, such athletes may have stroke volumes in excess of 200 ml, and maximal cardiac outputs greater than 40 L/min.

Equations can estimate maximal cardiac output and stroke volume (with heart rate data) (23) owing to the linearity of $\dot{V}O_2$ and cardiac output, where:

$$\text{cardiac output (L/min)} = 5.31 + 4.6\,(\dot{V}O_2 L/min)$$

Table 4   Classification of Aerobic Power

	Age	Low	Fair	Average	Good	High
				$\dot{V}O_{2\,max}$ (ml/kg/min)		
Men:						
	20–29	<25	25–33	34–42	43–52	>53
	30–39	<23	23–30	31–38	39–48	>49
	40–49	<20	20–26	27–35	34–42	>43
	50–59	<18	18–24	25–33	34–42	>43
	60–69	<16	16–22	23–30	31–40	>41
Women:						
	20–29	<24	24–30	31–37	38–48	>49
	30–39	<20	20–27	28–33	34–44	>45
	40–49	<17	17–23	24–30	31–41	>42
	50–59	<15	15–20	21–27	28–37	>38
	60–69	<13	13–17	18–23	24–34	>35

Source: Modified from *Exercise Testing and Training of Apparently Healthy Individuals: A Handbook for Physicians*. The Committee on Exercise. American Heart Association, Dallas. 1972.

Table 5 Classification of Functional Impairment

Class	Severity	Aerobic power ($\dot{V}O_{2\,max}$) ml/kg/min	Ventilatory threshold (ml/kg/min)
A	Mild to none	>20	>14
B	Mild to moderate	16–20	11–14
C	Moderate to severe	10–16	8–11
D	Severe	6–10	5–8
E	Very severe	<6	<4

Source: From Ref. 55; used with permission.

Safety of Exercise Testing

The risks associated with exercise testing are relatively low. Stuart and Ellestad (49a) summarized data obtained from close to 2000 clinical facilities and accounting for some 500,000 exercise tests. They reported an incidence of less than one death and four myocardial infarctions per 10,000 tests. In nonclinical settings, it is likely the risks are even lower. When testing those suspected of coronary disease, risks can be reduced through physician attendance, pretest history and examination, resting 12-lead ECG, continuous ECG monitoring during and after exercise, ensuring the availability of emergency resuscitation and drug kits, and full cool-down prior to showering (15). In certain cases, the risks of exercise testing may outweigh the potential benefits, and unless unusual circumstances dictate, exercise testing should be avoided in such cases. Absolute and relative and contraindications for exercise testing are presented in Table 6.

The Electrocardiogram and Exercise Testing

Preparation and Lead Configuration

Accurate monitoring of the electrocardiogram during exercise testing is assured by adequate skin preparation and choice of lead configuration. Typical problems observed during ECG monitoring include those caused by changes in body position or respiratory motion. Changes in body position will alter the QRS axis deviation and R-wave amplitude, whereas respiratory movements can influence Q-waves, R-wave amplitude, baseline voltage, and T-wave orientation.

Motion and impedance artifact are common problems during exercise testing. Improvement of the signal-to-noise ratio and baseline drift is best achieved by preparing the skin surface by abrasion of the

Table 6   Contraindications to Exercise Testing

Absolute:

   Recent myocardial infarction
   Unstable angina
   Uncontrolled cardiac arrhythmias compromising LV function
   Severe heart failure
   Severe aortic stenosis
   Dissecting aortic aneurysm
   Recent systemic or pulmonary emboli or acute thrombophlebitis
   Acute pericarditis
   Acute infection or fever

Relative:

   Resting DBP > 120 torr; SBP > 200 torr
   Left main coronary artery disease obstruction
   Fixed-rate pacemakers
   Cardiomyopathies
   Dangerous LV irritability
   Ventricular aneurysm
   Moderate valve disease
   Conduction defects
   Uncontrolled metabolic diseases
   Neuromuscular or musculoskeletal limitations

Abbreviations: DBP = diastolic blood pressure; SBP = systolic blood pressure; LV = left ventricle.

skin, removing the dry surface keratin. Various abrasion pads (fine-grain emery) and electrical devices (Quick Prep) are available and provide simple and expedient preparation. Impedance (ohms) is tested against a common electrode, and rotation of the abrading drill continues until the skin impedance is less than the maximum recommended value of 5000 Ω (17). Alcohol swabs aid in cleansing the skin of oil and in reducing impedance. Proper grounding with maintenance of lead attachments and cables will also minimize 60-Hz electrical interference.

A standard 12-lead ECG should be performed prior to any diagnostic or screening exercise test. The ideal number of leads to monitor during exercise is still not agreed. The V5 position has the greatest sensitivity for detecting ST-segment depression and is therefore routinely used, with Frank's X, Y, and Z leads advocated by some.

More recently, use of equipment providing digitization of the ECG signal has become widespread and economical for many clinical settings. The basic principle involves the conversion of continuous analogue signals to the corresponding digital voltages, providing (a) identification of ECG complexes, (b) temporal landmarking, (c) averaging, (d) waveform recognition, and (e) noise filtering (17). Use of computerized ECG should only be used routinely once the digitally averaged signals have been systematically checked against standard analogue output. For a more detailed account of computerized ECG analysis, the reader is directed to an excellent summary by Froelicher (17).

In the case of athlete testing and those previously assessed as free of cardiovascular disease, the modified lead II or CM5 lead is preferred. The ECG signal should be obtained every minute during exercise, and for a period of 5–10 min following exercise. Oscilloscopic monitoring throughout exercise is of particular advantage for instantaneous waveform analysis.

If subjects are suspected of having coronary artery disease, sensitivity in detecting myocardial ischemia is enhanced by supine recovery. But in normal circumstances, recovery should be active (25–30% $\dot{V}O_{2\,max}$) to minimize orthostatic hypotension, cramping, and rapid removal of blood lactate. Systemic blood pressure should be measured concurrently with the ECG; if movement and noise prevents this, resting, peak exercise, and recovery measures are essential.

Analysis of the Exercise Electrocardiogram

Analysis of the exercise should follow a basic nine-point evaluation including: (a) rate, (b) rhythm, (c) P-waves, (d) PR interval, (e) QRS complex, (f) ST-segment, (g) T-waves, (h) U-waves, (i) QT interval. These are well summarized by Blair et al. (5). Briefly, the normal response to exercise includes a reduction in the QT interval, an upsloping ST-segment at the j point, superpositioning of the P- and T-waves, reduction in the R-wave, and an increased amplitude of the Q- and T-waves. Common abnormal ECG criteria (ischemic) during exercise testing include (a) ST-segment changes, (b) U-wave inversion, (c) R- and Q-wave amplitude changes, and (d) T-wave changes. These are summarized in Table 7.

Apparently normal or abnormal responses must be assessed relative to the *sensitivity* and *specificity* of the test (Table 8). Sensitivity reflects the percentage of diseased patients who demonstrate positive test results; a large number of false-negative tests therefore reflects poor test sensitivity. Specificity reflects the ability of the test to rule out disease in a healthy population; false-positive tests reduce specificity.

Causes of false-positive and false-negative tests are presented in Table 9. Froelicher (17) reports treadmill ECG testing to yield an

Table 7 Ischemic Electrocardiographic Criteria

Segment or Wave	Pattern
ST segment	1. Horizontal 0.1 mV >80 ms 2. Upsloping "ST-delay" >0.1 mV >80 ms 3. Downsloping >0.1 mV >80 ms at J-point 4. Elevation >0.1 mV above resting ST-segment
T-wave	Inversion
U-wave	Inversion
R-wave	Diminished amplitude

Table 8 Diagnostic Value of Testing: Calculations and Definition

Calculation		Definition
Specificity	$= \dfrac{TP}{TP + FN} \times 100$	Percentage of normal (undiseased) subjects who show negative tests. Reduced by FP test results.
Sensitivity	$= \dfrac{TN}{FP + TN} \times 100$	Percentage of patients with documented CAD who show positive test results. Reduced by FN test results.
Predictive value of abnormal test	$= \dfrac{TP}{TP + FP} \times 100$	Percentage of individuals with an abnormal test who *have* disease.
Relative value	$= \dfrac{\dfrac{TP}{TP + FP}}{\dfrac{FN}{TN + FN}}$	Relative rate of occurrence of disease in groups with abnormal tests versus those with a normal test.

Abbreviations: TP = true positive (positive test result and documented disease); FP = false positive (positive test result but no disease); TN = true negative (negative test result and no disease); FN = false negative (negative test result but disease present)
Source: From Ref. 17; used with permission.

Table 9 Causes of False-Positive and False-Negative Tests

False-negative Tests:

  Inadequate work rate achieved
  Limited ECG leads
  Absence of ancillary data (blood pressure, heart rate)
  Single vessel disease
  Adequate collateral circulation (CAD without ischemia)
  Other exercise limitations
  Observer or technical error
  Postbypass surgery patients

False-positive tests:

  Female sex
  LV hypertrophy
  Digitalis
  Hypokalemia
  Preexisting ST-segment depression at rest
  Sudden intense exercise
  Valvular disease
  Anemia
  Cardiomyopathy
  Pectus cavatum
  Pericardial disease
  Vasoregulatory asthenia
  Conduction defects (Wolff-Parkinson-White syndrome/BBB)
  Hypertension
  Hyperventilation

Abbreviations: CAD = coronary artery disease; ECG = electrocardiogram; BBB = bundle branch block; LV = left ventricular.

overall specificity of 90% and sensitivity of 70%, with details of test methodology contributing significantly to the wide range reported for each variable (specificity: 35–90%; sensitivity: 40–100%).

Atypical Electrocardiographic Responses in Healthy Subjects

Well-trained athletes often exhibit ECG abnormalities (including abnormal waveforms and dysrhythmias) during and after exercise, many of which mimic alterations found in disease. Abnormalities in the ECG are common in the athletic population (Table 10); it is likely that rhythm disturbances are related to the increased parasympathetic activity which accompanies chronic training, with waveform abnormalities likely being due to various forms of cardiomegaly (37). Using proper diagnostic criteria, most training-induced irregularities can be differentiated from true pathological conditions (43).

Termination of an Exercise Test

Exercise tests should normally be terminated if maximal oxygen uptake is achieved, or if medical/and or safety factors compromise the health of the subject (Table 11). Warnings of potential medical problems include mild to moderate myocardial ischemia and/or nonspecific abnormalities in the ECG. Absolute indications dictate immediate termination of an exercise test. During treadmill testing, caution is necessary when subjects approach maximal effort. If subjects are attached to a mouthpiece, a signal system should be established prior to exercise to indicate impending exhaustion (e.g., 1 min). This may not only prevent injury, but also encourage the subject to complete a final work rate, yielding valuable data that might otherwise have been lost.

Table 10 Common Electrocardiographic Abnormalities During Exercise in Well-Trained Athletes

Conduction and Rhythm Abnormalities:	Possible physiological cause:
sinus bradycardia	
AV dissociation	
wandering atrial pacemaker	increased parasympathetic activity
AV block	
premature atrial contractions	
premature ventricular contractions	
supraventricular contractions	
Waveform Abnormalities:	
increased P-wave amplitude	atrial dilation and/or hypertrophy
QRS criteria for hypertrophy	LVH, RVH
increased QRS duration and notching	conduction defects, bundle branch blocks
ST-segment elevation	increased vagal tone
increased T-wave amplitude, inversion, biphasical	increased RV volume
increased U-wave voltage	bradycardia

Abbreviations: LVH = left ventricular hypertrophy; RV = right ventricle.

Table 11   Reasons for Terminating an Exercise Test

Absolute:

   Severe angina or progressing angina (to 3+ on angina scale)
   Severe dyspnea
   Marked ST-segment depression (>4 mm)
   Multifocal PVC (couplets, triplets)
   Excessive increase in BP (SBP >250 torr; DBP >120 torr)
   Drop in SBP with increasing work rate
   Second- or third-degree block
   Sustained SVT
   Confusion, pallor, cyanosis, cold clammy skin
   Patient request
   Equipment failure

Relative:

   ECG abnormalities including ST-segment depression >2mm
   Appearance of BBB or conduction abnormalities
   Hypertensive response
   SVT
   PVC (multifocal)
   Leg fatigue and/or cramps
   Increased chest pain

Abbreviations: DBP = diastolic blood pressure; SBP = systolic blood pressure; BP = blood pressure; BBB = bundle branch block; SVT = supraventricular tachycardia; PVC = premature ventricular contraction.

Assessment of Flexibility

Static flexibility is defined as the maximal range of motion at a single joint or a series of joints. Dynamic flexibility reflects the opposition (resistance) of a joint to motion (16). Also described as the inverse function of resistance encountered throughout a normal range of motion (46), the practical significance of dynamic flexibility is small, difficult to measure, and will not be covered in this chapter.

While flexibility is often an overlooked component of fitness, in certain sports it is essential and is linked to both prevention of (53) and recovery from various acute injuries. The factors that limit flexibility include joint structural characteristics (e.g., hinge, gliding, ball-and-socket), opposition of soft tissues, and joint pathologies and/or injuries. Johns and Wright (29) have suggested the relative contributions to joint rigidity are for the joint capsule (47%), muscle (41%), tendon and ligaments (10%), and skin (2%).

The tests of flexibility fall within two broad categories: *indirect* and *direct* methods. Indirect methods, while simple and expedient to administer, are limited by the confounding influence of various anthropometric factors (e.g., limb length), and may involve muscle compartments not directly tested in a specific protocol. Direct methods are relatively precise, but are more time consuming, and suffer from a paucity of available normative scores.

Indirect Methods to Assess Flexibility

Cureton's Test of Minimal Level of Flexibility. Two tests are administered: First, the subject performs straight-legged toe-touching (males: fingers must reach floor; females: palms must touch floor); A second test involves a simple sit-and-reach procedure with the legs extended; the distance from the forehead to the floor is measured in inches.

Wells and Dillon. The Wells and Dillon sit-and-reach test for hamstring and upper- and lower-back flexibility uses a fixed scale mounted 30 cm above the ground; the subject is instructed to lean forward as far as possible along the scale, pointing the fingers. The Canadian Standardized Test of Fitness (19) utilizes a modified Wells and Dillon flexometer to assess flexibility. The subject sits with legs fully extended, with the soles of the feet against the crossbars of the flexometer, which is adjusted vertically according to foot length. With legs fully extended, the subject reaches forward, sliding a marker along the measuring scale as far as possible. Maximal forward flexion is measured to the nearest cm, and is compared to available normative scores (Table 12).

Shoulder Elevation and Trunk Extension. Shoulder elevation is tested with the subject prone and the arms extended a shoulder width apart. A measuring stick is raised while the chin remains on the floor. The score is equal to the distance measured times 100, divided by the arm length (Table 13). Trunk extension is tested by positioning the subject in the prone position with the hands placed on the lower part of the back. The tester stabilizes the lower body of the subject during upward extension, and the maximal height up from the floor is measured from the suprasternal notch. The score is multiplied by 100, and the product is divided by the trunk length (measured from the suprasternal notch to the floor while the subject is seated) (Table 13).

Direct Methods to Assess Flexibility

Direct techniques to assess flexibility are best for athletic populations when specific assessments of joint flexibility are required during training or rehabilitation.

Table 12   Modified Wells and Dillon Sit-and-Reach Scores

	Trunk flexion (cm)				
Male:					
Age	20–29	30–39	40–49	50–59	60–69
Excellent	>39	>37	>34	>34	>32
Above average	34–39	33–37	29–34	28–34	25–32
Average	30–33	28–32	24–28	24–27	20–24
Below average	25–29	23–27	18–23	16–23	15–19
Poor	<25	<23	<18	<16	<15
Female:					
Excellent	>40	>40	>37	>38	>34
Above average	37–40	36–40	34–37	33–38	31–34
Average	33–36	32–35	30–33	30–32	27–30
Below average	28–32	27–31	25–29	25–29	23–26
Poor	<28	<27	<25	<25	<24

Source: Modified from Ref. 9; used with permission.

Table 13   Standard Values for Shoulder and Trunk Extension Tests of Flexibility in Adults (20–30 years)

	Shoulder extension	Trunk extension
Men		
Excellent	106–123	50–65
Good	88–105	43–46
Average	70–87	37–42
Fair	53–69	31–36
Poor	35–52	28–30
Women		
Excellent	105–123	48–63
Good	86–104	42–47
Average	68–85	35–41
Fair	50–67	29–34
Poor	31–49	23–28

Source: Modified from Ref. 30; used with permission.

Goniometer. This involves the use of a protractorlike device; the arms are placed along the limbs of the device, and the center of the goniometer is placed at the axis of rotation of the joint. The electrogoniometer uses a potentiometer in the place of a protractor, and can assess joint mobility during physical activity. The problems associated with goniometric measurements include identification of the axis of rotation of the joint, and precise positioning of the protractor arms along the limbs (24).

Leighton Flexometer. The Leighton flexometer uses a device encorporating a rotating needle that is sensitive to gravity. The device is fixed to a limb, and is capable of measuring the range of motion in several joints in various planes of orientation (32). This technique has a high test-retest reliability coefficient, and provides a standardized starting position with direct quantification of joint flexibility (24). Furthermore, it can be used on a wide number of joints and is relatively inexpensive.

Assessment of Muscle Strength and Endurance

Techniques used in the assessment of muscle strength and endurance vary considerably. The method that is chosen depends on the type of strength (isometric, isotonic, isokinetic) and the *specificity* desired for assessment and performance. Simple, yet practical field tests may provide a coarse measure of muscle strength, whereas laboratory tests can provide sophisticated data for athletes or for those undergoing neuromuscular and/or musculoskeletal rehabilitation. While the test-retest variation of usual methods is around 10%, the degree of specificity depends largely on the similarity of the test to the sport or activity under consideration (44).

Isotonic Strength Assessment
Isotonic strength testing elicits a muscular contraction against a force (resistance), while allowing muscle shortening. For instance, the investigator may measure the heaviest weight that can be lifted during a single attempt (1 RM, or repetition maximum). Either free weights or lifting machinery (e.g., Universal Gym) may be used. Jackson et al. (25) suggest the tests of upper- and lower-body strength should include the 1-RM bench press (upper body) and leg press (lower body) tests on the Universal Gym. Test scores are usually expressed as 1 RM N/body weight N (18).

Calisthenic exercise testing has been widely employed. However, strict adherence to testing procedures and guidelines is essential if reliable data are to be obtained. The most commonly used field tests include speed *sit-ups* (maximum per minute), and total *push-ups*. Typically, the push-up test is administered differently for males and females. Males must be "straight out," must lower the upper body to a level equal to a fist height above the ground, and must extend with straight arms. For females, the knees are bent and on the floor. Note is taken of the total number performed while maintaining the required position. The 1-min speed sit-up test requires the subject to perform the maximum number of bent-knee sit-ups possible in the allocated time (1 min), keeping the hands locked behind the head. The tester holds the ankles secure as the subject sits up touching elbow to knee. Various standards have been published for each test (Tables 14 and 15). Although this test can provide a simple measure of abdominal

Table 14 Normative Scores for Push-ups, Sit-ups, and Hand-grip Tests of Strength: Males

	Age (years)				
	20–29	30–39	40–49	50–59	60–69
Combined Left and Right Hand Grip (newtons)					
Excellent	>1129	>1120	>1083	>1000	>927
Above average	1037–1129	1037–1120	1010–1083	936–1000	854–927
Average	973–1028	963–1028	936–1000	881–927	789–845
Below average	890–964	890–955	863–927	799–872	725–780
Poor	<890	<890	<863	<799	<725
Push-Ups (total performed)					
Excellent	>35	>29	>21	>20	>17
Above average	29–35	22–29	17–21	13–20	11–17
Average	22–28	17–21	13–16	10–12	8–10
Below average	17–21	12–16	10–12	7–9	5–7
Poor	<17	<12	<10	<7	<4
Sit-Ups (total in 60 s)					
Excellent	>42	>35	>31	>26	>23
Above average	37–42	31–35	26–30	22–25	17–22
Average	33–36	27–30	22–25	18–21	12–16
Below average	29–32	22–26	17–21	13–17	7–11
Poor	<29	<22	<17	<13	<7

Note: 1 kg = 9.18 newtons
Source: Modified from Ref. 9; used with permission.

Table 15 Normative Scores for Push-ups, Sit-ups, and Hand-grip Tests of Strength: Females

	Age (years)				
	20–29	30–39	40–49	50–59	60–69
Combined Left and Right Hand Grip (newtons)					
Excellent	>643	>661	>661	>588	>542
Above average	579–643	606–661	597–661	542–588	496–542
Average	560–588	560–597	542–588	505–532	<568–587
Below average	505–551	514–551	505–532	468–496	441–459
Poor	<514	<505	<505	568	<441
Push-Ups (total performed)					
Excellent	>29	>26	>23	>20	>16
Above average	21–29	20–26	15–23	11–20	12–16
Average	15–20	13–19	11–14	7–10	5–11
Below average	10–14	8–12	5–10	2–6	1–4
Poor	<10	<8	<5	<1	<1
Sit-Ups (total in 60 s)					
Excellent	>35	>28	>24	>18	>15
Above average	31–35	24–28	20–24	12–18	12–15
Average	25–30	20–23	15–19	5–11	4–11
Below average	21–24	15–19	7–14	3–4	2–3
Poor	<21	<15	<7	<3	<1

Note: 1 kg = 9.18 newtons
Source: Modified from Ref. 9; used with permission.

muscle strength, extended practice of this exercise may lead to lower-back pain, and sit-ups should be performed while the legs are bent, the feet are unrestrained, and the small of the lower back is well supported.

Isometric Strength Assessment

Forearm isometric strength can be tested using the handgrip dynamometer (Harpenden) adjusted for hand size. A combined right and left hand (age-specific) score is usually reported (see Tables 14 and 15). In addition to this technique, calibrated force transducers or strain gauges can be used in conjunction with a hard-copy device, providing a record of force, rate of force development, and the force-time integral (44). Unfortunately, true isometric movements are rare in physical activity, and the value of conclusions drawn from this method of strength testing is therefore limited. Endurance tests can be performed, holding a certain percentage of maximum voluntary force (e.g., 50–70%) over a fixed period of time (e.g., 1 min); a fatigue index (FI) is then determined as the percent decline in force.

Isokinetic Strength Assessment

Isokinetic ("constant velocity") strength testing is usually performed in a laboratory, and is typically confined to elite athletes or those undergoing serial assessment during rehabilitation. Strength is usually measured during concentric muscle contraction, and is expressed as peak torque $(N \cdot m)$. The advantages of isokinetic testing over isometric or isotonic testing include: (a) the strength curve matches the range of motion for any specific movement and joint; therefore, *maximal* strength is measured throughout a specified range of movement; (b) specific of muscles are tested; (c) a range of angular velocities is easily assessed (e.g., 0–300°/s); (d) eccentric strength testing possible using certain types of equipment (Biodex isokinetic dynamometer).

Assessment of Body Composition

Numerous indirect methods to assess body composition (lean mass and fat mass) are available, including hydrostatic weighing, soft-tissue radiography, potassium (^{40}K) counting, total body water (isotope dilution), photon absorptiometry, bioelectric impedance analysis (BIA), total body electrical conductivity (TOBEC), ultrasound, and anthropometic techniques (18,42). Both the BIA and ultrasound methods have become popular in recent years, but their reliability and accuracy remain questionable and more validation is required before wide acceptance is gained. Potassium-40 counting (which determines lean body mass in terms of the natural γ-irradiation emitted by muscle tissue), TBW, and TOBEC are costly techniques, and are not practical basic assessment of body composition.

Hydrostatic Weighing

This technique uses Archimedes' principle of water displacement. At a specified temperature, the loss of weight of a submerged body is equal to the weight of water displaced, and thus to body volume. Residual volume of the lungs must be measured (for instance, by helium dilution) or it must be estimated using equations based on body mass, height, age, and sex (10). The volume of gastrointestinal gas is assumed to be 100 ml, and body density is then determined according to the formula:

$$\text{Density} = \frac{\text{weight in air}}{\dfrac{W\,(\text{air}) - W\,(\text{water})}{(\text{density of water})} - (RV + GI\ \text{gas})}$$

where W, RV, and GI are weight, residual volume, and volume of gastrointestinal gas, respectively. Body fat (%) is then calculated on the assumption that fat and lean tissue densities are constant throughout the general population. Two equations widely used are that of Brozeck et al. (7): %fat = (457/D) − 414.2; and that of Siri (49): %fat = (495/D) − 450. This technique is likely the best method to assess percentage of body fat, although sources of error include the determination of residual volume, underwater weighing measurement, and assumptions of uniformity of fat and lean tissue density.

Skin Fold and Girth Measurements

These can be used to assess fat mass indirectly. Using calipers that exert a uniform pressure (10 g/mm^2), the thickness of the skinfold is determined in millimeters within 2 s of applying the caliper. All measures are made on the right side of the body. A mathematical relationship is assumed between subcutaneous fat stores and body density. Generalized equations have been developed for men and women using various skinfold sites (26), with early reports suggesting a good correlation to the hydrostatic method. Common sites for measurements include the triceps, biceps, suprailiac crest, subscapular region, abdomen, and upper thigh folds, although many more sites have been used. Durnin and Womersley (12) use a logarithmic transformation of biceps, triceps, suprailiac, and subscapular skin folds, where body density (D_B) is given by:

Males: D_B = 1.1765 − (0.0744 × log sum of total skin folds)

Females: D_B = 1.1567 − (0.0717 × log sum of total skin folds)

Jackson and Pollock (26) have developed generalized equations using a quadratic sum of skin folds. For women, triceps, suprailiac, and thigh folds are measured, whereas in men, chest, abdominal, and thigh skin folds are used. Body density is determined according to the following equations:

Males: D_B = 1.109380 − 0.0008267 (sum of chest, abdomen, and thigh folds) − (0.0000016 [sum of chest, abdomen, and thigh folds]) 2 − 0.0002574 (age, years)

Females: D_B = 1.0994921 − 0.0009929 (sum of suprailiac, tricep, and thigh folds) + (0.0000023 [sum of suprailiac, tricep, and thigh folds]) 2 − 0.0001392 (age, years)

Sources of error using anthropometric techniques are numerous, and may contribute to spurious results. High interindividual variation (technique), proper identification of skin fold sites, and unreliable calipers can all contribute to error, in addition to the weaknesses inherent in the basic assumptions of skin fold assessment.

Based upon body composition assessment, other indices can be calculated, such as absolute fat mass (% fat/100 × body mass), lean body mass (body mass − absolute fat mass), and desirable mass ([lean body mass/1.00 − desirable %fat]). Although there is a wide range of normality, some suggest an ideal %fat range of 12–18% for men and 20–28% for women, depending on age. Standards of percent of body fat (Table 16) and the sum of skin folds (Table 17) provide a basis for weight management, although it may be more accurate simply to sum the skin folds and use these measures serially over time to assess changes in body composition. Use of nomograms describing body mass index (BMI) should also be incorporated in such determinations.

PRESCRIPTION OF EXERCISE

Precautions

Contraindications to an increase of physical activity and limiting factors to training may be identified by means of various screening

Table 16 Percentage Body Fat—Standard Values

	Age				
Score	20–29	30–39	40–49	50–59	>60
Men					
excellent	<10	<11	<13	<14	<15
good	11–13	12–14	14–16	15–17	16–18
average	14–20	15–21	17–23	18–24	19–25
fair	21–23	22–24	24–26	25–27	26–28
poor	>24	>25	>27	>28	>29
Women					
excellent	<15	<16	<17	<18	<19
good	16–19	17–20	18–21	19–22	20–23
average	20–28	21–29	22–30	19–22	20–23
fair	29–31	30–32	31–33	32–34	33–35
poor	>32	>33	>34	>35	>36

Source: Adapted from Jackson, A. S., Pollock, M. L., Generalized equations for predicted body density of men. Br. J. Nutr. 40: 497–504, 1978., and Jackson, A. S., Pollock, M. L., Generalized equations for predicted body density of men. Med. Sci. Sports Exerc. 12: 175–182; used with permission.

Table 17   Sum of Skin Folds[a]: Percentile Scores

Percentile score	Age group									
	20–29		30–39		40–49		50–59		60–69	
	M	F	M	F	M	F	M	F	M	F
95	26	37	28	40	28	42	31	48	33	45
90	29	40	32	45	37	48	36	54	38	54
85	30	43	35	48	40	51	40	60	41	61
80	32	46	38	52	44	56	44	65	45	65
75	34	49	41	55	46	59	46	69	48	67
70	36	51	44	58	48	62	48	73	50	70
65	38	53	46	61	51	66	51	75	52	72
60	40	56	49	63	53	69	53	78	54	76
55	43	58	52	66	56	73	55	81	56	80
50	46	60	55	69	58	77	58	84	58	82
45	49	63	58	72	60	81	60	87	59	85
40	52	65	60	76	63	86	62	90	61	87
35	55	69	63	79	66	90	65	93	63	93
30	58	72	67	83	69	94	68	97	65	98
25	62	76	71	88	72	98	71	101	69	100
20	68	81	76	93	75	105	74	106	72	103
15	74	86	82	99	79	113	77	112	76	112
10	82	95	89	109	86	125	81	121	81	123
5	94	111	101	128	97	150	88	138	91	139

[a] Sum of: triceps + biceps + subscapular + iliac crest + medial calf (mm)
Based on Canada Fitness Survey, 1981.
Source: Modified from Ref. 9; used with permission.

options. Self-administered questionnaires, such as the Par-Q (Fig. 6), medical examination, and clinical stress testing are used as screening devices prior to the writing of an exercise prescription. Medically supervised stress testing in apparently health and "risk-free" individuals is not recommended. Such testing is advised for those with multiple primary risk factors and/or symptoms of coronary heart disease, in addition to those in the coronary-prone age group (males, 40–49), and/or who are grossly overweight. Healthy patients should be encouraged to undergo a submaximal exercise testing and generalized fitness assessment. Such evaluations provide valuable information for quantification of the exercise prescription, and motivation toward program compliance.

'NAME OF PARTICIPANT

DATE _____

PAR Q & YOU

PAR-Q is designed to help you help yourself. Many health benefits are associated with regular exercise, and the completion of PAR-Q is a sensible first step to take if you are planning to increase the amount of physical activity in your life.

For most people physical activity should not pose any problem or hazard. PAR-Q has been designed to identify the small number of adults for whom physical activity might be inappropriate or those who should have medical advice concerning the type of activity most suitable for them.

Common sense is your best guide in answering these few questions. Please read them carefully and check (√) the ☐ YES or ☐ NO opposite the question if it applies to you.

YES NO

☐ ☐ 1. Has your doctor ever said you have heart trouble?

☐ ☐ 2. Do you frequently have pains in your heart and chest?

☐ ☐ 3. Do you often feel faint or have spells of severe dizziness?

☐ ☐ 4. Has a doctor ever said your blood pressure was too high?

☐ ☐ 5. Has your doctor ever told you that you have a bone or joint problem such as arthritis that has been aggravated by exercise, or might be made worse with exercise?

☐ ☐ 6. Is there a good physical reason not mentioned here why you should not follow an activity program even if you wanted to?

☐ ☐ 7. Are you over age 65 and not accustomed to vigorous exercise?

If You Answered

YES to one or more questions

If you have not recently done so, consult with your personal physician by telephone or in person BEFORE increasing your physical activity and/or taking a fitness appraisal. Tell your physician what questions you answered YES to on PAR-Q or present your PAR-Q copy.

programs

After medical evaluation, seek advice from your physician as to your suitability for:
● unrestricted physical activity starting off easily and progressing gradually;
● restricted or supervised activity to meet your specific needs, at least on an initial basis. Check in your community for special programs or services.

NO to all questions

If you answered PAR-Q accurately, you have reasonable assurance of your present suitability for:
● A GRADUATED EXERCISE PROGRAM – a gradual increase in proper exercise promotes good fitness development while minimizing or eliminating discomfort;
● A FITNESS APPRAISAL – the Canadian Standardized Test of Fitness (CSTF).

postpone

If you have a temporary minor illness, such as a common cold.

* Developed by the British Columbia Ministry of Health. Conceptualized and critiqued by the Multidisciplinary Advisory Board on Exercise (MABE). Translation, reproduction and use in its entirety is encouraged. Modifications by written permission only. Not to be used for commercial advertising in order to solicit business from the public.
Reference: PAR-Q Validation Report, British Columbia Ministry of Health, 1978.
* Produced by the British Columbia Ministry of Health and the Department of National Health & Welfare.

Figure 6 The Par-Q Physical Activity Readiness Questionnaire, used for screening prior to exercise testing and participating in an exercise program.

Absolute contraindications for exercise training include conditions that seriously alter the normal cardiovascular response to exercise, thereby dangerously compromising the patient's health. "Relative" contraindications should also be considered, both when determining the potential benefits of exercise training relative to the associated risks, and when deciding the necessary extent of control and monitoring. Patients in this category should undergo a supervised exercise test and enter a supervised program (Table 18).

Table 18   Absolute and Relative Contraindications for Exercise Training

Absolute:
1. Recent myocardial infarction (<6 weeks)
2. Unstable angina at rest
3. Severe sinus arrhythmias and conduction disturbances
4. Congestive heart failure
5. Aortic stenosis—severe
6. Diagnosed or suspected aortic aneurysm
7. Myocarditis or disease induced cardiomyopathy (recent)
8. Thrombophlebitis, recent emboli (systemic or pulmonary)
9. Fever
10. Uncontrolled metabolic disorders
11. Severe hypertension with exercise (SBP > 250; DBP > 120)

Relative:
1. Frequent ectopic beats and/or uncontrolled supraventricular arrhythmias
2. Pulmonary hypertension—untreated
3. Moderate ventricular aneurysm and/or aortic stenosis
4. Severe myocardial obstructive syndrome
5. Mild cardiomyopathy
6. Toxemia or complicated pregnancy

Conditions requiring a supervised program:
1. Myocardial infarction; postaortocoronary bypass surgery; documented CHD
2. Pacemakers—fixed rate or demand
3. Cardiac medication—chronotropic or inotropic
4. Morbid obesity in conjunction with multiple risk factors
5. ST-Segment depression at rest
6. Severe hypertension
7. Intermittent claudication

Source: Adapted from Ref. 21; used with permission.

Additional conditions, both medical and environmental, may merit caution in the prescription of exercise, or a temporary moderation of activity (Table 19). If activity is curtailed for a long period of time (>3–4 weeks), a subsequent modification of the exercise prescription may be necessary.

Intensity of Aerobic Exercise

The intensity of exercise is the most important issue when prescribing exercise. Exercise yielding a heart rate less than a "target" level (Fig. 7) may be insufficient to elicit a training effect; the threshold commonly lies at 60% of the difference between maximal and resting heart rate, although the level can vary from 50 to 80% of $\dot{V}O_{2\,max}$.

Typically, intensity is expressed as (a) a percentage of maximal heart rate or heart rate reserve (the maximum minus the resting value), or (b) functional capacity (% of $\dot{V}O_{2\,max}$ or metabolic equivalents, or METS). The initial prescription is highly dependent upon the initial level of fitness. Unconditioned patients have a low threshold for improvement in functional capacity, whereas conditioned patients require a high intensity. However, as intensity increases, the incidence of musculoskeletal injuries rises. A dose-response relationship has been suggested (15), with the required dosage relative to response increasing (in addition to risk of injury) as fitness improves (Fig. 8).

Determining Intensity by Heart Rate

This method requires the measurement or estimation of maximal heart rate. Assuming a linear relationship between heart rate and $\dot{V}O_2$, this technique is an indirect method of expressing intensity as a percentage of functional capacity. Intensity is expressed as a percentage of maximal heart rate (HR_{max}), where HR_{max} = 220 − age, or 210 − 0.65 (age). Thus, the absolute work level varies with the individual's age. Intensities 60–75% maximal heart rate ("target zone") are usually sufficient to induce a training effect; these correspond to approximately 65–85% of functional capacity (see Fig. 7). Potential errors in the estimation of maximal heart rate amount to ±15 beats (15).

In the Karvonen method, the heart rate reserve (HRR) = HR_{max} − HR_{rest}; and the training heart rate (THR) is calculated as:

$$THR = 0.60-0.85\,(HR_{max} - HR_{rest}) + HR_{rest}$$

where 0.60–0.85 represents a range of intensity. Intensity should begin at low levels (0.6), increasing gradually as fitness improves (Table 20). This method accounts for training-induced bradycardia, and is preferred over simple measures of maximal heart rate.

Table 19 Conditions Requiring Precaution in the Exercise Prescription and Moderation of Activity

Conditions requiring precaution in exercise prescription:
1. Viral infection or cold
2. Chest pain
3. Irregular heart beat
4. Exercise induced asthma
5. Prolonged, unaccustomed physical activity
6. Conduction disturbances (left bundle branch block, complete AV block, biphasicular block with or without 1-degree block, rare conduction syndromes

Conditions requiring moderation of activity:
1. Extreme heat and relative humidity
2. Extreme cold, especially when strong winds present
3. Following heavy meals
4. Exposure to high altitudes (>1700 m)
5. Musculoskeletal injuries

Source: Adapted from Ref. 21; used with permission.

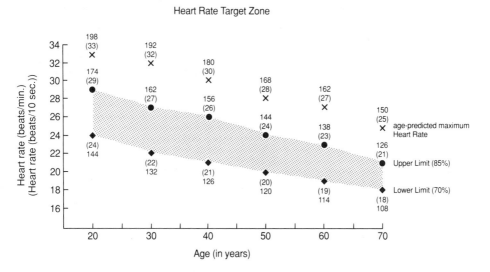

Figure 7 The "target zone" for exercise training. Pulse rates (per min and per 10 s) are illustrated, showing the decline in maximal heart rate with age, and the corresponding slope of the optimal training intensity with increasing age. (Modified from Ref. 9; used with permission.)

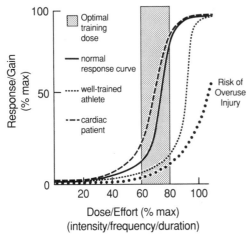

Figure 8 The dose-response relationship between training intensity (dosage), changes in cardiorespiratory fitness (response), and probability of musculoskeletal injury. Low dosage or stimulus is required at the initial stage of training, with smaller gains observed at high levels of conditioning. The stimulus requirements are lowest in deconditioned or pathological states, and are greatest in well-conditioned athletes. Lower intensity and duration will yield lower injury rates. (Modified from M. M. Dehn and C. B. Mullins, "Physiologic Effects and Importance of Exercise in Patients with Coronary Artery Disease," in: *Cardiovascular Medicine*, 2:365, 1977, Group Medicine Pub. Inc., N.Y., N.Y.; H. K. Hellerstein and B. A. Franklin, "Exercise Testing and Prescription," in: *Rehabilitation of the Coronary Patient, 2nd Ed.* N. K. Wenger and H. K. Hellerstein, Eds. John Wiley and Sons, N.Y., N.Y., 1984; and Fardy, P. S. Train for aerobic power. In: *Toward an Understanding of Human Performance.* E. J. Burke, ed. Ithaca, Mouvement Publication, 1977, N.Y., N.Y.)

Exercise Prescription Using METS

Intensity of exercise may be prescribed in MET units, once functional capacity has been determined. This method allows for the prescription of various activities with documented energy requirements (Table 21). Expressing work output in METS (1 MET = 3.5 ml/kg/min) is comparable to expressing work output by heart rate, since both variables tend to be linearly related. Prescriptions often utilize both units, with a range from 60 to 85% maximum METS (MMET), corresponding to low and peak conditioning intensities, respectively (2). An average training intensity may be calculated by (a) adding the MMET as a base value to 60%, (b) dividing this value by 100, and (c) multiplying by MMET. Thus, for an individual with a maximal functional capacity = 15 METS, the average conditioning intensity = [(60 + 15)/100] ×

Table 20 Recommended Target Heart Rates for Healthy Individuals
(assuming resting heart rate = 75)

	Age							
	20–24	25–29	30–34	35–39	40–44	45–49	50–54	55–59
HR_1	198	193	188	183	178	173	168	163
HR_2	186	181	177	172	168	168	158	154
HR_3	161	158	154	151	147	143	140	136
HR_4	149	146	143	140	137	133	131	128

HR_1 = maximal heart rate (220 − age)
HR_2 = peak training heart rate
  $= 0.9\,(HR_{max} - HR_{rest}) + HR_{rest}$
HR_3 = average training heart rate
  $= 0.7(HR_{max} - HR_{rest}) + HR_{rest}$
HR_4 = low training heart rate
  $= 0.6(HR_{max} - HR_{rest}) + HR_{rest}$
Source: Adapted from Ref. 21; used with permission.

MMETS = 11.25 METS. Since 1 MET = 4.19 kJ/kg/min (1 kcal/kg/h), energy expenditure per activity session can be also determined. Hence a 70-kg male exercising at this intensity for 30 min would expend 1651 kJ (394 kcal). In addition, the metabolic cost (METS or $\dot{V}O_2$) can be estimated from horizontal walking and running (Table 22), thereby assisting in the prescription and monitoring of exercise.

Use of the Ventilatory Threshold

Exercise should be set well below the VT in untrained adults, since this intensity corresponds to a rapid increase in blood lactate, probably brought about by increased anaerobiosis. As described earlier, those with a greater aerobic power will have a higher relative threshold level (greater % of $\dot{V}O_{2\,max}$), with a correspondingly greater intensity requirement. The prescribed exercise intensity is typically set at a heart rate corresponding to 5–15% below the threshold.

Exercise Duration

The duration of exercise is the second most important factor in prescription, with a minimum recommended energy expenditure of 1200–1300 kJ/session (300 kcal).

Very short periods of exercise (5–10 min) are sufficient to induce a cardiovascular training effect if performed at a high intensity (90–95% of functional capacity) (12). However 20–60 min of continuous aerobic

Table 21 Energy Costs of Various Activities

Activity		METS	kJ/kg/min
Walking			
	4.8 km/h (81 m/min)	3.0	6.3
	6.4 km/h (107 m/min)	4.6	9.7
Running			
	7.5 min/km (134 m/min)	8.7	18.3
	6.2 min/km (161 m/min)	10.2	21.4
	5.0 min/km (201 m/min)	12.5	26.5
	3.7 min/km (268 m/min)	16.3	34.4
Cycling			
	50W	3.7	7.8
	75 W	5.0	10.5
	100 W	6.0	12.6
	125 W	7.0	14.7
	150 W	8.5	17.9
	Pleasure	7-8+	14.7+
	16.1 km/h	7.0	114.7
Swimming (front crawl)			
	20 m/min	6.0	12.6
	40 m/min	12.0	25.2
Golf		5.1	10.7
Hiking		3-7	6.3-12.6
Cross-country skiing		6-12+	12.6-25.2+
Squash		8-14	16.8-25.2
Tennis		6-10	12.6-21

Note: 1 kcal = 4.19 kJ

activity at a moderate intensity is ideal for conditioning (1). Initially, the stimulus period should remain relatively short (15–20 min), gradually extending as cardiovascular endurance improves. Fat utilization increases significantly after approximately 20 min of light to moderate exercise (46), thereby enhancing weight control and fat loss. Furthermore, favorable changes in the blood lipid profile, including a reduction in triglyceride, increases in high-density lipoprotein cholesterol (HDL-C), and the HDL-C:total cholesterol ratio are associated with longer periods of exercise duration (46).

Table 22 Estimation of Energy Requirements in METs for Horizontal Walking and Running

Horizontal walking:						
min/km	28	19	15	12	11	10
min/mile	35	30	24	20	17.6	16
km/h	2.7	3.2	4	4.8	5.5	6
mph	1.7	2.0	2.5	3.0	3.4	3.75
m/min	45.6	53.7	67.0	80.5	91.2	100.5
$\dot{V}O_2$[a]	8.1	8.8	10.2	11.6	12.6	13.7
METs	2.3	2.5	2.9	3.3	3.6	3.9
Horizontal running:						
min/km	7.5	6.2	5.3	5	4.7	4.1
min/mile	12:00	10:00	8:34	8:00	7:30	6:40
km/h	8	9.7	11.3	12.1	12.9	14.5
mph	5	6	7	7.5	8	9
m/min	134	161	188	201	215	241
$\dot{V}O_2$[a]	30.1	35.7	41	43.8	46.6	51.8
METs	8.6	10.2	11.7	12.5	13.3	14.8

[a] ml/kg/min
Source: Adapted from Ref. 2; used with permission.

Frequency of Exercise Sessions

The optimal frequency of training is dependent upon the intensity and duration of the exercise program. A training threshold of two sessions per week is rquired for an improvement in aerobic power, but the exercise intensity must be relatively high for conditioning to occur (39). The recommended frequency for normal adults (3–10 METs functional capacity) is three sessions per week, with sessions scattered evenly through the week. This is optimal at the initial stage of the exercise program, as it allows for sufficient rest between exercise bouts and for musculoskeletal adaptations to occur.

In obese subjects and adults with very low functional capacities (less than 3 METs), it may be more practical to recommend frequent (>4) and short (5 min) sessions daily. As functional capacity improves to 3–5 METs, there can be a transition to one to two daily sessions.

Five days per week is adequate to attain optimal fitness levels. Progression from 3 to 5 days per week should occur gradually over a 4-week period, and no more than three intense exercise sessions should occur per week. Activity on the remaining days should be of reduced intensity and duration. Exercising 7 days per week does not further improve aerobic power significantly (27); any gains of 1–2% are only relevant for the competitive athlete.

If strength fitness or isotonic resistance training activities are to be incorporated into the regular aerobic exercise program, these should be undertaken no more than 2–3 days per week, as the recouperative period is longer for heavy resistance work than for lower intensity aerobic activities.

Exercise Mode

Activities that utilize large muscle groups in a rhythmic and continuous manner are the preferred mode of aerobic exercise. Theoretically, there should be no difference between modalities in terms of conditioning effect, providing the criteria of intensity, frequency, and duration are met (15). Most investigations have shown that a similar cardiovascular training effect is generated by jogging/running, swimming, bicycling, and cross-country skiing programs. Less intense activities (e.g., golf, bowling) offer little training stimulus, since heart rates rarely exceed 100 beats/min, well below the target heart rate (see Fig. 7). Certain indoor racquet sports (e.g., squash) involve rapid starts, thereby increasing systemic blood pressure and myocardial O_2 demand; they should thus be prescribed only in healthy, risk-free patients.

Sustained isometric (static) activities with heavy resistance is strongly discouraged in unconditioned, hypertensive, and/or coronary-prone patients; little or no improvement of $VO_{2\,max}$ is observed when the resistance exercise employs heavy weights and a low number of repititions. The mode of activity should be of sufficient intensity to elicit a cardiovascular training effect, minimizing both musculoskeletal strain and blood pressure response.

Type of Exercise

Exercise training can include either continuous or intermittent (interval) exercise. The advantage of interval training (high intensity, short duration, with rest intervals) is that more energy expenditure is possible without a progressive accumulation of blood lactate. In the case of an athlete, increased speed is often the objective, whereas in highly deconditioned patients, total work can be accomplished with less physiological stress. Therefore, it may be advantageous to prescribe exercise on an alternating run-walk basis initially, and as functional capacity improves, a higher energy output may be performed on a more continuous basis. Activities which are continuous and elicit constant heart rate response (walking, jogging or running, cross-country skiing, swimming, and cycling) are preferred when both duration and control of the exercise intensity are desired.

Muscular Strength Activities

Enhancement of muscle strength through dynamic, high-resistance, low-repetition exercise is strongly discouraged for patients who are unconditioned, hypertensive, at risk to cardiovascular disease, or with documented cardiovascular disease. Dynamic and static strength exercises, especially when performed with the Valsalva maneuver, may cause an excessive rise of systemic blood pressure, thereby reducing venous return, and increasing ventricular afterload. Light weights, preferably in the form of a circuit training session, may be the optimal method of combining cardiorespiratory fitness and muscle strength training (16).

The Exercise Session

Each exercise session should include three components: a warm-up period, an endurance phase (stimulus period), and a warm-down. The warm-up should be relatively short (5–10 min), consisting of light calisthenics, static stretching exercises, slow jogging and walking; such activities facilitate a more favorable response to subsequent, more intense exercise. Increases in muscle and general body temperature, as brought about by warming-up, will increase local muscle blood flow, reduce muscle viscosity, and enhance both O_2 dissociation and enzymatic reactions (Law of Arrhenius). There is also evidence suggesting that sudden bursts of intense exercise without a warm-up may precipitate ventricular fibrillation, and that a warm-up reduces the likelihood of unfavorable electrocardiographic responses (see Tables 7 and 10).

The definitive stimulus period, consisting of the specified intensity and duration of activity (see above) should be initiated slowly and should immediately follow the warm-up period.

A gradual warm-down of approximately 5–10 min, utilizing exercises similar to those used during the warm-up period, is recommended following the stimulus period. An abrupt cessation of exercise, particularly in a warm and humid environment, may cause orthostatic hypotension, precipitating myocardial ischemia in those with latent coronary disease. Thus, hot showers, saunas, and whirlpools are strongly discouraged until long after the warm-down period, and are contraindicated in patients with coronary heart disease (CHD).

Monitoring Exercise

A 10-s pulse is taken immediately (within 5 s) following exercise. The first beat is counted as zero, and the observed value is compared to recommended target levels (see Fig. 7). As individuals become accustomed to the perception of the appropriate intensity of exercise, pulse rates can be counted once during and after the stimulus period. In addition, Borg's linear or nonlinear rating of perceived exertion (RPE) scale (Table 23) can be used to monitor exercise intensity in selected situations or patients. Scores of 12-16 on the old (nonlinear scale) represent the target zone HR for most age groups (60–85% $\dot{V}O_{2\,max}$); they provide reproducible self-ratings of effort (6).

Progression of Exercise Prescriptions

Intensity, frequency, and duration can be adjusted to a higher level over time, but the *rate* of progression is often difficult for the practitioner to determine. The individual patient and training environment must be considered when planning progression. Three phases can be identified (2). The initial stage covers the first to the fifth week of training. It concludes an introduction to stretching, light calisthenics, and low-intensity aerobics. The duration of the aerobic session should be kept at 12-15 min, with aim to achieve an energy expenditure of 830–

Table 23   Borg's (1982) Rating of Perceived Exertion Scales

Original scale		Linear scale	
6		0	nothing at all
7	very, very light	0.5	very, very weak
8		1	very weak
9	very light	2	weak
10		3	moderate
11	fairly light	4	somewhat strong
12		5	strong
13	somewhat hard	6	
14		7	very strong
15	hard	8	
16		9	
17	very hard	10	very, very strong
18			maximal
19	very, very hard		

850 kJ/session (200 kcal) during the first week of training, and eventually 1200–1300 kJ/session (300 kcal).

Two types of variable indicate that the participant can progress to the next level. Objective measures include: (a) a 3–8 beats/min decrease in HR during the aerobic phase exercise, (b) a slightly faster voluntary jogging or walking pace, and (c) an improvement of functional capacity ($\dot{V}O_{2\,max}$, steady-state $\dot{V}O_2$, METs). Subjective measures include the level of fatigue, facial expression, breathing, RPE scores, and biomechanical form.

The second phase is the improvement stage. It lasts from 6 to 24 weeks, and is characterized by the progression of intensity (from 60% in the first phase, to 70–80%), duration, and frequency.

In certain individuals in whom functional capacity is low, the transition from walking to jogging might best be accomplished by initially using discontinuous walk/run aerobic exercise, and progressing toward continuous steady-state exercise. Duration should be increased before increasing the intensity.

The third phase of progression is the maintenance stage. Participants should now be exercising at the full 70–80% of estimated functional capacity for at least 30–45 min, four to five times per week.

Compliance with Exercise Programs

Compliance, defined as the degree to which someone's behavior matches medical or health advice (36), is a key factor in the long-term success of exercise programming. Exercise compliance is usually expressed as a defined number of sessions completed per week or month. A wide range of compliance rates have reported for programs of primary prevention. Before long-term compliance is sought, strategies should maximize adoption and maintenance of the new behavior (36).

The willingness to adopt and comply with exercise on a regular basis typically ranges from 30 to 60% of a population sample. Unfortunately, some studies report that fewer than 50% of those who begin exercise programs will be complying sufficiently after 4 weeks. There are a number of factors which have been identified to enhance compliance, including (a) convenience of sessions or proximity to the exercise facility, (b) spousal support and/or participation (c) freedom from musculoskeletal injury, particularly early in the programs, (d) group exercise programs, and (e) desire to improve fitness (33,36). The last point appears obvious. However, it is unlikely that compliance will remain high if personal motivation is not present. Freedom from musculoskeletal injury is a key factor, particularly early in the program, underscoring the importance of slow progression.

The time course of adaptation (changes in $\dot{V}O_{2\,max}$) is initially rapid. A 10- to 11-day half-time has been reported for improvement of $\dot{V}O_{2\,max}$ (22). The initial improvement provides considerable motivation and can greatly influence compliance (36). Further improvements are less dramatic, and at this stage maintenance of fitness must be stressed.

During the third phase, compliance-oriented goals become particularly important. New activities can be introduced to provide variety, while holding the energy expenditure, duration, and intensity at the necessary levels to maintain aerobic fitness. Periodic reassessment of cardiovascular fitness will provide on-going feedback and aid in sustaining compliant behavior.

EQUATIONS USED FOR CALCULATING EXERCISE INTENSITY

Intensity Based on Heart Rate

$$HR_{train} = HR_{rest} + 0.6 - 0.8(HR_{max} - HR_{rest})$$

$$HR_{max} = 210 - 0.65\,(age)\ or\ = 220 - age$$

(also see Fig. 7).

Walking, Jogging, Running Speeds Using METs

METs to speed of walking, jogging:

$$<6.4\ km/h \qquad v = \frac{(TMETs - 1\,MET)}{0.88} - 1.01$$

$$6.4 - 8.0\ km/h \qquad v = \frac{(TMETS - 1\,MET)}{3.37} + 8.51$$

$$>8\ km/h \qquad v = \frac{(TMETS - 1\,MET)}{1.37} - 1.85$$

where v-speed (km/h) and TMETs = calculated training METs.

Walking or Jogging Speed Based on % $\dot{V}O_{2\,max}$ (ml/kg/min)

$$jogging\ velocity\,(km/h) = \frac{I\,(\dot{V}O_{2\,max}\,ml/kg/min) - 3.5}{8.63}$$

$$walking\ velocity\,(km/h) = \frac{I\,(\dot{V}O_{2\,max}\,ml/kg/min) - 3.5}{4.31}$$

where I = desired training intensity.

O_2 Costs of Walking, Jogging, and Running

$$\dot{V}O_2 = 2.97(v) + 6.57$$

where v = running speed (1.6–4.8 km/h).

$$\dot{V}O_2 = 7.36(v) - 29.8$$

where v = walk/jog speed (5.6–8 km/h)

$$\dot{V}O_2 = 1.94(v) + 3.5$$

where v = walking speed (8–16.1 km/h)

Cycle Ergometry

$$\dot{V}O_2 \, ml/min = 10.7 \, (W) + 300$$

$$\dot{V}O_2 \, ml/min = (kpm/min \times 2 \, ml/kpm) + 3.5 \, ml/kg/min \times kg \, (wt)$$

REFERENCES

1. American College of Sports Medicine—Position Statement, *Med. Sci. Sports, 10*: vii (1978).
2. American College of Sports Medicine, *Guidelines for Exercise Testing and Prescription*. 3rd Ed. Lea & Febiger, Philadelphia (1986).
3. Åstrand, P.O., and Rodahl, K., *Acta Physiol. Scand., 49* (Suppl.): 169 (1960).
4. Balke, B., and Ware, R.W., *U.S. Armed Forces Med. J., 10*: 675 (1959).
5. Blair, S.N., *Resource Manual for Guidelines for Exercise Testing and Prescription* (S.N. Blair, P. Painter, R.R. Pate, L.K. Smith, and C.B. Taylor, eds). Lea & Febiger, Philadelphia (1988).
6. Borg, G.V., *Med. Sci. Sports Exerc., 14*: 377 (1982).
7. Brozek, J., Grande, F., Anderson, J.T., and Keys, A., *Ann. N.Y. Acad. Sci., 110*: 173 (1963).
8. Bruce, R.A., Kusumi, F., and Hosmer, D. *Am. Heart J., 85*: 346 (1973).
9. *Canadian Standardized Test of Fitness (CSTF)*. Operations Manual. 3rd Ed. Minister of Supply and Services Canada, Ottawa (1987).
10. Crapo, R.O., *Bull. Eur. Physiopathol. Resp., 18*: 419 (1982).
11. Cunningham, D.A., and Rechnitzer, P., *Arch. Phys. Med. Rehab., 55*: 296 (1974).
12. Durnin J.V., and Womersley, J., *Br. J. Nutr., 32*: 77 (1974).
13. Durnin, J.G., Brockway, J.M., and Whitcher, H.W., *J. Appl. Physiol., 15*: 161 (1960).
14. Ellestad, M.H., Allen, W.A., Wan, M.L.K., and Kemp, G.L., *Circulation, 39*: 517 (1969).
15. Fardy, P.S., Yanowotz, F.G., and Wilson, P.K., *Cardiac Rehabilitation,*

Adult Fitness, and Exercise Testing. 2nd Ed. Lea & Febiger, Philadelphia, p. 41 (1988).

16. Fox, E.L., Bowers, R.W., and Foss, M.L., *The Physiological Basis of Physical Education and Athletics.* 4th Ed. Saunders College, Toronto (1988).

17. Froelicher, V.F., *Exercise and the Heart: Clinical Concepts.* Year Book, Chicago (1987).

18. Gettman, L.R., *Resource Manual for Guidelines for Exercise Testing and Prescription* (S.N. Blair, P. Painter, R.R. Pate, L.K. Smith, and C.B. Taylor, Eds.). Lea & Febiger, Philadelphia, p. 161 (1988).

19. Goodman, J., PhD dissertation, University of Toronto, Canada (1987).

20. Goodman, J., Lefkowitz, C., Shurvell, B., McLaughlin, P., and Plyley, M., *Clin. Invest. Med., 8 (Suppl. B)*: B32 (1986).

21. Goodman, J., and Goodman, L., *Current Therapy in Sports Medicine* (R.P. Welsh and R.J. Shephard, eds.). B.C. Decker, Philadelphia, p. 17 (1985).

22. Hickson, R.C., Hagberg, J.M., Ehsani, A.A., and Holloszy, J. O., *Med. Sci. Sports and Exerc. 13*: 17 (1981).

23. Hossack, K.F. (1980). *Am. J. Cardiology. 46*: 204.

24. Hubley, C., *Physiological Testing of the Elite Athlete* (J. D. MacDougall, H.A. Senger, and H.J. Green, eds.). Canadian Association of Sport Sciences, Ottawa, p. 7 (1981).

25. Jackson, A., Watkins, M., and Patton, R., *Med. Sci. Sports Exerc., 12*: 274 (1980).

26. Jackson, A.S., and Pollock, M.L., *Can. J. Appl. Sports Sci., 7*: 187 (1982).

27. Jackson, J.T., Sharkey, B.J., and Johnston, P., *Res. Quart. Exers. Sports, 39*: 295 (1968).

28. Jette, M., Campbell, J., Mongeon, J., and Routhier, R., *Can. Med. Assoc. J., 114*: 685 (1976).

29. Johns, R., and Wright, W., *J. Appl. Physiol., 17*: 824 (1962).

30. Johnson, B.L., and Nelson, J.K. *Practical Measurements for Evaluation in Physical Education.* Burgess, Minneapolis, p. 74 (1969).

31. Jones, N.L., and Campbell, E.J.M. *Clinical Exercise Testing.* Saunders, Toronto, p. 113 (1982).

32. Leighton, J.R., *Res. Quart., 13*: 205 (1942).

33. Massie, J.F., and Shephard, R.J., *Med. Sci. Sports Exerc., 3*: 110 (1971).

34. Moffat, R.J., *Resource Manual for Guidelines for Exercise Testing and Prescription* (S.N. Blair, P. Painter, R.R. Pate, L.K. Smith, and C.B. Taylor, eds.). Lea & Febiger, Philadelphia, p. 263 (1988).

35. Naughton, J., Sevellus, G., and Balke, B., *J. Sports Med. 31*: 201 (1963).

36. Oldridge, N.B., *Prevent. Med., 11*: 56 (1982).

37. Park C.R., and Crawford, M.H., *Curr. Prob. Cardiol., 10(5)*: 38 (1985).

38. Plyley, M.J., *Current Therapy in Sports Medicine—2* (J. S. Torg, R.P. Welsh, R.J. Shephard, eds.). B.C. Decker, Toronto, p. 139 (1990).

39. Pollock, M.L., *Ex. Sports Sci. Rev., 1*: 155 (1973).

40. Pollock, M.L., Broida, J., Kendrick, Z. Miller, H.S., Janeway, R., and Linnerud, A.C. *Med. Sci. Sports, 4*: 1972 (1972).

41. Pollock, M.L., Cureton, T.K., and Greninger, L. *Med. Sci. Sports, 1:* 70 (1969).
42. Powers, S.K., and Howley, E.T., *Exercise Physiology: Theory and Application.* W.C. Brown, Dubuque, Iowa (1990).
43. Rost, R., *Athletics and the Heart.* Year Book, Chicago (1986).
44. Sale, D.G., and Norman, R.W., *Physiological Testing of the Elite Athlete* (J.D. MacDougall, H.A. Wenger, and H.J. Green, eds.). Canadian Association of Sport Sciences, Ottawa, p. 7 (1981).
45. Sharkey, B.J., *Med. Sci. Sports, 2:* 197 (1970).
46. Shephard, R.J., *Physiology and Biochemistry of Exercise.* Praeger, New York (1982).
47. Shephard, R.J., *Endurance Fitness.* 2nd Ed. University of Toronto Press, Toronto, (1977).
48. Siconolfi, S.F., Cullinane, E.M., Carleton, R.A., and Thompson, P.D., *Med. Sci. Sports Exerc., 14:* 335–338 (1982).
49. Siri, W.E., in *Techniques for Measuring Body Composition* (J. Brozek and A. Henschel, eds.). National Academy of Sciences National Research Council, p. 223 (1961).
49a. Stuart, R.J., Ellestad, M.H., *Chest., 77:* 94–97 (1980).
50. Taylor, H.L., Buskirk, E., and Henschel, A., *J. Appl. Physiol., 8:* 73 (1955).
51. Teraslinna, P., Partanen, T., Aja, P., and Koskela, A., *J. Sports Med. Phys. Fit., 41:* 491 (1970).
52. Thoden, J.S., Wilson, B.A., and MacDougall, J.D., *Physiological Testing of the Elite Athlete* (J.D. MacDougall, H.A. Wenger, and H.J. Green, eds.). Canadian Association of Sport Sciences, Ottawa, p. 7 (1981).
53. Tiption, C.M., Matthes, R.D., Maynard, J.A., and Carey, R. A., *Med. Sci. Sports, 17:* 175 (1975).
54. Wasserman, K., Hanson, J.E., Sue, D.Y., and Whipp, B.J., *Principles of Exercise Testing and Interpretation.* Lea & Febiger, Philadelphia (1987).
55. Weber, K.T., and Janicki, J.S., *Cardiopulmonary Exercise Testing: Physiologic Principles and Clinical Applications.* p. 153 (1986).
56. Weiner, J.S., and Lourie, J.A., *Practical Human Biology.* Academic Press, New York (1981).

3

Children and Exercise

Linda D. Zwiren

Hofstra University
Hempstead, New York

INTRODUCTION

Childhood has been considered a naturally active part of one's life. However, an increasingly urbanized environment and an increasingly mechanized existence may be counteracting the child's innate drive for physical activity. It is hard to establish accurately whether the physical fitness level of present day children has actually declined, since comparable baseline data do not exist (102). Some surveys, however, have indicated that children are spending large amounts of time watching television and/or playing video games, and this may be contributing to an increase in childhood obesity (32,50,102). On the other hand, a case has been made that most children are active enough to maintain health (16).

While many are concerned with the health risks of physical inactivity and advocate increased activity levels for those children who are developing sedentary lifestyles, there is concern, also, about the possible harmful effects on children who participate in competitive sports at a progressively younger age and with ever-increasing intensity. This chapter will review research on the effects of both regular physical activity and extremely intense exercise on growth and sexual maturity (especially the age of menarche).

If one accepts the assertion that less active adults benefit from an increase in physical activity be reducing their risk of chronic disease, can one make the same assumption for children? This chapter will explore research indicating the link between physical inactivity in childhood and the presence of disease risk factors. Evidence of whether disease risk factors found in children track into adulthood will also be explored. Physiological differences between adults and children will be summarized, and research concerning the trainability of children will be reviewed. The procedures and problems of exercise testing and exercise prescription for children will finally be presented.

While this chapter is a review of physical activity and its effects on children, the word *child* encompasses a very broad category of subjects. It is most often used to refer to the prepubescent period, whereas the word *youth* refers to the adolescent (pubescent period), and *young adult* refers to the postpubescent period. Unfortunately, the studies reviewed have infrequently used a maturational index when selecting subjects. Most authors have simply used chronological age to determine whether subjects were prepubescent, pubescent, or postpubescent. Since the age of maturation is so variable (covering ages 9–16 years), it is unclear whether subjects were truly prepubescent when classified solely by chronological age.

The studies discussed in this chapter are drawn mainly from the United States, Canada, and Western Europe. The literature examining any aspect of children and exercise from the Third World is unfortunately very sparse.

The words *physical activity*, *exercise*, and *physical fitness* describe different concepts. However, these phrases have sometimes been used interchangeably and the terms are often confused with one another in the literature. This review will use a modification of the model of Caspersen et al. (24). Physical activity is defined as any production of energy by skeletal muscles. This energy has historically been expressed in terms of kilocalories (a measure of heat), but is more accurately expressed in kilojoules (a measure of energy expenditure): 1 kcal = 4.184 kJ. Caspersen et al. (24) define physical activity as any bodily movement produced by skeletal muscles. The term *movement* was deliberately left out of the definition used in this chapter in order to include isometric contraction (where no movement takes place). One's physical activity level is a continuous variable ranging from low (minimal energy expenditure above basal metabolic rate and diet-induced thermogenesis) to high.

Exercise is treated as a subcategory of physical activity. Exercise is defined as any physical activity that is planned, structured, repetitive, and purposive in the sense that improvement or maintenance of one or more components of physical fitness or of sport skill attainment is an objective (see Ref. 24, p. 128). Training and conditioning are used as synonyms for exercise.

Physical fitness has been defined as (94):

the ability to carry out daily tasks with vigor and alertness, without undue fatigue and with ample energy to enjoy leisure-time pursuits and to meet unforeseen emergencies.

The World Health Organization, alternatively, has defined physical fitness as an ability to perform muscular work satisfactorily (118).

Whereas physical activity is related mainly to movements people perform, physical fitness is a set of attributes that people currently have or are doing exercises to improve. Since this chapter is written from the point of view of health and disease reduction, the components of physical fitness will be limited to health-related fitness (as opposed to components that improve athletic ability such as agility and speed). The components of health-related fitness are: (a) cardiovascular endurance, (b) muscular endurance, (c) muscular strength, (d) flexibility, and (e) body composition (attainment of an appropriate body mass with a healthy proportion of body fat).

EFFECT OF PHYSICAL ACTIVITY ON GROWTH AND MATURATION

There is a distinction between maturation and growth (see Ref. 71, p. 229).

Maturity implies progress toward the mature state, which varies with the biological systems considered. Skeletal maturity, for example, is a fully ossified skeleton; sexual maturity is reproductive capability; somatic maturity is often defined as adult stature. Growth on the other hand, refers to changes in the size of the organism or of its parts. All individuals attain adult stature, skeletal maturity, and sexual maturity. However, the age of attaining each is variable. Thus progress toward maturity implies time or variation in rate, whereas growth is size oriented.

Although there is a fundamental difference between the two terms, maturation and growth are often used interchangeably in the literature. While the two processes are under separate genetic control, one is related to the other. Children advanced in biological maturity tend to be taller and heavier than children who are delayed in maturity (71).

Stature and Skeletal Maturity

The prevailing consensus is that regular physical activity has no effect on the stature of the growing individual (8,9,74,116,117,139). However, earlier studies indicated an increase of stature with regular exercise (74). The maturity status of the subjects was not determined in these studies, therefore, it is difficult to determine whether the suggested increase in stature with regular exercise was actually related to activity or to the athlete's earlier maturation.

Kato and Ishiko (58) found that the children who engaged in extremely hard labor in the remote areas of Japan had retarded growth. In this case, the retarded bone development may not have been the result of intensive physical activity, but it may rather have reflected poor nutritional status.

Malina (74) points out that whether an individual reaches his or her growth potential is a product of genetic and environmental influences. Linear body measurements (stature) tend to have a large genetic factor. Theintz et al. (125) studied the potential effect of intensive and regular physical training (exercise) on growth potential in elite female gymnasts and moderately trained swimmers. The apparent "shortness" of female gymnasts who had been intensely exercising for a minimum of 5 years was nevertheless still appropriate for their parental height. Their results did not eliminate the possibility that intense training may lead to a loss of growth potential in young children. However, Theintz et al. (125) point out that patterns of parental development are important and should be considered when studying the potential long-term effects of intensive exercise on growth.

Skeletal maturity is most commonly assessed from x-rays of the hand and wrist bones, using the Greulich-Pyle atlas (14). The x-rays of a specific child are matched as closely as possible to one in a series of standard hand-wrist x-ray plates, corresponding to successive levels of skeletal maturation at a given chronological age (70). The Tanner-Whitehouse method, also used in research, entails matching features of individual bones from the x-ray to a series of written criteria.

Shephard (117) points out that several factors limit the precision of the radiograph-matching procedure, resulting in interobserver errors of up to 6 months. A newer method of assessing skeletal maturity (the Fels method) may reduce interobserver errors, since the criteria for matching have been refined, redundant indicators have been eliminated, and calculations include a standard error for the film evaluated (100).

Studies examining the effect of physical activity on skeletal maturity (the majority of which used the Tanner-Whitehouse or the Greulich-Pyle method) generally indicate that skeletal maturity is not affected by regular physical training (9,72,74). "Although regular activity functions to enhance mineralization of bone tissue, it does not accelerate or delay skeletal maturation of the hand or wrist" (see Ref. 70, p. 254).

There is some evidence, however, that young athletes who are exposed to extreme compression forces may be at risk of damage to growing bones. The Trois-Rivieres longitudinal experiment followed 546 primary school children from ages 6 to 12 (117). The experimental group was in a special physical education program (5 h/week or required physical education taught by a physical educator), whereas the control group followed a normal program (a 40-min period of physical activity per week taught by a nonspecialist). Body dimensions, such as height and arm span, were found to be very similar in both experimental and control groups during the 6 years of the study. Comparison of the wrist radiographs, however, suggested that skeletal maturation of experimental subjects was retarded by an average of 3.6 months. Shephard and colleagues (119) suggest that this represented a local mechanical response, since the maturation of the teeth and mandible of the experimental groups was accelerated by 1.5 months. It was also suggested that if these children had been observed into their adolescent growth spurt, or if the experimental group had been exposed to the very rigorous exercise program of some young athletes, a larger effect on skeletal maturity might have been found.

The theory that exposure to excessive stresses at young ages may have detrimental effects on bone maturation is supported by studies on young competitive gymnasts (76,108). Roy et al. (108) identified radiographic evidence of stress changes in the distal radial epiphysis of young gymnasts. Mandelbaum et al. (76) examined the ulnar variance of 38 college-aged gymnasts. Ulnar variance was designated as positive if there was radiographic evidence that the caput ulna was distal to the radius. In this study and in a follow-up study of 43 gymnasts with a mean age of 11 years (85), wrist x-rays showed significantly greater ulnar variance in the gymnasts than in an age- and gender-matched control group. The authors theorized that the strenuous inherent weight-bearing stresses of compression, rotation, and distraction of gymnastic movements (especially on the pommel horse) may have had detrimental effects on wrist growth and injury patterns.

An often stated concern is that the skeletally immature child may be susceptible to injury of the growth cartilage. Growth cartilage is located at three sites in the children's bones—at the apophysis (the site of insertion of a tendon into the bone), at the growth plate of the epiphysis, and at the ends of the bones (articular cartilage). The incidence of serious growth plate injuries in skeletally immature athletes is quite small (80). However, the presence of growth tissue in children and the growth process itself may both increase the child's vulnerability to "overuse" injuries (repetitive microtrauma) (78). Although not researched at present, intense, repetitive running may prove to have implications for growth.

Somatic Maturity

Somatic maturity (the progress toward adult stature) is usually indicated by the age at peak height velocity (PHV). The PHV is the age of maximal growth in stature during the adolescent spurt. Frequent longitudinal observations are required to estimate the age at PHV. The mean values reported for North American and European children range from 11.4 to 12.2 years for girls and 13.5 to 14.4 years for boys (15), with standard deviations of 0.7–1.2 years for both sexes. The age at PHV does not appear to be affected by regular training (70,91).

In summary, there is no strong evidence that regular physical activity affects growth. The majority of evidence also supports the view that regular physical activity does not influence the skeletal or somatic maturity of children, although young competitive gymnasts, who experience repetitive compressive impacts on the epiphyseal structures of the forearm, may experience a cumulative slowing of normal growth.

Sexual Maturation

Adolescent development is often determined by the Tanner method, where children are categorized by physical examination into one of five categories (101). Children of both sexes are categorized by the extent of pubic hair development. In addition, girls are evaluated for breast changes and boys for testicular and phallic development. The greatest variation is in the age of onset of pubertal development (usually indicated by breast budding in females). Most girls experience menarche between 2.0 and 2.5 years after the onset of breast budding. Puberty may be considered delayed in girls (and one should be suspicious of a developmental abnormality) if they have not achieved breast budding by 13 years, or if more than 5 years has elapsed between breast budding and menarche (101).

Sexual maturity in girls has usually been determined by the age of onset of menarche (AOM). Menarche, however, is a relatively late component of the pubertal process, and it is attained well after the PHV (the indicator of somatic maturity). Puberty, on the other hand, covers the entire period of transition from childhood to adulthood. Puberty involves the activation of the hypothalamic-pituitary-adrenal axis (adrenarche), activation of the hypothalamic-pituitary-ovarian axis (gonarche), breast development (thelarche), and the appearance of pubic and axillary hair (pubarche) (91,136).

Since adolescent development is based on fairly similar hormonal and physiological changes in both males and females, it is illogical to assume that physical activity will affect females and not males. The research literature, however, has almost exclusively examined the effect of intensive regular exercise on female adolescent development. "Little attention has been paid to the sexual maturation of young male athletes, despite the fact that males may be more sensitive to environment influences than females during growth and development" (see Ref. 91, p. 304).

Menarche and Physical Activity

Menarche usually occurs at a significantly later age in the young female athlete than in her nonathletic counterpart (9,75,91,136). Two earlier studies had reported an earlier menarche in athletic females than in inactive controls (7,36). However, these two studies were conducted in an era when training programs were not as intensive as at present.

Two popular explanations of the apparent association between strenuous physical exercise and late menarcheal age are the critical lean/fat ratio (44,45) and the two-part hypothesis (75). Frisch and colleagues have reasoned that since fat tissue converts androgen into estrogen, and this conversion accounts for one-third of blood estrogen in premenopausal women, a minimal critical lean/fat ratio is necessary for menarche. Frisch et al. (45) have found that the earlier a girl starts training, the later her menarche and the authors have, therefore, attributed the delay in menarche in athletes to environmental effects. Malina (75), on the other hand, has proposed a two-part theory which includes genetic selection and socialization:

1. A later age of menarche is associated with certain physical characteristics (e.g. a more linear physique; less weight for height). The physical characteristics found in late maturers are the same characteristics that are generally more suitable for athletic performance.
2. Early maturing girls are socialized away from sports partici- pation, whereas late-maturing girls are socialized into sport participation.

Malina's hypotheses implies that age of onset of menarche can ulti- mately be attributed to the phenotypic expression of an inherited trait (122).

Frisch's fatness hypothesis has been vigorously challenged. Trussell (126) criticized the index of fatness used by Frisch, suggesting that the estimates of fatness were so imprecise as to render her evi- dence invalid. Others have also criticized both Frisch's methodology and the use of correlational statistics to imply cause and effect (14,136). On the other hand, Malina's two-part explanation does not constitute a complete hypothesis (75). Other factors such as diet, family size, sociocultural phenomena, body composition, and somatotype need to be considered (14,67,91).

No one theory adequately explains the relationship between training and menarche. Stager and Hatler (122) conducted a cross- sectional study to determine whether the delayed menarche observed in competitive swimmers should be attributed to genetic factors or to intense prepubertal training. The age of onset of menarche (AOM) in competitive swimmers and their sisters was ascertained by a recall questionnaire. The AOM of the swimmers and siblings were then com- pared to nonathletes and their sisters. Their results indicated that at menarche the athletes were significantly older than all other groups, but that the sisters of athletes were also significantly older than con- trols and their sisters. The interpretation of the data is complicated by the fact that the sisters of the athletes were likely to be athletes (75%), whereas the sisters of the control group tended to be nonathletes (74%). The authors concluded that the data could be interpreted as supporting the importance of both inherited characteristics and intense prepubertal activity.

Warren (131) followed ballet dancers (aged 12–15 years) and a control group (aged 13–15 years) for 4 years, distinguishing between menarche and adrenarche. The ballet dancer's menarche (mediated by ovarian steroid hormones) was delayed, but breast development (mediated by adrenal steroid hormones) was unaffected. Warren concluded that the energy drain from intensive exercise may affect the hypothalamic-pituitary set point (the lowering of the sensitivity of the hypothalamus to circulating gonadal steroid hormones which is thought to initiate pubertal development), and in combination with a low percentage of body fat, may prolong the prepubertal state.

Liu et al. (65) assessed body composition and sexual maturation in a cross-sectional comparison of athletes and nonathletes. Body fat was determined by hydrostatic weighing and heavy water analysis. Sexual maturation (in terms of breast and pubic hair development) was self-assessed, using Tanner stages. This determination may lack precision because of the self-assessment and because the development of secondary sex characteristics is a continuous process which has to be categorized into discrete stages. The female athletes, ranging in age from 7 to 15 years, had less body fat than nonathletes at all stages of development, but nevertheless progressed at the same rate through the stages of breast and pubic development as the nonathletes.

In summary, no one theory seems to explain the relationship between training and menarche. The assumption is that the mechanism is hormonal in nature; however, studies involving the hormonal response to prepubertal training are extremely limited and contain flaws in research design (72,91). An explanation which integrates genetic and various environmental factors is needed. Stager and Hatler (122) suggest that athletes may have inherited tendencies to slower maturation and that this tendency is reinforced by early athletic training.

It is yet to be established whether the delay in menarche has any long-term effects on bone density or on future reproductive capabilities. There is no conclusive evidence that athletes who have experienced delayed menarche are more susceptible to secondary amenorrhea later on (91), or that sexual maturation is impaired in athletes (92). Loucks (69) considers osteoporosis a pediatric disease, and recommends regular activity, including weight training, for adolescent girls in order to increase the rate of bone deposition. It is wise to monitor pubertal development, since a delay in menarche beyond 16 years may jeopardize bone mineralization. However, Plowman (91) suggests that further research is needed before any alarm is sounded. "There is need of longitudinal study in which young athletes are followed from prepubescence through puberty, where several maturity indictors are monitored, the training stimulus is monitored, and both boys and girls are included" (see Ref. 72, p. 136). Until such data are available, children should be encouraged to engage in regular physical activity, with a monitoring of maturational progress in those who are involved in strenuous competitive training (91).

EFFECT OF PHYSICAL ACTIVITY ON FITNESS COMPONENTS

Aerobic Power

Maximal aerobic power ($\dot{V}O_{2max}$, the maximal amount of energy the aerobic metabolic system can produce per minute) is measured by a graded exercise test. In adults, maximal aerobic power serves as an indicator of cardiovascular efficiency and of one's ability to perform endurance-type exercise. It has been questioned whether $\dot{V}O_{2max}$ has the same implication for children, especially prepubescent children, as it does for adults (103,140). Maximal oxygen intake may not limit the child's capacity to perform aerobic activities. Performance on aerobic-type events is difficult to predict from $\dot{V}O_{2max}$ data, especially in the younger child (135,140). In addition, boys increase their endurance performance with maturation, but no qualitative improvement in VO_{2max} is seen beyond the changes expected from growth (103). The increase in endurance performance during maturation may be due to increased running efficiency with growth, geometric (surface area/body mass ratio) changes with growth, or increased anaerobic capacities which allows children to run closer to their maximal aerobic power (11,103).

Growth and Aerobic Power

Up to the age of 12 years, untrained children increase their absolute aerobic power with age (11,61) (Fig. 1). Since absolute aerobic power increases as a result of growth alone, a relative term has been used to compare the peak aerobic power of children who differ in body size and mass. When expressed relative to body mass, there are minimal age-related changes in the peak oxygen intake of boys from ages 6 to 16, whereas girls have a declining VO_{2max} (ml/kg/min) from the age of about 6 years (11,61). The decline of relative $\dot{V}O_{2max}$ in adolescent girls may be attributed to an increase in adiposity (with a corresponding decrease in the percentage of lean tissue), a decrease in habitual physical activity, and/or a reduced haemoglobin concentration (9,11).

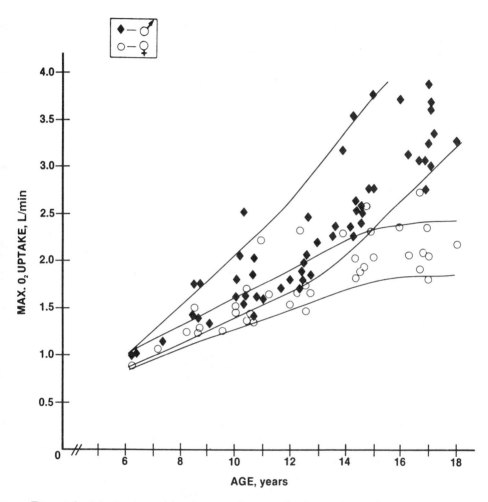

Figure 1 Maximal aerobic power and age. Absolute values of maximal O_2 uptake in girls (n = 1730) and boys (n = 2180) 6 to 18 years old. Each dot represents a mean of a group. The shaded areas were constructed by eye-ball technique to indicate a general trend. Taken from Bar-Or. *Pediatric Sport Medicine*, 1983 p. 4.

Several authors have challenged the expression of $\dot{V}O_{2\,max}$ values relative to body mass as the best indicator of changes in aerobic power beyond that expected from maturation and growth (9,11,117). Scaling against a linear dimension such as height has been suggested as an alternative (8,117). Height has the advantage of being largely independent of extrinsic environmental factors (9), but expressing $\dot{V}O_{2\,max}$ relative to body mass remains the most common way to express $VO_{2\,max}$ when examining changes with growth.

Changes of Aerobic Power and Physical Training: Design Problems

Exercise training studies in children have generally adopted one of three designs:

1. Longitudinal studies of more than 6 months in duration, where cardiorespiratory fitness measurements are compared between children who are active or athletes and those who are inactive or nonathletes.
2. Longitudinal studies of less than 6 months duration, where the amount or activity level of physical education classes is increased, or where the experimental group follows a prescribed training regimen. Measurements made before and after treatment are compared with results for other classes that did not have the physical education class modifications or to a control group which has maintained their normal activity level.
3. Cross-sectional studies where athletes or active children are compared with inactive children at a given time.

Longitudinal studies of long duration are difficult to conduct and include problems of subject recruitment, selectivity and adherence, and standardization of exercise and training dosages. In those studies which have used physical education classes, the difference of activity level between experimental and control groups has often been minimal, and activity levels outside of classes have not been controlled. Random-assignment longitudinal studies are usually of extremely short duration (9,110).

Bar-Or (11,12) points out that, in adults, changes in function before and after training can be evaluated easily. However, in children and adolescents, the effects of a training program may be confounded by changes due to growth, development, and maturation. In longitudinal studies, even with a control group, it is not always easy to determine if the training program has a significant effect on certain physiological variables which normally increase with growth and maturation. "In other physiological variables, training and physical development may induce changes in the opposite direction from those that accompany growth and development. . . . Physical development may indeed mask the training effect on these functions" (see Ref. 12, p. 66).

Longitudinal studies must include a carefully selected control group, since matching groups simply by chronological age may not be sufficient. Rutenfranz (109) pointed out that when he and his colleagues analyzed longitudinal data (collected on Norwegian and West German boys and girls) by chronological age, differences in physical activity level were concluded to be the reason for the noted differences in maximal oxygen intake between Norwegian and German children. However, when the data were reanalyzed as a function of somatic maturation (age at peak height velocity: PHV), the investigators concluded that the discrepancies in maximal oxygen intake were mainly a result of normal growth, with little or no additional effects from physical activity.

Cunningham et al. (30) pointed out that results of longitudinal studies may be confounded by differences in rates of maturation between active and inactive groups. Although aligned on PHV, boys who were early (as opposed to late) maturers show markedly different cardiovascular responses to exercise.

Cross-sectional data are subject to criticism that athletes may be initially selected into a sport on the basis of an "abnormal" pattern of growth or maturation. Male athletes tend to have average or advanced biological maturity, whereas female athletes are usually delayed in their maturation (14).

A further consideration is the possible role of heredity. Bouchard and colleagues (19) explored the variation in response to training within and between pairs of monozygous twins. The authors concluded that 7–77% of the variance in training response was genotype dependent (9,19).

Changes of Aerobic Power and Physical Training: Trainability

The response to training in pubescent and postpubescent children is similar to the response seen in adults. Increased activity of sufficient duration and intensity improves aerobic power by about 10%, with an increase in maximal cardiac output due to an increase in maximal stroke volume (11,61,110). Several articles have suggested that physical activity or training has little or no effect on the maximal aerobic power of prepubescent children (9,110,135,140). Review articles by Rowland (106), Krahenbuhl et al. (61), and Vaccaro and Mahon (127) have concluded, however, that when aerobic training is vigorous and of significant duration, prepubescents show an increase in $\dot{V}O_{2\,max}$ corrected for body mass.

In a recent review, Pate and Ward (88) selectively reviewed 15 studies (12 on prepubescents; three on adolescent youngsters) that met the following criteria:

1. A control group that was matched for age, gender, developmental status, initial fitness, and activity levels
2. A training protocol quantifiable in terms of mode, frequency, intensity, and duration of exercise sessions and overall length of the intervention.
3. Physiological measurements (preferably obtained during maximal exercise) that could be used to document training adaptations
4. A good methological design and statistical analysis

Longitudinal studies were included only if there was a clear exercise intervention, and an appropriate control group had been included.

While the authors tried to select those studies employing design and methodologies that met stringent, preestablished criteria, several constraints still existed in the studies that were reviewed. These included a lack of assessment of developmental status (if the maturational age was not determined, male subjects under the age of 13 years were considered to be prepubescent), extremely few female subjects, limited physiological observations, and a heterogeneous array of training protocols. With these limitations in mind, the authors concluded that both prepubescent and adolescent children could adapt to endurance training; older children were more likely to show increases of $\dot{V}O_{2\,max}$ than their younger counterparts; gender did not appear to be an important determinant of trainability; and children could increase their maximal aerobic power with systematic training regardless of their initial $\dot{V}O_{2\,max}$.

In summary, current knowledge concerning the effect of regular physical training on the aerobic power of children remains quite limited. However, while both pre- and post-pubescent children respond physiologically to regular physical activity (that is, with an improvement in $\dot{V}O_{2\,max}$), there may be a difference in the magnitude of the training response between pre- and postpubescent children. In addition, the $\dot{V}O_{2\,max}$ value may not have the same significance for prepubescents as for older children and adults. These factors need to be considered both when conducting research and when prescribing exercise programs.

The final verdict regarding the relative aerobic trainability of different maturation groups is still pending. It will require a controlled, randomized design with stratification for prepubescent,

pubescent, and postpubescent groups and a matched training dose (see Ref. 10, p. 75)

Muscular Strength

Growth and Muscular Strength

Muscular strength increases linearly with chronological age for both boys and girls from early age to about 14 years of age. After the age of 13–14 years, boys show a marked acceleration in the development of strength. In girls, strength improves linearly up to about the age of 15 years, with no clear evidence of an adolescent spurt (73). Similar chronological growth curves have been observed for isometric hand-grip strength and for composite scores of strength (17).

Longitudinal studies tracking strength development relative to somatic maturity have shown that the maximum strength development of boys occurs approximately 1.0–1.5 years after PHV (15). The accelerated increase in strength coincides with an increased secretion of male sex hormones. The peak of strength development is quite variable in girls (15); some have found the greatest increase in muscle strength during PHV (10,14), whereas others have seen a peak of strength development after PHV (73).

Boys have a rather small strength advantage compared to girls prior to ages 13–15 years; however, after the adolescent growth spurt, the separation in strength scores becomes much larger. After the age of 16 years, few females can generate more absolute strength than males (17). About half of the difference in strength between males and females is related to body size; the remainder reflects both hormonal and cultural factors (117).

Peak gains in strength have a better relationship with peak mass velocity (PMV) than with PHV.

> Thus, muscle tissue apparently increases first in mass and then in strength during male adolescence. This suggests changes in metabolic and contractile features of muscle tissue as adolescence progresses and/or, perhaps, neuromuscular maturation affecting the volitional demonstration of strength (see Ref. 15, p. 527).

Strength Training

In 1983, the American Academy of Pediatrics (2) issued guidelines regarding weight lifting and weight training for children. Weight training (also termed resistive, or strength, training) is the use of static (isometric) or dynamic (isotonic or isokinetic) contractions in order to increase strength. Weight training programs usually involve repetitive contractions with submaximal resistance (2,137). Submaximal resistance, in dynamic training, is a weight that can be lifted through the entire range of motion for a minimum of three or four continuous repetitions (137). Weight lifting is "a sport in which an individual attempts to lift his or her maximum amount of weight" (see Ref. 2, p. 157). The AAP (2) has recommended that if properly supervised, weight *training* can be endorsed for children. However, weight lifting as a competitive sport was not recommended for the preadolescent child.

The 1983 AAP guidelines contained statements that have apparently been contradicted by more recent research. Based primarily on the results of a study by Vrijens (129), the AAP stated that prepubertal boys could not significantly improve their strength or increase their muscle mass by means of weight training programs. This inability to gain strength was attributed to insufficient androgen levels. The Vrijens (129) study found no consistent pattern of strength gains in prepubescent boys after they had trained isometrically for 8 weeks, whereas pubescent boys gained strength in all muscle groups after a similar 8 week program. Weltman (137) points out that the conclusions of the Vrijens study (129) may have been invalidated by the lack of a control group, the low volume of work (only one repetition was performed), and because the subjects trained dynamically but had strength changes determined isometrically. In 1983, the number of studies on strength training in preadolescents was extremely limited. Therefore, the Vrijens study was often cited as the rationale for *not* conducting resistive weight training (RST) programs with prepubertal children.

Several more recent studies have shown that prepubescent boys and girls can increase their muscle strength, and that the increments are well beyond those expected from growth alone. Weltman et al. (138) examined the response of prepubertal boys to a 14-week concentric isokinetic RST program. The strength training program was closely supervised, utilized hydraulic resistive machines (Hydrafit), and included flexibility exercises. Subjects ranged in age from 6 to 11 years and were determined to be prepubertal based on (a) the Tanner classification using pubic and axillary hair, and (b) testicular volume and levels of serum testosterone and dihydroepiandrosterone sulfate (DHEAS). The experimental group (n = 16) significantly improved their isokinetic strength relative to the control group (n = 10). The control group did not weight train but continued to participate in organized sports activities. The safety of the program was evaluated by injury surveillance, scintigraphy, and creatine phosphokinase measurements (95). Effects on growth, development, and flexibility were also investigated. Results indicated a low injury rate with no evidence of damage to the epiphyses, bones, or muscles as a result of RST. In addition, the program did not adversely affect growth, development, or flexibility.

Sewall and Michelli (115) trained 10 subjects (eight boys, two girls; two Tanner stage I, 1 Tanner stage II) for 9 weeks utilizing variable resistance equipment (Nautilus and Cam II). The RST program consisted of three sets of 10 repetitions, preceded by stretching and a warm-up. Strength was determined isometrically prior to and after treatment. The prepubescent experimental group showed significant isometric strength gains over the control group (seven boys, one girl; one Tanner stage I, one Tanner stage II).

Several other studies have used dynamic weight-training programs of short duration with prepubescent children (111). Sale (111) in his review concludes that prepubescent children can increase voluntary strength significantly after RST.

There is less controversy over whether adolescent children respond to RST. Several studies have demonstrated increases in strength after isometric training, dynamic weight training, and stretch-shortening cycle ("plyometrics") training (11).

Pfeiffer and Francis (90) conducted a well-designed RST study on 80 subjects who were assessed for maturity level (Tanner staging). Subjects in stage I (n = 30) were classified as prepubescent, subjects in stages II–IV as pubescent (n = 30), and subjects in stage V as postpubescent (n = 20). Subjects were then randomly assigned to experimental and control groups. The former group trained isotonically (on machines with stacked weights) 3 days a week for 9 weeks. Three repetitions were performed, using 50, 75, 100% of 10 RM. Strength was determined isokinetically on a Cybex dynamometer prior to and after treatment. All three experimental groups increased muscle strength relative to the corresponding control groups. The upper body appeared to be more responsive than the lower extremities. Of the 16 strength measurements, only three posttest measures showed significance among the three maturity groups. In all three cases, the prepubescent group showed the greatest strength gains. The authors concluded that resistance exercises produced greater strength gains during pubescence than during other developmental stages.

Sale (111) reported recent unpublished studies conducted at McMaster University (Hamilton, Ontario). Prepubescent boys (10 years) were compared to young men (21 years) before and after a 20-week RST. The elbow and knee flexors were trained isotonically, using sets of 5 to 12 repititions at one repitition max. The training program was similar for both groups. Measurements were made to determine changes in isometric, isotonic, and isokinetic strength. Results were expressed both in absolute and relative terms. "Regardless of how the increases are expressed, however, the prepubescent boys were 'competitive' in their training response" (see Ref. 111, p. 173). The prepubescent boys, however, did not exhibit any increase in cross-sectional area of the trained muscles (as assessed by computed tomography scanning method). The Vrijens study (129) also found that adolescent boys showed significant increases in muscle mass (measured by radiography), whereas the prepubertal boys showed no muscle hypertrophy, even though the strength of the trunk muscles increased.

In summary, recent studies indicate that prepubescents can safely engage in *carefully supervised* weight-training programs. However, weight lifting (maximal lifts) is not recommended for prepubescents. Prepubescent children are capable of increasing their voluntary strength in response to RST and prepubescents are as trainable as adolescents. There is limited evidence, however, that prepubescents experience difficulty in increasing their skeletal muscle mass after short-term RST (129; unpublished data reported by Sale, 111). Increases in voluntary strength after RST could be a result of a combination of "neural" adaptations (increased ability to activate and coordinate relevant motor units); and "muscular" adaptations (increases in muscle size and the force generated per unit of muscle cross-sectional area). It remains to be determined whether the relative importance of neural and muscular adaptations to RST are similar in prepubescents as in older groups.

Body Mass, Body Composition, and Growth

Body mass, like body stature, follows a four-phase pattern: There is a rapid gain in infancy and early childhood, a slower, relatively constant gain in middle childhood, a rapid gain during the adolescent spurt, and a slow increase with eventual cessation of growth on attainment of adult size (70). Body mass can continue to increase after statural growth has stopped. Peak mass velocity (PMV), another indicator of somatic maturity, generally occurs after peak height velocity (PHV). Boys have a mean age difference between PHV and PMV of 0.2–0.4 years; in girls, the discrepancy varies from 0.3 to 0.9 years (15).

Body composition is frequently conceived as a two-compartment system (fat-free mass [FFM] and fat mass [FM]) (Fig. 2). The term lean body mass (LBM) is often used interchangeably with FFM, although, by definition, LBM consists of fat-free mass plus essential body fat (that is, structural fat as opposed to storage fat). Investigators have used both direct and indirect methods to determine children's body composition.

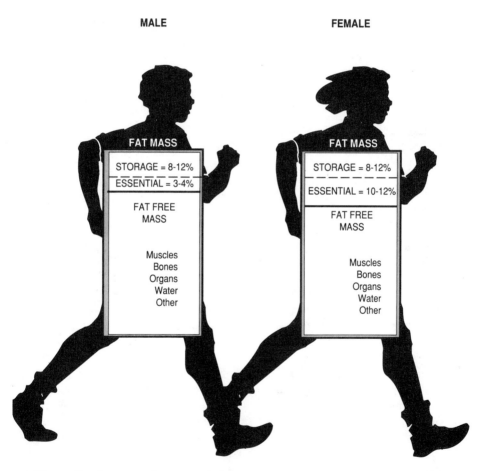

Figure 2 Conceptualization of body composition as a two component model: total body mass = fat − free mass + fat mass.

The most common direct methods include densiometry (body volume being estimated by underwater weighing) and hydrometry (total body water [TBW] determinations). Values obtained from body density have to be converted to estimates of FFM and FM using an equation which assumes that FFM and FM have different but consistent densities, whereas the TBW depends on assumptions about tissue hydration. Indirect methods include the use of anthropometric measurements (such as skin fold thickness, circumferences, and bone diameters) to estimate body density from regression equations developed by the use of direct methods. Forbes (39) provides a detailed description of the various direct and indirect methods appropriate to the determination of body composition in adolescence.

Lohman (68) has pointed out that children's body fat is often estimated inaccurately because equations used to predict FFM and FM have been based on adult models. The child is "chemically immature," the densities of FFM and FM are not the same as in adults, and densities are changing as the child matures.

Malina (70) compiled body density data from 32 studies and TBW data from eight studies of children, youth, and young adults. To allow for the changing chemical composition of the FFM during growth, estimates of density and water content at different ages (68) were used to derive FFM and FM from body density and TBW values. Malina (70) found that FFM followed a growth pattern similar to stature and body mass. Females tended to have a slightly higher FM and percent body fat than boys during prepubescence; however, the gender difference became clearly established during the adolescent growth spurt. For boys, the adolescent spurt reflected mainly gains in skeletal tissue and muscle mass, with fat mass remaining relatively stable at the time of PHV. Girls do not experience as intense an increase in stature or muscle mass as boys, but they have a continuous rise in fat mass (15). Malina (70) has estimated that from the ages of 10 to 18 years boys gain about 4.1 kg FFM and 0.4 kg FM, but there is a decrease of 0.3% fat per year; in contrast, females gain about 2.2 kg FFM, 0.9 kg FM and 0.6% fat per year. In late adolescence and young adulthood, males have, on the average, a FFM that is about 1.5 times larger than that of females, whereas females have, on the average, about 1.5–2.0 times the FM of males.

FFM and FM are gross estimates and do not reflect fat distribution.

Fat distribution refers to location of fat and not to the absolute or relative amount of fat. Adults with a more central distribution of fat, e.g., relatively more on the abdomen than on the extremities, are apparently more at risk for cardiovascular disease and non-insulin dependent diabetes.... The proportional distribution of trunk and extremity subcutaneous fat is rather stable during childhood and similar in boys and girls. Subsequently, sex differences in subcutaneous fat distribution occur. Females appear to gain relatively more subcutaneous fat on the trunk during early adolescence, but later they gain fat on the trunk and extremities at a similar rate. Males, on the other hand, accumulate relatively more fat on the trunk during adolescence, which is accentuated by reduction in subcutaneous fat on the extremities at the time (see Ref. 70, p. 233).

The genetic influence on skin fold thickness, circumferences, and body mass is lower than the genetic influence on stature and bone dimensions. The pattern of fat distribution, however, appears to be highly influenced by genetics (74).

Regular physical activity plays an important role in the regulation of body mass and body composition (9). Youngsters who engage in regular sports training or physical activity tend to have a larger FFM and less FM than children who are inactive (39). In cross-sectional studies, however, children who select vigorous activity may have a genetically different body composition.

Parizkova (87) followed a small sample of boys from ages 11 to 18 years. Three groups with varying physical activity levels were compared: (a) regularly trained (intensive exercise, 6 h/week; n = 8); (b) trained in sport schools, but not on a regular basis (about 4 h/week of organized exercise; n = 18); and (c) an untrained group (about 2.5 h/week of activity, including normal physical education classes; n = 13). The most active group had significantly more FFM and less FM throughout the study. The other two groups did not differ significantly in FFM, but the least active group had a greater relative fatness. These results suggest that physical activity is more likely to affect the fat mass, and to increase FFM during growth, a more intense training stimulus is needed. Parizkova (87) also followed 10 female gymnasts from ages 13 to 18 years. Those who trained most intensely had the lowest body fat and the highest body density. Fat levels were lowest during training, but increased again in the off-season.

Von Döbeln and Eriksson (128) found boys (ages 11–13 years; n = 9) who trained for 16 weeks in an endurance program gained about 4.0 kg in muscle mass and 0.5 kg in total body mass, but lost about 3.0 kg of body fat. Since the boys gained 3.5 cm in stature over the 16-

week program, it is likely that some of the subjects were experiencing their adolescent growth spurt. Therefore, the changes reported were probably the result of a combination of training and growth.

There is no information on the possible influence of physical activity on fat distribution in children. Studies are needed to determine if children who are regularly active can decrease trunk versus extremity subcutaneous fat, or internal fat versus subcutaneous fat, and whether there are gender-related differences. Nevertheless, it appears that regular physical activity can play an important role in the maintenance of a "healthy" amount of body fat.

PHYSICAL ACTIVITY AND THE RISK OF CORONARY HEART DISEASE

Growth and Risk Factors for Coronary Heart Disease (CHD)

"Atherosclerosis is a specific type of lipid accumulation in the intima and subintimal region of large elastic arteries such as the aorta and or medium-sized muscular arteries such as the coronary or carotid arteries" (see Ref. 27, p. 836). Fatty streaks and fibrous plaques have been found in the arteries of children by 10 years of age, and the presence of such lipid deposition in coronary arteries has been associated with adult atherosclerosis (77).

Risk factors for adults are listed in Table 1. Favorable changes in cardiovascular risk factors have been associated with a reduced progression of atherosclerosis. The primary modifiable risk factors commonly cited are hypercholesterolemia, systolic hypertension, and

Table 1 Coronary Heart Disease Risk Factors for Adults

Nonmodifiable	Modifiable	Treatable
Age	Physical inactivity	Hyperlipidemia
Gender	Obesity (abdominal)	Diabetes mellitus type II
Race	Hypertension	Hypertension
Family history	Cigarette smoking	Low levels of HDL-C
	Imprudent diet	Platelet aggregation and fibrinolysis
		Hyperuricemia
		Hypertension

Source: Adapted from Ref. 49; used with permission.

cigarette smoking (49). Powell et al. (93) found in those studies, which had evaluated physical activity levels with fairly strident methodology, that the risk of developing coronary heart disease (CHD) due to physical inactivity was just as great as for high blood cholesterol, hypertension, and smoking. However, physical inactivity was the most important community risk factor, since at least 60% of adults in the United States had too low levels of activity to protect against CHD, whereas only 20% of the United States population had any of the three supposed primary risk factors.

Risk factors for CHD do not have the same effect on the morbidity and mortality of children and youth as in adults. However, the presence of risk factors, especially when aggregated (as in the obese child), could lead, over many years, to the development of coronary atherosclerosis (31,121).

The Bogalusa Heart Study examined CHD risk factors in black and white children from birth to 26 years of age between 1973 and 1982. Using a combination of cross-sectional and longitudinal methods, data were collected on subsets of 5000 children. Measurements included anthropometric and demographic data, blood pressure, serum lipids and lipoproteins, nutrition, and behavior. The information gathered strongly substantiated the concept that atherosclerosis began in childhood and supported pediatric approaches to the primary prevention of atherosclerotic CHD (83,121). The tracking (that is, the persistence of a given condition identified in childhood into adult life) will be considered for blood lipid profiles, blood pressure, glucose tolerance and fasting insulin levels, and obesity.

Blood Lipid and Lipoprotein Profiles

The risk of CHD is related to three components of serum total cholesterol (Total-C): low-density lipoprotein cholesterol (LDL-C); high-density lipoprotein cholesterol (HDL-C); and very low–density lipoprotein cholesterol (VLDL-C). The role of apoproteins has also been investigated recently. Elevated LDL-C, VLDL-C, and apoprotein B are atherogenic, whereas higher levels of HDL-C and apoprotein A-I protect against coronary atherosclerosis. The ratio of LDL-C to HDL-C or the ratio of Total-C to HDL-C is more closely related to coronary morbidity and mortality than is Total-C.

At birth, Total-C, LDL-C, and triglycerides (TG) levels are very low, but there are sharp increases during the first year of life. After infancy, LDL-C, HDL-C, and TG levels remain relatively stable until puberty. The Bogalusa Heart Study (27) found that the mean Total-C was approximately 160 mg/dl from 2 years of age until the onset of sexual maturation (Fig. 3). This finding did not differ with race or gender. At all ages, LDL-C was the major component of Total-C. Therefore, youngsters with elevated Total-C usually had an elevated LDL-C as well. Both Total-C and LDL-C decline during adolescence but increased in later adolescence. There was a rise in the ratio of LDL-C to HDL-C; in VLDL-C and in TG in white adolescent males,

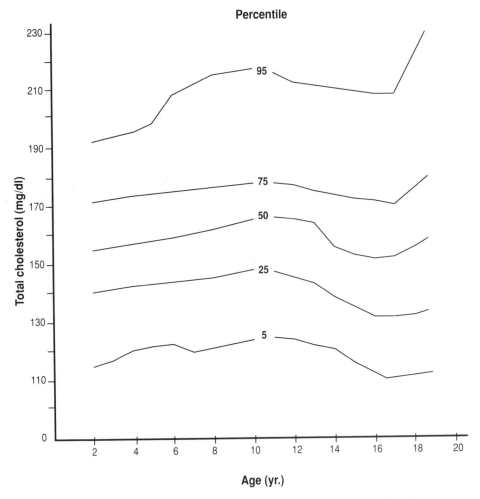

Figure 3 Norms for serum total cholesterol level in children aged 2–19 years in the Bogalusa Heart Study. From Cresanta, J. L., et al. (1984), p. 380. Reprinted with permission.

placing these individuals at an extremely high risk of premature CHD. This has been related to a greater body fat in white children of the Bogalusa region (27).

An 8-year follow-up study of lipid and lipoprotein levels (27) showed a high degree of tracking. Tracking of plasma lipid values into adulthood was most evident during and after puberty in those children with extreme plasma lipid values (133). Early identification of children who are at risk of CHD can be accomplished by measuring Total-C and LDL-C during puberty (62).

Blood Pressure

The systolic blood pressure (SBP) of children in the Bogalusa Heart Study was found to increase by 2 mm/year whereas diastolic blood pressure (DBP) increased by 1 mm/year, except for 2- to 4-year-old children (133). The increase in blood pressure reflected increases in body size; mainly an increase in height.

Blood pressure does not track as well as plasma cholesterol levels. In the Bogalusa Heart Study (133), a linear discriminant model was only moderately effective in distinguishing the characteristics of children who maintained a high blood pressure ranking from those who did not. The tracking was most persistent for those who had extreme high ranks in SBP.

Lauer et al. (63) noted that many longitudinal studies of children have shown a degree of peer rank order consistency for blood pressure. While there is indeed some tracking of blood pressure, there is also a considerable lability of blood pressure rank over time. If there is a persistent ranking above the 90th blood pressure percentile relative to age, height, and gender over 6–12 months and the parents are hypertensive, such children are particularly likely to become hypertensive as adults (63,99).

Fasting Insulin Levels and Insulin Sensitivity

Plasma insulin levels (decreased peripheral cell sensitivity and hyperinsulaemia) are related to the risk of CHD. In nondiabetic men, fasting insulin is a better predictor of CHD risk than postglucose-load insulin (121).

Fasting plasma insulin levels increase from 5 to 17 years of age. Insulin sensitivity is higher in 5–10 year olds than in adolescents and adults. A decrease of insulin sensitivity occurs in both boys and girls with puberty; in girls, the cause may be an increase in body fatness, whereas in boys, the explanation seems to be due to an increase in free testosterone (31).

A high fasting plasma insulin level after 10 years of age may be a useful indicator of CHD risk, since insulin insensitivity is an important determinant of plasma lipoprotein levels (23). Since puberty is associated with relative insulin resistance, since insulin insensitivity and obesity are significant correlates of hypertension, and since adiposity further exacerbates insulin hypersecretion, it may be important to pay attention to the obese adolescent when identifying those who are in greatest need of risk modification (31,133).

Obesity and Regional Tissue Distribution

The changes in body composition and regional fat distribution with growth have been discussed in a previous section (physical fitness). Although obesity has not been identified as an independent risk factor for CHD, its strong association with hypertension, hyperlipidaemia, hyperinsulaemia, and diabetes mellitus make it one of the most potentially modifiable risk factors (27). The prevalence of obesity increases sharply in late adolescence, with a particularly rapid rise in black females (133). Obese Bogalusa children were found to have a higher mean blood pressure, Total-C, LDL-C, VLDL-C, and plasma insulin and lower HDL-C when compared to nonobese children of similar age, race, and gender (27).

To assess the relationship of obesity to clustering of CHD risk factors (121), 3503 subjects were measured for obesity (subscapular and tricep skin fold thickness), SBP, LDL-C + VLDL-C to HDL-C ratio, and fasting insulin levels. Lean subjects (the lower tertile of the obesity distribution) showed less clustering of risk factors than expected. The more obese individuals (the upper tertile of the obesity distribution) had a greater clustering than expected, with trunk fat deposition (subscapular fold) having a greater impact on clustering than limb fat deposition (triceps fold). The authors concluded that since obesity was related to clustering of risk factors in children and young adults, the prevention of the onset of obesity in early life may be important to reducing the risk of CHD in later life.

A subset of the Bogalusa subjects were tracked over 8 years to determine if juvenile-onset obesity (as measured by triceps skin fold thickness and Rohrer index: body mass/height^3) persisted in a cohort of 1490 children aged 2–14 years (41). The results indicated that moderate, juvenile-onset obesity was malleable, but the child who was extremely obese over consecutive examinations was likely to become an obese adult. About 43% of initially obese children remained obese after 8 years, but 13% fell below the 50th percentile at follow-up. Tracking of obesity was found to increase with age and tracking was strongest in black females.

Since a substantial proportion of obese children do not necessarily become obese, the following criteria can be considered in identifying those who are likely to become obese adults:

1. Familial aggregation: the fatness level of siblings, parents, and grandparents (46).
2. Age of onset of obesity: children older than 5 years are more likely to remain obese and the tracking of obesity increases with age (20,41).
3. Severity of obesity (greater than 95th percentile): obese children who are *not* at the extreme end of the distribution do not necessarily become obese adults (84).

PHYSICAL ACTIVITY AND CORONARY HEART DISEASE RISK FACTORS

Physical inactivity is not usually considered as an independent or primary risk factor. However, as previously mentioned, physical inactivity has been gaining increased recognition as a major risk factor in adults because of the increase in the risk of CHD with inactivity and the growing prevalence of a sedentary lifestyle (93). Physical inactivity is often considered as an indirect risk factor because of its potential effect on hypertension, blood lipid and lipoprotein profiles, insulin sensitivity, and control of body mass (particularly the accumulation of body fat).

Consistency (tracking) of physical activity levels into adulthood has not been studied extensively. A few studies have shown that children who were athletes during their school years did not remain active as adults (22,34,86). Perusse et al. (89) concluded that there is a substantial genetic predisposition toward being physically active in children. However, a significant fraction of children's participation in activity was also acquired from the parents' behavior toward exercise.

Familial aggregation or familial similarities (the combination of genetic and environmental influences within a family) have only recently been studied. Sallis et al. (112) observed 33 preschool children during free play and found that select familial variables accounted for 39% of the variance in children's level of moderate activity. Evenson and Freedson (37) examined physical activity levels of 5- to 9-year-old children (n = 30) and their biological parents. Activity levels were determined by the Caltrac monitor (physical activity counter), which was worn by each family member for three consecutive 12-h days. Results clearly implied familial trends; while inactive parents were likely to have an inactive child, highly active parents did *not* necessarily have a highly active child. The authors suggested that physical *in*activity tracked more readily than physical activity. Both studies (37,112) found a slightly higher association aggregation of physical activity with the mother (than with the father) of the child. The promotion of physical activity at the family level should be considered a useful strategy for exercise promotion in children.

A child who is considered fit is usually a child with a high aerobic energy capacity ($\dot{V}O_{2\,max}$). This value is sometimes measured directly during maximal work, but more frequently, it is predicted from exercise duration or variables measured in submaximal exercise. Unfortunately, submaximal predictions, especially those using physical work capacity at a heart rate of 170 beats/min (PWC_{170}) do not predict maximal values accurately (38,60). Physical fitness depends on both levels of physical activity and inherited characteristics. Physical activity is usually measured by recall questionnaires. Less frequently, activity levels are obtained from heart rate monitoring, activity monitors, direct observation, or the use of double-labeled water (113).

Several investigations have failed to show a relationship of physical fitness to physical activity (38). However, such studies may have been limited by difficulties in assessing both aerobic power and habitual exercise. Recently, Fenster et al. (38) showed that aerobic power (as measured by peak $\dot{V}O_{2\,max}$ during a maximal exercise test) and level of activity (as measured by the Large Scale Integrated Activity Monitor) correlate moderately well ($r = 0.59$, $p < 0.05$) in 6- to 8-year old children ($n = 18$).

Attempts to relate physical activity and/or physical fitness with the coronary risk factors cited in the previous section have had equivocal results (31,64,81). Cross-sectional studies comparing athletes and nonathletes suggest that physically fit and active adolescents have lower TG (more evident in girls) and higher HDL-C levels (more evident in boys) (31). There is some evidence that habitual physical activity lowers blood lipid and lipoprotein more effectively in adolescent black children (64). Short-term (6–12 weeks) activity programs have shown limited, and sometimes opposite, effects on blood lipid and lipoprotein levels (31,81). The inconsistency of findings may be due to the fact that:

1. Cross-sectional studies are confounded by subject selection.
2. The levels of some risk factors, especially blood lipid and lipoprotein levels in young children, are very low. Changes in CHD risk factors are more likely in those who are at high risk.
3. Longitudinal studies have been of too short a duration and/or too low an intensity.

4. Habitual activity levels are extremely hard to determine, especially in young children.
5. Physical fitness has a large genetic component that may be underestimated because children are unwilling to give an all-out effort.
6. Genetic variation influences the response to increased activity and its effect on CHD risk factors (31).

Hagberg et al. (52) found that hypertensive (BP persisting above the 95th percentile for age and sex) adolescents (n = 25) who exercised for 6 months at 60–65% of $\dot{V}O_{2\,max}$ significantly lowered both SBP and DBP without any body fat weight loss.

Fripp and colleagues (43) found that the aerobic fitness of 289 tenth graders (as determined by exercise duration) was associated with atherosclerotic risk factors (BP, TG, HDL-C). However, obesity (measured by BMI) explained the largest portion of variance in the risk factors evaluated. The authors recommended that when aerobic conditioning is used to modify atherosclerotic risk factors in adolescents a reduction of body mass be the primary focus of the increased activity in order to maximize change in CHD risk factors. Sallis et al. (112) found that physical fitness was highly correlated with CHD, but BMI accounted for a large portion of the correlation between fitness and CHD risk factors (BP and blood lipids) in children. These authors concluded that the findings from their study "reinforce recommendations for regular exercise and suggest that increased activity and fitness in childhood may enhance CHD risk profile" (see Ref. 112, p. 939).

In summary, the evidence of changes in CHD risk with increased physical activity is equivocal. The American Heart Association (98) recommends physical activity as a prophylactic for CHD. An increase in large muscle dynamic exercise (for instance, jogging, swimming [laps], and stationary cycling) is especially recommended for children with sedentary lifestyles. An increase of regular physical activity is particularly important in modifying risk factors for the obese child, and the activity behaviors of parents may be a significant modeling factor for children's physical activity.

Conclusions

The following variables have been identified as risk factors for CHD in children: family history, poor blood lipid profile, hypertension, obesity, diet (a high fat intake and a large intake of snack foods), cigarette smoking, carbohydrate intolerance (hyperinsulinemia), physical inactivity, and behavioral responses to stress (27). No single childhood

CHD risk factor increases the morbidity and mortality from CHD in adulthood. Obesity is a large factor in the clustering of CHD risk factors in children and adolescents (31,121). The obese child is often hyperinsulinemic, hypertensive, and hyperlipidemic. The obese child who increases daily energy expenditure is likely to lower his or her BP, increase insulin sensitivity, increase HDL-C, and/or lower LDL-C (31).

With obese children, the main avenue for a reduction of CHD risk factors seems to be a decrease of body mass, since metabolic risk factors can be lowered without changes of aerobic fitness. "However it is important to remember that a substantial amount of exercise is essential to substantially alter energy balance and that the duration of the prescribed exercise session must be high" (31). It is not easy to achieve weight loss by increased physical activity. To improve the chances of success, the increase of physical activity must be accompanied by dietary modification (a reduction of fat, simple sugar, and sodium intake), parental involvement, and other behavioral modifications (for instance, smoking cessation).

Després et al. (31) have suggested that there is a specific genetic component which allows some individuals to respond more easily to the lowering of CHD risk factors with exercise. Identification of children who are sensitive to exercise training (perhaps by deoxyribonucleic acid [DNA] polymorphism of certain genes) will help to determine those individuals who require only an increase in their habitual activity level. Resistive children would require a more rigorous multifactorial intervention.

Whether or not increased energy expenditure leads to a decrease of body fat or increased physical fitness, the development of an active lifestyle has been hypothesized to help obese children. Shephard (117) suggested that since catecholamine secretion has been reported to increase with training in both children and adolescents, regular physical activity would lead to enhanced fat utilization. Bray (20) postulated that when obesity developed between the ages of 4 and 11 years, an increase in the number of fat cells occurred, making it likely that obesity would persist into adulthood. Physical activity may help to limit such adipocyte hyperplasia.

Oscai (84) has suggested that animal studies indicate an important role for the prevention of obesity in the early stages of development. Oscai (84) hypothesized that adipose tissue lipoprotein lipase (LPL) played a regulatory role in the etiology of obesity. Increased circulating insulin levels were linked to increases in adipose tissue LPL. Regular physical activity has a profound effect on insulin sensitivity, and may, therefore, reduce obesity by reducing circulating insulin levels and, therefore, decreasing LPL.

To help identify those children with increased risk of CHD, the following suggestions can be made for the child's periodic medical examinations. Besides a good family history and use of the standard height and weight percentile grids to record linear growth and weight increments, physicians should use a simple grid to assess serum total cholesterol levels by age, and a height-, age-, and gender-specific grid to examine blood pressures (82) (Fig. 4). Children who continually remain in the 90th to 95th percentile can then be easily identified, and they are the ones who are most likely to track their risk factors into adulthood (27).

Since the waist-to-hip circumference ratio provides a useful guide to abdominal fat deposition, clinicians and clinical investigators are encouraged to add this measurement as well as subscapular and abdominal skin fold thickness to their measurments of height and body mass (21).

EXERCISE PRESCRIPTION

Exercise prescription for improving one's aerobic power (that is, cardiovascular fitness) has been fairly well established for the adult population (5). For the younger population, however, the guidelines for exercise prescription for increasing $\dot{V}O_{2\,max}$ have been established by default (140). The exact duration, intensity, and frequency needed to improve aerobic capacity has not received positive scientific verification; therefore, the existing adult recommendations have been followed for children, adolescents, and young adults (11,106,110).

While for adults, exercise prescription emphasizes improving cardiovascular fitness, various issues surround whether exercise prescription for children should be mainly concerned with increasing $\dot{V}O_{2\,max}$:

1. $\dot{V}O_{2\,max}$ may not have the same meaning for children: The connection between $\dot{V}O_{2\,max}$ and positive health status may not be the same as for adults, and $\dot{V}O_{2\,max}$ in children may not be indicative of cardiovascular endurance.
2. High-intensity repetitive exercise needed to increase aerobic power has been cited as the reason for the increase in microtrauma (overuse) injuries seen in children (80).
3. Motivation: If the physical activity is repetitive and a negative association may be made with the exercise experience and affect future activity habits.

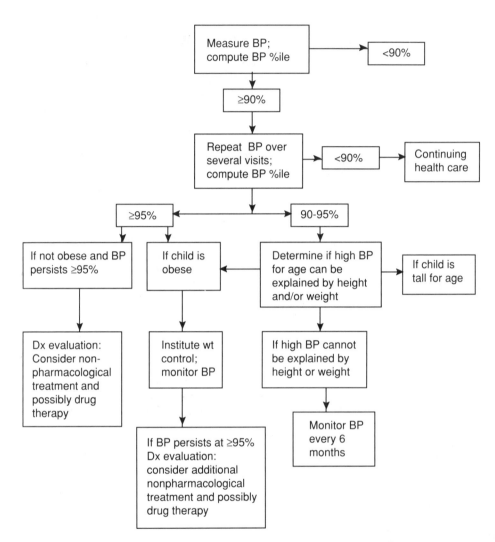

Figure 4 Algorithm for identifying children with high BP. From the *Report of the second task force on blood pressure control in children—1987*, developed by the Task Force on Blood Pressure Control in Children at the National Heart, Lung, and Blood Institute, Bethesda, Maryland. *Pediatrics* 79(1), 1987, p. 8. Reprinted with permission. Note: Whenever BP measurement is stipulated, the average of at least two measurements should be used. Age-specific percentiles of BP for children ages birth to 12 months appear in the Report.

Controversy exists as to whether children are becoming less fit and less active. Gilliam and colleagues (47) found that few children spontaneously participate in activity with enough intensity (elevation of heart rate to 160 bpm), duration (20–60 min), or frequency (3–5 days a week) to maintain cardiorespiratory fitness. However, Blair and colleagues (16) make the case that 80–90% of children are expending enough calories per day to lower CHD risk. Whether or not children, *in general*, are fit and active, it is extremely important to identify the child who is *not* maintaining a positive health status. The child who is obese, disabled, and/or who is leading a sedentary life needs to be motivated to engage in life-long activity for cardiovascular health (that is, physical activity of a sustained nature which may not be of a minimal intensity to increase aerobic power [cardiovascular fitness] but has been linked to health).

Motivation, Adherence, and Compliance

It is generally accepted that participation patterns, quality of physical activity and perception of physical activity formed during childhood will determine whether a habit of daily activity will persist into adulthood (116,134). Negative experiences with physical activity in childhood may create a life-long aversion to an active lifestyle (105). Motivational factors that are important in getting children interested in a regular physical activity program and maintaining compliance have largely been unexplored. Little is known about the determinants and health outcomes of physical activity patterns among children under 18 years of age. As a result, the information needed to guide effective interventions in children to increase physical activity as an adult is not available (33).

Limited research, however, has identified some key motivational factors which can influence adherence and compliance to an activity program and may, therefore, influence activity levels as an adult:

1. Internal rather than external rewards:

    If the habit of regular activity is to persist into adult life, motivation must become internal. It cannot be dependent upon parent, coach, or school teacher. One criticism of competitive sport, with its external rewards, is that it tends to inhibit the development of such internal motivation (see Ref. 116, p. 9).

2. Fun: If enjoyment is experienced the child "owns" the experience.

3. Influence of parents: Parents need to encourage and, more importantly, be role models for exercise behavior. However, parents
should not pressure children to participate in sports or activity,
since this may be viewed as a stress and may contribute to negative feelings about physical activity (134).

Rowland (105) conducted a study to compare compliance rates in
two exercise programs: a well-structured 12-week aerobic exercise program for diabetic children aged 9–14 years of age, and a home running
program prescribed by a physician for inactive children who attended,
with their parents, a group pediatric practice for well child care (aged
8–13 years). The highly structured program had a more successful
enrollment compliance than did the home-based program. Peer competition and achievement of tangible rewards (T-shirts, certificates)
were *not* important factors in the compliance rate of either group. For
the diabetic children, the influence of the physician stressing the
importance of exercise was critical. Other factors identified as effecting
compliance to the structured exercise program were:

1. Location: geographical proximity of the exercise site.
2. Time of year: spring seemed to be a better time of year, since outdoor running could sometimes be substituted for indoor running.
   In the summer, vacation plans interfered with attendance at exercise sessions.
3. Enthusiastic leadership: The personality of the leader was a factor
   in motivating children to attend exercise classes.
4. Parental support: Parental support was exhibited by parents
   attending exercise sessions and clearly expressing their encouragement.
5. Goals and achievement of realistic goals: If the exercise capacity of
   the child was identified, then goals could be more readily designed
   for improvement and success and provided a sense of self-worth
   for the child.

Although self-concept was not formally evaluated in the Rowland
(105) study, several parents indicated that their *nonathletic* children had
experienced a great deal of self-satisfaction in participating in physical
activity.

Dishman (33) stated that correlational studies and clinical observations of children and adolescent have generally shown a positive
relationship between physical fitness, body image (the cognitive and
affective representation a person has about themselves), and self-
image (expression of qualities, attitudes, and values that a person

consciously experiences as his or hers). However, the influence of physical fitness and activity was mediated by the initial level of body image or self-image, by the probability of eventual success in performance, and by the duration and intensity of the training.

Self-esteem is the value that individuals learn to place on themselves (33). It is developed through the interaction between the person and his or her environment/social experiences. Gruber (51), in a meta-analysis of 84 correlational, case, and experimental studies (mainly involving prepubescent children) concluded that physical fitness activities contribute to the development of self-esteem. When normal children and children who were classified as handicapped (emotionally disturbed, trainable and educable mentally retarded, economically disadvantaged, and perceptually handicapped) were compared, the handicapped children showed the greatest gains in self-esteem with an increase in activity levels.

Gruber (51) also found that the teaching method used in the school setting was an important factor. Allowing children to interact with teachers and share in decision making showed a somewhat greater effect than the traditional instructor-dominated style. Shephard (116) stated that ''. . . a cognitive internalization of the desired movement patterns does much to ensure lasting interest. A good instructor thus seeks not only to improve a child's performance, but also to stress clearly the resulting implications for health'' (see pp. 9–10).

Gruber (51) also noted that the most marked effect on self-esteem occurred when physical activity was given in a clinical setting or with clinical groups.

In summary, while there is no definitive research to help determine how to best instill physical activity as a life-long habit, some key motivational factors to get children to participate in activity have been identified. Undue emphasis on external rewards may detract from internal motivational factors. An environment needs to be provided which allows children to achieve a sense of competence, to feel they have some control over their actions, and to develop a sense of reward from within the activity itself. Positive competency attitudes are very important, since what one thinks of himself/herself may be the prime determinant of future behavior (51). Enjoyment is an important component. A key variable is understanding the sources of enjoyment, which probably changes throughout various stages of the lifespan. Outdoor settings may produce a more positive attitude toward activity than in indoor setting. The physician may play an extremely important role in promoting physical activity as a positive health measure, especially for the clinical patient.

Parents should encourage children in their participation in physical activity and should become role models for their children by participating in regular physical activity

Physiological Aspects

Major differences in physiological responses to exercise exist between children and adults. These differences and their implications for exercise are presented in Table 2. Apart from the low economy of locomotion and limitations upon exercising in climatic extremes, no underlying physiological factor has been identified that would make children less suitable than adults for prolonged, continuous activities. The American Academy of Pediatrics (AAP) stated, ''. . . if children enjoy the activity and are asymptomatic, there is no reason to preclude them from training for and participating in such events'' (see Ref. 1, p. 800).

Although children can perform exercise over a wide variety of intensities and durations, children spontaneously prefer short-term intermittent activities with a high recreational component and variety rather than monotonous, prolonged activites. In accordance with both their phsiological and their psychological profile, children seem best suited for repeated activities that last a few seconds interspersed with short rest periods. The least suitable forms of exercise for children, from a physiological viewpoint, are highly intensive activities lasting 10–90 (11).

Precautions When Exercising in Climatic Extremes

Because children have a higher metabolic level at a given submaximal walking or running speed, children produce excessive amounts of body heat. A combination of this higher metabolic load and a poor sweating capacity along with an immature cardiovascular system (see Table 2) causes children to have a shorter tolerance of exercise in hot climates and a greater susceptibility to heat stress despite a large surface-to-mass ratio (11). The AAP recommends: ''Clothing should be light weight, limited to one layer of absorbent material in order to facilitate evaporation of sweat and to expose as much skin as possible. Sweat-saturated garments should be replaced by dry ones. Rubberized sweat suits should never be used to produce loss of weight'' (3).

Children have low tolerance to extreme heat. They thermoregulate as effectively as adults, however, when exercising in neutral or moderately warm climates (55). The AAP recommends that activities lasting 30 min or more should be reduced whenever relative humidity and air temperature are above critical levels (Table 3) (3).

Acclimatization

Children tend to lag behind adults in physiological acclimatization to a hot environment, and therefore they should be involved in a longer and more gradual program. The AAP recommmends: "... that intensity and duration and exercise should be restrained initially and then gradually increased over a period of 10 to 14 days to accomplish acclimatization of the effects of heat" (3). Children can acclimate, to some extent, when they exercise in neutral environments, and when they rest in hot climates; however, acclimatization is subjectively faster than in adults. Therefore, children, especially at the early stages of acclimatization, may feel quite capable of performing physical exercise in the heat despite a marked liability to physiological heat stress (55).

Fluid Replacement

Children have a smaller plasma pool from which to lose water. Fluid replacement is, therefore, critical, since a given amount of water loss has greater physiological significance for children (139). During continuous activity of more than a 30-min duration, fluid should be replaced at a rate of 100–150 ml every 15–30 min, even when the child is not thirsty (3,11). Bar-Or (11) recommends that replacement fluids for children should not exceed 5 mEq/L Na^+ (0.3 g/L NaCl), 4 mEq/L K^+ (0.28 g/L KCl), and 25 g/L sugar (11). There may not be any great merit in additives, and Haymes and Wells (53) suggest that a child weighing 40 kg should ingest 150 ml of cold tap water every 30 min during activity.

Overuse Injury

Recent increases in overuse injuries in children have been attributed to the growing number of children who compete and train intensively. Overuse injuries seem attributable to training and *not* to the actual playing situation, since injuries are not seen in free play situations (80).

Risk factors include:

Abrupt change in the intensity, duration, or frequency of training (the intensity should not be increased more than 10% per week)
Musculotendinous imbalance in strength and flexibility
Anatomical malalignment of the lower extremities
Poor footwear or an inappropriate running surface

Gender Differences

Most studies of physiological differences between children and adults have used male subjects. Rowland and Green (107) compared the

Table 2 Comparison of the Physiological Response of Children to Exercise

Function	Compared to adults	Implications for exercise
Metabolic:		
Aerobic:		
$\dot{V}O_{2\,max}$ L · min^{-1}	Lower (function of body mass)	
$\dot{V}O_{2\,max}$ ml · kg^{-1} · min^{-1}	Similar	Can perform endurance tasks reasonably well.
Submaximal oxygen demand (economy)	Cycling: similar (18–30% mechanical efficiency) Walking and running: Higher metabolic cost	Greater fatigability in prolonged high-intensity tasks (running and walking): Greater heat production in children at a given speed of walking or running.
Anaerobic:		
Glycogen stores	Lower contraction and rate of utilization of muscle glycogen	Ability of children to perform *intense* anaerobic tasks that last 10–90 sec is distinctly lower than adults.
PFK concentration	Glycolysis limited because of low level of PFK.	Same ability to deal metabolicallly with very brief intense exercise.
Phosphagen stores	Stores and breakdown of ATP and CP the same	
LA$_{max}$	Lower maximal blood lactate levels	
LA$_{submax}$	Lower at given precent of $\dot{V}O_{2\,max}$	May be reason children perceive a workload as easier.
HR at lactate threshold	Higher	
Oxygen transient	Faster reaching of steady state than adults. Shorter half-time of oxygen increase in children	Children reach metabolic steady state faster. Children contract a lower oxygen deficit. Faster recovery. Children, therefore, well suited to intermittent activities.

Cardiovascular:

$\dot{Q}_{max}$	Lower due to size difference	Immature CV system means child is limited in bringing internal heat to surface for dissipation when exercising intensity in the heat.
$\dot{Q}$ at a given $\dot{V}O_2$	Somewhat lower	
SV_{max}	Lower due to size and heart volume difference	
SV at a given $\dot{V}O_2$	Lower	
HR_{max}	Higher	Up to maturity HR_{max} is between 195 and 215 bpm. Higher HR compensates for lower SV.
HR_{submax}	At given absolute power output and at relative metabolic load, child has higher HR	
Oxygen-carrying capacity	Blood volume, Hemoglobin conc., Total Hb lower in children	
$C_{aO_2} - C_{vO_2}$	Somewhat higher	
Muscle blood flow to active muscle	Higher	Potential deficiency of peripheral blood supply during maximal exertion in hot climates.
SBP and DBP	Lower maximal and submaximal	No known beneficial or detrimental effects on working capacity of child.

Pulmonary responses:

$\dot{V}_{Emax} L \cdot min^{-1}$	Smaller	Early fatigability in tasks that require large respiratory minute volumes.
$\dot{V}_{Emax} ml \cdot kg^{-1} \cdot min^{-1}$	Same as adolescents and young adults	
$\dot{V}_{Esubmax}$	$\dot{V}_E$ at any given $\dot{V}O_2$ is higher in children	Less efficient ventilation would mean a greater oxygen cose of ventilation. May explain the relatively higher metabolic cost of submaximal exercise.
Ventilatory Equivalent		
Respiratory frequency and tidal volume	Marked by higher rate and shallow breathing response	Children's physiological dead space is smaller than adults, therefore, alveolar ventilation is still adequate for gas exchange.

Table 2 (Continued)

Function	Compared to adults	Implications for exercise
VT	VT occurs at a higher % of $\dot{V}O_{2\,max}$ in children	Additional indicators that children may relay more on aerobic metabolism to meet energy demands.
$R_{max}(VCO_2/\dot{V}O_2)$	Lower in children	
Perception:		
RPE	Exercising at a given physiological strain is perceived to be easier by children.	Implications for initial phase of heat acclimatization.
Thermoregulatory:		
Surface area (SA)	Per unit mass is approximately 20–40% greater in children (Percentage is variable and depends on size of child)	Greater rate of heat exchange between skin and environment. In climatic extremes, children at increased risk of stress.
Sweating rate	Lower —absolute amount —per unit of SA Greater increase in core temp. to start sweating	Greater risk of heat-related illness on hot humid days due to reduced capacity to evaporate. Lower tolerance time in extreme heat.
Acclimatization to heat	Slower physiologically Faster subjectively	Children require longer and more gradual program of acclimatization. Special attention during early stages of acclimatization.
Body cooling in water	Faster cooling due to: —higher SA per heat-producing unit mass —lower thickness of subcutaneous fat	Potential hypothermia
Body core heating during dehydration	Greater	Prolonger activity: Well-hydrated prior to and enforced fluid intake during activity.

Source: Adapted from Ref. 141; used with permission.

Table 3 Weather Guide for Prevention of Heat Illness

Air temperature		Danger zone (% RH[a])	Critical zone (% RH[a])
°F	°C		
70	21	80	100
75	24	70	100
80	26.5	50	80
85	29.5	40	68
90	32	30	55
95	35	20	40
100	38	10	30

[a] Relative humidity.
Source: Adapted from Ref. 53; used with permission.

findings indicated that pre- and postmenarcheal females exhibited similar differences in physiological responses to those previously observed in males. Cooper (26) states, "It appears that from a functional point of view, the integration of cardio-respiratory and musculoskeletal growth is the same in boys and girls" (see p. 78). Telford et al. (124) examined echocardiographic data on approximately 200 children aged 9–12 years old. When the data were analyzed by gender, little difference of the cardiac dimensions was found between boys and girls. Ventilatory threshold (considered an indicator of anaerobosis) is reached at a lower exercise intensity in girls than boys (97). "Clinical observations have suggested that, at the prepubescent level, the relative risk of injury is similar in boys and girls" (see Ref. 80, p. 283).

Bar-Or (10) and Pate and Ward (88) have both concluded that gender is not an important determinant of aerobic or anaerobic trainability. Such conclusions are limited, however, by the fact that extremely few studies have used female subjects.

Exercise Prescription for Increasing Cardiovascular Fitness (Maximal Oxygen Uptake)

To improve cardiovascular fitness one has to exercise above a certain threshold intensity for a minimum duration and frequency. For adults, the intensity zone has been established at 50–85% of $VO_{2\,max}$ for a minimum of 15–20 min within the intensity training zone, for three to five times per week (4). The range of the intensity zone is quite large. Individuals in poor or fair condition should exercise at the lower end of the zone (e.g., 50–65%), whereas those in good to excellent condition should exercise in the upper range (75–85%). Whether one is exercising in their intensity zone, in a practical setting, is usually determined by heart rate (HR), and/or rated perceived exertion (RPE). Exercise prescription can also be done using metabolic equivalent units (METs) (5). Heart rate is either measured during exercise with an ECG machine or a heart rate monitor; or by palpation taken for 10 s immediately after stopping exercise. Two methods to establish intensity zone limits have been used with HR. The Karvonen method uses heart rate reserve(HRR), that is maximal heart rate minus resting HR, to determine training zones. Maximal HR is either determined from an exercise tolerance test (ETT) or is predicted by subtracting one's age from the number 220. The intensity range used with HRR is the same as $\dot{V}O_{2\,max}$ (50–85%). The Karvonen formula to establish HR training zones is:

$$\%(HHR) + HR_{rest}$$

For example, the training zone for a 20 year old in poor physical condition with a resting HR of 70 beats/min would be (HR_{max} is predicted from age and the percent range is 50–65).

$$0.50\,(200 - 70) + 70 = 65 + 70 = 135\,bpm$$
$$0.65\,(200 - 70) + 70 = 84.5 + 70 = 155\,bpm$$

The heart rate maximal method establishes target HR limits by calculating a percentage of the HR_{max}. However, when using the maximal HR method, the intensity zone limits are 60–90%, since the slope of the relationship between HR and HRR with $\dot{V}O_{2\,max}$ are different. Therefore, for the same 20 year old the target HR zone (using 65–75%) would be:

$$0.65\,(200)^* = 130\,bpm \quad *[HR_{max}\ predicted\ from\ age]$$
$$0.75\,(200)^* = 150\,bpm$$

The same training zone ranges established for adults have been used for adolescents and young adults. There is very little information concerning the appropriate intensity, duration, and frequency needed for prepubescents to improve their aerobic power. As previously discussed in the section on trainability, there is some question as to whether children can increase $\dot{V}O_{2\,max}$ beyond the increase expected from growth. Some evidence exists to suggest that the intensity of work must be quite vigorous for prepubescents to show increase in aerobic power (104). Rowland (104) suggests that children need to train at an intensity equal to the anaerobic threshold (AT: the intensity level of exercise where blood lactate concentration begins to increase) to appropriately tax the oxygen delivery system. Washington and his colleagues (132) using ventilatory anaerobic threshold (VAT: the intensity of exercise where there is an increase in $\dot{V}_E/\dot{V}O_2$ without a change in $\dot{V}_E/\dot{V}CO_2$ as an indicator of AT) found that prepubescent boys and girls, when exercising on a cycle ergometer, had a mean HR value of 85% of maximal HR at VAT. Heart rate at VAT was quite variable, with HR values ranging from 130 to 197 bpm. Therefore, Rowland (104) suggests that the target HR for prepubescents to improve cardiovascular fitness should be set at 85% of maximal HR.

The use of RPE has become a valid tool in the monitoring of intensity in exercise training programs. Borg (18) developed a rating scale from 6 to 20 for individuals to rate how they perceive the exercise to be (Table 4). For adults, after being trained in using RPE or after using RPE as an adjunct to HR, RPE alone can be used to establish that an individual is exercising within his or her training intensity zone. The range of intensity is usually from a rating of 12 (somewhat hard) to 16 (hard) for asymptomatic individuals (5). In certain patient populations where precise knowledge of heart rate may be critical to the safety of the program (4), RPE is not recommended.

Bar-Or and Ward (12) indicate that research on the use of RPE with children has shown that at any given HR level or at a given percentage of HR_{max}, children rate their exercise intensity lower than adolescents and adults. Although no cause and effect relationship has been established between RPE and lactate levels, it is possible that the lower ratings reflect that at any given percentage of their maximal aerobic power children have lower levels of muscle and blood lactate.

When exercising at intensities greater than 50% of maximal aerobic power, children who were 9 years or older showed good test-retest reproducibility in their perception of exercise and had RPE to HR (or % HR_{max}) correlations similar to those found in adults (12). In addition, mildly to moderately obese children (aged 9–15 years) have been found to also rate their perceived exercise intensity accurately and consistently (130). In these obese children, when exercising at a certain percentage of maximal aerobic power, the ratings of perceived exertion were similar to those of the general child population. When exercising at the same work rate, however, obese children tended to give a higher perceived effort rating.

Ward and Bar-Or (130) also examined whether RPE could be used for exercise prescription in obese children. The children were found to be able to discriminate among four different cycle work rates using RPE. However, the children selected too narrow a range of intensities for cycle exercise, and consistently underestimated the intensity of walking/running tasks. While this one study indicated that RPE may *not* be appropriate for exercise prescription in children, the authors suggested that with feedback training, they could be taught to select appropriate intensities using RPE (12).

A newer RPE scale was also developed by Borg (18) using a 0–10 scale (Table 4). This scale is a combination of a category-scale and a ratio scale. While this newer scale has been used with adults to rate specific symptoms during exercise, it has not been evaluated for use with children (11).

Exercise Prescription for Increasing Health Benefits

Exercise prescription for prepubescent children should emphasize an increase in physical activity by level. The quantity and quality of exercise needed to attain a positive health status may differ from the exercise recommendations for improving maximal oxygen uptake. Blair et al. (16), after reviewing epidemiological studies on physical activity and mortality, found that in adults an energy expenditure of approximately 11–13 $kJ \cdot kg^{-1} \cdot d^{-1}$ was consistently associated with lower risk

Table 4   The Borg Category Scales for Rating of Perceived Exertion

6		0	Nothing at all
7	Very, very light	0.5	Very, very weak (just noticeable)
8		1	Very weak
9	Very light	2	Weak (light)
10		3	Moderate
11	Fairly light	4	Somewhat strong
12		5	Strong (heavy)
13	Somewhat hard	6	
14		7	Very strong
15	Hard	8	
16		9	
17	Very hard	10	Very, very strong (almost maximal)
18			Maximal
19	Very, very hard		
20			

Source: From Ref. 18; used with permission.

of all-cause and CHD mortality. Precise guidelines for the appropriate amount of exercise for children and youth to lower chronic disease risk, however, does not exist. This is partly due to the difficultly in assessing exercise habits and because longitudinal data must be obtained from children followed into middle ages. Therefore, until research indicates otherwise, the recommendation of 11–13 KJ/kg of body weight per day is proposed as a reasonable standard for energy expenditure associated with health-related changes in children (16).

Exercise prescription for children, therefore, to increase positive health status, should stress the increase of energy expenditure with physical activity of lower intensity than is recommended for increasing maximal aerobic capacity but of longer duration and greater frequency. Energy expenditure for an individual can be calculated from the oxygen uptake measured during physical activity. In most cases, unless an exercise tolerance test (ETT) was administered and oxygen intake measured at submaximal loads, this data is not available for a given individual. The amount of energy expended for several activities can be approximated from caloric equivalent tables (see Ref. 11, Appendix IV).

Exercise prescription for increasing energy expenditure is especially important for children at risk:

1. Children with at least one major CHD risk factor
2. Obese children
3. Children leading a sedentary lifestyle, including the disabled child

A safe, well-supervised strength training program of moderate intensity (see previous section on strength training) should be included in the exercise prescription for increasing positive health status. Although resistive training does *not* involve a high caloric expenditure, low to moderate resistive training may help to maintain lean body mass in those children who are trying to lose fat mass. While there is no direct evidence that strength training will reduce the incidence of musculoskeletal injury, it appears logical that a stronger muscle is less susceptible to injury (42). In addition, there is some evidence that dynamic resistive training which involves light to moderate resistance and high repetition with short rest intervals (such as circuit training) may improve insulin sensitivity, blood lipoprotein profiles, and blood pressure in adults (49).

General guidelines for resistance training in children include (42,111):

1. Program should be closely supervised and monitored. Emphasis should be placed on proper lifting and breathing techniques.

2. Each work-out should be preceded by a warm-up (stretching and unloaded or very lightly loaded resistance exercises).
3. Two to three sessions per week are recommended with at least 1 day of rest between workouts. Workouts should include six to 10 different exercises where both upper and lower body are stressed in an alternating sequence. Emphasis should also be placed on strengthening antagonist muscle groups (for example, hamstring/ quadriceps; pectoralis major/trapezius and rhomboids), since muscle imbalance has been cited as a reason for injury (80).
4. The resistance training should emphasize a high number of repetitions and low resistance (two or three sets of eight to 15 repetitions). To increase overload, repetitions should be increased first and when the upper limit of repetitions is attained, then absolute resistance should be increased.

Exercise Guidelines for Pediatric Cardiac Patients

Exercise prescription for children with heart disease is difficult, since there is tremendous variability in the severity of heart problems and difficulty in quantifying the cardiovascular stress of various recreational and sport activities. The effect of competition and the training programs used to get children ready for participating in competitive sports activity are variables which may increase the cardiovascular risk of sports participation. Children with cardiac conditions, however, should *not* automatically be eliminated from sports participation or from participating in regular physical activity. Many parents and physicians are overprotective and tend to dismiss physical activity for pediatric cardiac patients even though participation in regular physical activity could increase health status and improve prognosis (11,116).

Children with lesser degrees of congenital and acquired heart disease such as mild pulmonary stenosis, small atrial or ventricular septal defects, and mild mitral or aortic regurgitation can participate with minimal or no restriction of recreational or competitive sports except perhaps those sports requiring very prolonged exertion such as cross-country running and skiing (40,116). On the other hand, those with severe heart disease such as aortic stenosis with ischemic changes, obstructive or nonobstructive cardiomyopathy and Marfan's syndrome with a dilated aortic root are at real risk of sudden death with exercise (40). Strenuous competitive or recreational activity would be contraindicated for these children. However, participation in moderate strenuous habitual physical activity or nonstrenuous recreational activities can be allowed with negative yearly exercise tolerance tests (40). Children with serious conditions such as myocarditis, congestive heart failure with ischemic changes, cardiac dilation of more than 20%, and incipient heart failure should not be allowed to participate in any physical activity (40,116). More specific recommendations for various heart conditions can be found in the articles by Freed (40) and Strauzenberg (123) and in the books by Bar-Or (11) and Shephard (117).

Graded exercise testing can provide clues to the mechanisms that limit physical work capacity in children with heart disease and can be helpful in estimating cardiac reserve (40). Exercise prescription should be based on the results of the ETT, limitations of specific disease conditions, desired goals (such as weight loss, increase in cardiovascular fitness, socialization, and reduction of CHD risk factors), and information obtained from an activity questionnaire which elicits information on the child's activities, activity habits of other family members, and parental attitudes toward activity (see Ref. 11, Appendix II, for an example of such a questionnaire).

EXERCISE TESTING

Maximal exercise testing has advantages over submaximal testing in most circumstances. However, the reason for testing should dictate what type of test is employed and what measurements are taken. Exercise tolerance tests involve bringing an individual to an intensity of effort where fatigue or symptoms prohibit further exercise, a plateau of oxygen intake ($VO_{2\,max}$) is achieved and no further increase in heart rate occurs (5). Most protocols use a graded exercise procedure, with gradual increments in work intensity during a continuous exercise bout or at successive stages of discontinuous exercise.

Rationale for Exercise Testing

Reasons for using exercise testing in pediatric diagnosis are listed in Table 5. "Exercise testing has been used in a wide variety of cardiac problems in children and adolescents. . . . A well-designed exercise test allows not only an objective measurement of the effect of medical treatment or operation but also insight into the mechanisms of change induced by treatment" (see Ref. 35, pp. 230–231).

In many cases, the ETT is used most successfully to show the child and parents that exercise can be performed at high intensity with no ill effects (11). Exercise testing is used infrequently to detect a specific defect, or a specific disease process, but it is used to assess the

Table 5 Rationale for Exercise Testing in Pediatric Diagnosis

1. Measure physical working capacity
   a. Assess daily function—establish whether a child's daily activities are within the child's physiological functioning level
   b. Identify deficiency in specific fitness component—muscular endurance and strength may limit daily performance rather than aerobic capacity (e.g., muscular dystrophy)
   c. Establish a baseline before the onset of an intervention program
   d. Assess the effectiveness of an exercise prescription
   e. Chart the course of a progressive disease (e.g., cystic fibrosis, Duchenne's muscular dystrophy)
2. Exercise as a provocation test
   a. Amplify pathophysiological changes
   b. Trigger changes otherwise not seen in the resting child
3. Exercise as an adjunct diagnostic test
   a. Noninvasive exercise test can be used for screening to determine the need for an invasive test
   b. Assessing the severity of dysrhythmias
   c. Assessing the functional success of surgical correction
   d. Assessing the adequacy of drug regimens at varying exercise intensities
4. Assessment and differentiation of symptoms: chest pains (asthma from MI), breathlessness (bronchioconstriction from low physical capacity), coughing, easy fatigability.
5. Instill confidence in child and parent
6. Motivation or compliance in intervention program

Source: Adapted from Bar-Or, O., *Scand. J. Sport. Sci.*, 7: 35–39 (1985); used with permission.

effects of a known disease process or treatment upon maximal aerobic power and the cardiorespiratory response to exercise (35). Patients at risk of hypertension may be screened and identified by an atypical exercise response. The ETT has also been used to reassure hypertensive adolescents that they are not at significant cardiovascular risk when participating in dynamic exercise training programs (59).

Exercise tolerance tests (or graded exercise testing [GXT]) have proven effective in measuring the efficacy of cardiac operations in the following conditions (35):

Pulmonary valvotomy
Aortic Valvotomy
Repair of tetralogy of Fallot
Transposition of the great arteries

Ebstein's anomaly of the tricuspid valve single ventricle
Pulmonary atresia with ventricular septal defect
Mechanical pacemaker systems
Arrythmias

Detailed application of exercise tolerance testing for specific diseases or problems is beyond the scope of this chapter, and the reader is referred to other references for more information (11,35, 48,57,59).

> Exercise testing should not replace sound clinical judgement in the rationale and orderly workup of patients, but it provides valuable information . . . there has been increasing applicability of ETT in the evaluation of the child with heart disease. It is likely that the next decade will bring together exercise testing performed simultaneously with other noninvasive modalities, such as two-dimensional echocardiography/Doppler to give the clinician a more complete and realistic picture of the hemodynamic status of the cardiac patient (see Ref. 59, pp. 546, 558).

Ergometers

The same types of ergometers can be used with children and adults, although children younger than 7 years of age would preferably be tested on a treadmill. Premature local muscle fatigue and an inability to maintain a specific cadence prevent many children from reaching a maximal value on the cycle ergometer. Cardiorespiratory measurements must be directly assessed on the treadmill. Prediction of maximal values from a submaximal VO_2 are not applicable in children, because the efficiency of a child's gaits is so variable (11).

If a cycle ergometer is used, an electronically braked cycle ergometer is preferred because power output is then independent of pedal rate (29). On mechanically braked ergometers, pedal rates of 50–60 rev min^{-1} are recommended (11). If children aged 8 or 9 years old or younger are to be tested, special pediatric models should be used, or existing cycle ergometers should be modified. The handlebars should be lengthened, the seat height must be adjusted so that the angle of the knee joint at extension is 15°, and the pedal crank length should be reduced (13 cm for age 6 years; 15 cm for ages 8–10 years) (11,141). In addition, smaller resistance increments may be needed, and resistance indicators should be calibrated in 5-W steps. Testing of children with diseases that involve the legs may require the use of arm ergometers.

Protocol

A variety of exercise protocols are available for children who are symptomatic (6,11,29,48). Some protocols are very similar to those used
with adults. In some instances, protocols are modified so that the initial power output and subsequent increments are smaller. The specific
protocol selected depends on the question(s) to be answered, the
measurements to be obtained, whether submaximal and/or maximal
data are needed, and on the abilities and limitations of the patient. An
ETT is not required when evaluating asymptomatic children.

Supervisory Personnel

During ETT, a technician and/or nurse should be present, and a physician should be available within 30 to 60 s. For the following conditions,
a physician should be actively involved in the testing (11,29):

Serious rhythm disorders
Aortic stenosis with anticipated pressure gradients of over 50 torr
Cyanotic heart disease
Advanced pulmonary vascular disease
Ventricular dysrhythmia with heart disease
Coronary arterial disease

Contraindications

In addition to the contraindications listed in the ACSM Guidelines (5)
(Table 6), specific contraindications for testing pediatric patients follow
(6):

1. Asthmatic child who is dyspneic at rest or whose 1-min forced
    expiratory volume (FEV_1) or peak expiratory flow is less than 60%
    of the predicted value
2. Acute renal disease
3. Hepatitis
4. Insulin-dependent diabetic who did not take prescribed quantity of
    insulin or who is ketoacidotic (11)

Criteria for Termination of a Test

Criteria for halting an exercise test are similar to those for adults, as
included in the Guidelines (5) (Table 7).

Attainment of Maximal Values

Maximal Oxygen Intake ($\dot{V}O_{2\,max}$)
The evidence of an oxygen plateau is less common in children than in

Table 6 Contraindications to Exercise Testing

Recent acute myocardial infarction
Unstable angina
Uncontrolled ventricular dysrhythmia
Uncontrolled atrial dysrhythmia which compromises cardiac function
Congestive heart failure
Severe aortic stenosis
Suspected or known dissecting aneurysm
Active or suspected myocarditis
Thrombophlebitis or intracardiac thrombi
Recent systemic or pulmonary embolus
Acute infection
Third-degree heart block
Significant emotional distress (psychosis)
A recent significant change in the resting ECG
Acute pericarditis

Relative contraindications to exercise testing
Resting diastolic blood pressure over 120 torr or resting systolic blood pressure
  over 200 torr
Moderate valvular heart disease
Digitalis or other drug effect
Electrolyte abnormalities
Fixed-rate artificial pacemaker
Frequent or complex ventricular irritability
Ventricular aneurysm
Cardiomyopathy, including hypertrophic cardiomyopathy
Uncontrolled metabolic disease (diabetes, thyrotoxicosis, myxedema, etc.)
Any serious systemic disorder (mononucleosis, hepatitis, etc.)
Neuromuscular, musculoskeletal, or rheumatoid disorders which would make
  exercise difficult

Source: From Ref. 5; used with permission.

adults (11,61). Data on intraindividual variation in $\dot{V}O_{2\,max}$ indicate, however, that acceptable data can be obtained even if the normal criteria for identifying an oxygen plateau are not always satisfied (61).

Maximal Heart Rate

Alterations in myocardial and sympathetic catecholamine stores; damage to the sinus node and conduction system as a result of cardiac operation will limit the use of maximal heart rate as an indicator of maximal stress (29). Children with congenital complete heart block (and a number of other congenital heart defects); and children receiving β-blocker therapy may have reduced maximal heart rates (11,29).

Table 7 Indications for Stopping an Exercise Test

Subject requests to stop.
Failure of the monitoring system.
Progressive angina (stop at 3 + level or earlier on a scale of 1 + to 4 +)
2 mm horizontal or downsloping ST-depression or elevation.
Sustained supraventricular tachycardia.
Ventricular tachycardia.
Exercise induced left or right bundle branch block.
Any significant drop (10 torr) of systolic blood pressure, or failure of the
    systolic blood pressure to rise with an increase in exercise load after the
    initial adjustment period.
Lightheadedness, confusion, ataxia, pallor, cyanosis, nausea, or signs of
    severe peripheral circulatory insufficiency.
Excessive blood pressure rise: Systolic greater than 2SD torr: diastolic greater
    than 120 torr.
R on T premature ventricular complexes.
Unexplained inappropriate bradycardia—pulse rise slower than 250 below
    age-adjusted normals.
Onset of second- or third-degree heart block.
Multifocal PVCs.
Increasing ventricular ectopy

Source: From Ref. 5; used with permission.

Alternative Exercise Test: Ventilatory Threshold

Since a reliable and reproducible measurement of maximal aerobic
power (i.e., $\dot{V}O_{2\,max}$) is dependent on the subject's ability to reach a
plateau of oxygen uptake during the last loads of an incremental exercise test to exhaustion, a suggestive alternative is to use the ventilatory
threshold (VT) as a predictor of $\dot{V}O_{2\,max}$ and maximal endurance performance (97). Assessment of cardiorespiratory endurance capacity by
VT may be more useful in a pediatric group, since it is independent of
a child's motivation to perform maximal exercise.

Ventilatory threshold can be measured with a submaximal exer-
cise test, where increments in exercise intensity are made very minute.
Gas exchange is measured breath-by-breath, and the criteria to detect
VT are:

1. An increase in ventilatory equivalent ($\dot{V}_E/\dot{V}O_2$) without a concomi-
    tant increase in ($\dot{V}_E/\dot{V}CO_2$)
2. An increase in end-tidal PO_2 without an increase in end-tidal PCO_2

Reybrouck (97) has cited studies which indicate that in children with congenital heart disease and left-to-right shunt, or in children after total repair of the tetralogy of Fallot, the determination of VT is a more sensitive indicator of subnormal exercise performance than other indices of exercise performance (such as the oxygen uptake at heart rate of 170 beats/min).

The VT may not be readily detected in children who have irregular breathing patterns. In such cases, Reybrouck (97) has suggested that the exercise test consists of several discontinuous constant intensity bouts. During each exercise bout (lasting 6 min at a given intensity) ventilation is measured from the third to the sixth minute. The VT is determined as the highest exercise level at which no difference of ventilation is found between the third and sixth minute.

REFERENCES

1. American Academy of Pediatrics (AAP), Committee on Sports Medicine, *Pediatrics*, 86(5):799–800 (1990).
2. American Academy of Pediatrics (AAP), *Physician Sport Med.*, 11: 157–161 (1983).
3. American Academy of Pediatrics (AAP), *Physician Sport Med.*, 11: 153, 159 (1983).
4. American College of Sports Medicine (ACSM), *Med. Sci. Sport Exerc.*, 22: 265–274 (1990).
5. American College of Sports Medicine (ACSM), *Guidelines for Exercise Testing and Prescription*. Lea & Febiger, Philadelphia (1990).
6. American Heart Association (AHA), *Circulation, 66*: 1377A–1397A (1982).
7. Åstrand, P.O., Engstrom, L., Eriksson, B., Karlberg, P., Nylander, I., Saltin, B., and Thoren, C., *Acta Pediatr. Scand., 147* (Suppl.): 1–75 (1963).
8. Bailey, D.A. and Mirwald, R.L., in *Young Athletes: Biological, Psychological, and Educational Perspectives* (R.M. Malina, ed.). Human Kinetics, Champaign, Illinois, pp. 33–48 (1988).
9. Bailey, D.A., Malina, R.M., and Mirwald, R.L., in *Human Growth: A Comprehensive Treatise*. Vol. 2 (F. Falkner and J.M. Tanner, eds.). Plenum Press, New York, pp. 147–170 (1986).
10. Bar-Or, O., *Physician Sport Med., 17*(5): 65–82 (1989).
11. Bar-Or, O., *Pediatric Sports Medicine for the Practitioner*. Springer-Verlag, New York (1983).
12. Bar-Or, O., and Ward, D.S., *Advances in Pediatric Sport Sciences*.Vol. 3, *Biological Issues* (O. Bar-Or, ed.). Human Kinetics, Champaign, Illinois, pp. 151–168 (1989).
13. Becque, D.M., Katch, V.L., Rocchini, A.P., Marks, C.R., and Moorehead, C., *Pediatrics, 81*(5): 605–612 (1988).

14. Beunen, G., *Advances in Pediatric Sport Sciences*. Vol. III. Human Kinetics, Champaign, Illinois, pp. 1–40 (1989).
15. Beunen, G., and Malina, R.M., *Exerc. Sport Sci. Rev.*, *16*: 503–540 (1988).
16. Blair, S.N., Clark, D.G., Cureton, K.J., and Powell, K.E., in *Perspectives in Exercise Science and Sports Medicine. Youth, Exercise, and Sport*, Vol 2, (C.W. Gisolfi and D.R. Lamb, eds.). Benchmark Press, Indianapolis, pp. 401–422 (1989).
17. Blimkie, C.J.R., *Perspectives in Exercise Science and Sports Medicine*. Vol. 2, *Youth, Exercise, and Sport* (C.V. Gisolfi and D.R. Lamb, eds.). Benchmark Press, Indianapolis, pp. 99–163 (1989).
18. Borg, G. *Med. Sci. Sports Exerc.*, *14*: 377–381 (1982).
19. Bouchard, C., Boulay, M.R., Simoneau, J.A., Lortie, G., and Pérusse, L., *Sports Med.*, *5*: 69–73 (1988).
20. Bray, G.A., *Med. Clin. North Am.*, *73*(1): 160–181 (1989).
21. Bray, G.A., and Bouchard, C., *Am. J. Clin. Nutr.*, *47*: 551–552 (1988).
22. Brill, P.A., Buckhalter, H.E., Kohl, H.W., Blair, S.N., and Goodyear, N.N., *Res. Quart. Exerc. Sport*, *60*(3): 209–215 (1989).
23. Burke, G.L., Webber, L.S., Srinivasan, S.R., Radhakrishramurthy, B., Freedman, D.S., and Berenson, G.S., *Metabolism*, *35*: 441–446 (1986).
24. Caspersen, C.J. Powell, K.P., and Christenson, G.M., *Publ. Health Rep.*, *100*(2): 126–131 (1985).
25. Clarke, W.R., Schrott, H.G., Leaverton, P.E., Connor, W.E., and Lauer, R.M., *Circulation, 58*: 626–634 (1978).
26. Cooper, D.M., In *Advances in Pediatric Sport Sciences* (O. Bar-Or, ed.). Vol. 3. Human Kinetics, Champaign, Illinois, pp. 67–100 (1989).
27. Cresanta, J.L., Hyg, M.S., Burke, G.L., Downey, A.M. Freedman, D.S. and Berenson, G.S., *Pediatr. Clin. North Am.*, *33*(4): 835–858 (1986).
28. Cresanta, J.L., Srinivasan, S.R., Webber, L.S., and Berenson, G.S., *Am. J. Dis. Child. 138*: 379–387 (1984).
29. Cumming, G.R., in *Current Therapy in Sport Medicine*. (R.P. Walsh and R.J. Shephard, eds.). Mosby, Toronto (1985).
30. Cunningham, D.A., Paterson, D.H., and Blimkie, C.J.R. in *Advances in Pediatric Sport Sciences* (R.A. Boileau, ed.). Human Kinetics, Champaign, Illinois, pp. 85–116 (1984).
31. Després, J.P., Bouchard, C., and Malina, R.M., in *Exercise and Sport Science Reviews*. Vol 18. Macmillan, New York: pp. 243–262 (1990).
32. Dietz, W.H., Jr., and Gortmaker, S.L., *Pediatrics, 75*: 807–812, 1985.
33. Dishman, R.K., in *Perspectives in Exercise Science and Sports Medicine, Vol. 2: Youth, Exercise and Sport* (C.V. Gisolfi and D.R. Lamb, eds.). Benchmark Press, Indianapolis, pp. 47–95 (1989).
34. Dishman, R.K., *Am. J. Prevent. Med. 4*: 153–160 (1988).
35. Driscoll, D.J., in *Advances in Pediatric Sport Sciences*. Vol 3. (O. Bar-Or, ed.). Human Kinetics, Champaign, Illinois, pp. 223–251 (1989).

36. Erdelyi, G.J., *J. Sports Med. Physical Fit.*, 2: 174–179 (1962).
37. Evenson, S.K., and Freedson, P.S., *Med. Sci. Sports Exerc.* 21(2): S94, (abst.) (1989).
38. Fenster, J.R., Freedson, P.S., Washburn, R.A., and Ellison, R.C., *Pediat. Exerc. Sci.*, 1(2): 127–136 (1989).
39. Forbes, G.B., in *Human Growth*. Vol 2, Postnatal Growth; Neurobiology (F. Falkner and J.M. Tanner, eds.). Plenum Press, New York, pp. 119–145.
40. Freed, M.D., *Pediat. Clin. North Am.*, 31(6): 1307–1320 (1984).
41. Freedman, D.S., Shear, C.L., Burke, G.L., Srinivasan, S.R., Webber, L.S., Harsha, D.W. and Berenson, G.S., *Am. J. Pub. Health*, 77: 588–592 (1987).
42. Freedson, P.S., Ward, A., and Rippe, J.M., in *Advances in Sports Medicine and Fitness*. Vol. 3, (W.A. Grana, J.A. Lombardo, B.J. Sharkey, and J.A. Stone, eds.). Year Book, Chicago, pp. 57–65 (1990).
43. Fripp, R.R., Hodgson, J.L., Kwiterovich, P.O., Werner, J.C., Schuler, G., and Whitman V., *Pediatrics*, 75: 813–818 (1985).
44. Frisch, R.E., and McArthur, J.W., *Science*, 185: 949–951 (1974).
45. Frisch, R.E., Gotz-Welbergen, A.V., McArthur, J.W., and Albright, T., Witschi, J., Bullen, B., Birnholz, J., Reed, R.B., and Hermann, H., *J.A.M.A.*, 246: 1559–1563 (1981).
46. Garn, S.M., and LaVelle, M., *Am. J. Dis. Child.*, 139: 181–185 (1985).
47. Gilliam, T.B., and MacConnie, S.E., in *Advances in Pediatric Sport Sciences*. Vol. 1, *Biological Issues*. (R.A. Boileau, ed.). Human Kinetics, Champaign, Illinois, pp. 171–188.
48. Godfrey, S., *Exercise Testing in Children: Applications in Health and Disease*. W.B. Saunders, Philadelphia (1974).
49. Goldberg, A.P., *Med. Sci. Sport Exerc.*, 21(6): 669–674 (1989).
50. Groves, D., *Physician Sports Med.*, 16(11): 117–122 (1988).
51. Gruber, J.J., in *Effects of Physical Activity on Children, American Academy of Physical Education Papers #19* (G.A. InStull and H.M. Eckert, eds.). Human Kinetics, Champaign, Illinois, pp. 30–48 (1986).
52. Hagberg, J.M. Goldring, D., Ehsani, A.A., Health, G.W., Hernandez, A., Schectman, K., and Holloszy, J.O., *Am. J. Cardiol.*, 763–768 (1983).
53. Haymes, E.M., and Wells, C.L., *Environment and Human Performance*. Human Kinetics, Illinois (1986).
54. Hughson, R., *Can. J. of Appl. Sport Sci.*, 11: 162–172 (1986).
55. Inbar, O. (1985). in *Current Therapy in Sport Medicine 1985–1986* (R.P. Walsh and R.J. Shephard, ed.) Mosby, Toronto.
56. Inbar, O., and Bar-Or, O., *Med. Sci. Sport Exer.*, 18: 264–269 (1986).
57. James, F.W., in *Exercise and the Heart* (N.K. Wenger, ed.). Cardiovascular Clinics 15/2. Davis, Philadelphia (1986).
58. Kato, S., and Ishiko, T., in *Proceedings of International Congress of Sport Sciences* (K. Kato, ed.). Japanese Union of Sports Science, Tokyo, p. 479.

59. Klein, A.A., *Pediatr. Ann.*, *16*(7): 546-549, 554-556, 558 (1987).
60. Koch, G., Karlegard, L., and Frannson, L., *Pediatr. Exerc. Sci.*, *1*(2): 175 (Abst.) (1989).
61. Krahenbuhl, G.S., Skinner, J.W., and Kohrt, W.M., in *Exercise Sport Science Review.* Vol. 13. Macmillan, New York, pp. 503-538 (1985).
62. Kunze, D., *Prevent. Med.*, *12*: 806-809 (1983).
63. Lauer, R.M., Burns, T.L., Mahoney, L.T., and Tipton, C.M., in *Perspectives in Exercise Science and Sports Medicine.* Vol. 2, *Youth, Exercise, and Sport* (C.V. Gisolfi and D.R. Lamb, eds.). Benchmark Press, Indianapolis, pp. 431-459 (1989).
64. Linder, C.W., and DuRant, R.H., *Pediatr. Clin. North Am.*, *29*(6): 1341-1354 (1982).
65. Liu, N., Plowman, S., and Wells, C., *Med. Sci. Sport Exerc.*, *20*(2) (Suppl.): S31, (Abstr.) (1988).
66. Liu, N.Y., Plowman, S.A., and Wells, C.L., *Hum. Biol.*, *61*(2): 227-247 (1989).
67. Lloyd, T., Buchanan, J.R., Bitzer, S., Waldman, C.J., Myers, C., and Ford, B.G., *Am. J. Clin. Nutr.*, *46*: 681-684 (1987).
68. Lohman, T.G., *Exerc. Sport Sci. Rev. 14*: 325-357 (1986).
69. Loucks, A.B., in *Competitive Sports for Children and Youth* (E.W. Brown and C.F. Branta, eds.). Human Kinetics, Champaign, Illinois, 213-224 (1988).
70. Malina, R.M., in *Perspectives in Exercise Science and Sports Medicine.* Vol. 2, *Youth, Exercise, and Sport* (C.V. Gisolfi and D.R. Lamb, eds.). Benchmark Press, Indianapolis, pp. 223-265 (1989).
71. Malina, R.M., in *Competitive Sports for Children and Youth* (E.W. Brown and C.F. Branta, eds.). Human Kinetics, Champaign, Illinois, pp. 227-246 (1988).
72. Malina, R.M., in *Young Athletes: Biological, Psychological, and Educational Perspectives* (R.M. Malina, ed.). Human Kinetics, Champaign, Illinois, pp. 121-140 (1988).
73. Malina, R.M., in *Human Growth.* Vol. 2, *Postnatal Growth, Neurobiology* (F. Falkner and J.M. Tanner, eds.). Plenum Press, New York, pp. 77-99 (1986).
74. Malina, R.M., in *Advances in Pediatric Sports Sciences* (R.A. Boileau, eds.). Human Kinetics, Champaign, Illinois, pp. 59-84 (1984).
75. Malina, R.M., *Ann. Hum. Biol.*, *10*: 1-24 (1983).
76. Mandelbaum, B.R., Bartolozzi, A.R., Davis, C.A., Teurlings, L., and Bragoner, B., *Am. J. Sports Med.*, *17*(3): 305-317 (1989).
77. McGill, H.C., Jr., in *Childhood Prevention of Arteriosclerosis and Hypertension* (R.M. Lauer and R.R. Shekelle, eds.). Raven Press, New York, pp. 41-49 (1980).
78. Micheli, L.J., *Pediatr. Exerc. Sci.*, *1*(4): 329-335 (1989).
79. Micheli, L.J., in *Competitive Sports for Children and Youth* (E.W. Brown and C.F. Branta, eds.). Human Kinetics, Champaign, Illinois, pp. 99-106 (1988).

80. Micheli, L.J., in *Competitive Sports for Children and Youth* (E.W. Brown and C.F. Branta, eds.). Human Kinetics. Champaign, Illinois, pp. 279–284 (1988).
81. Montoye, H.J., in *American Academy of Physical Education Papers*, No. 19 (G.G. Stull and H.M. Eckert, eds.). Human Kinetics, Champaign, Illinois, pp. 127–152 (1986).
82. National Institutes of Health (NIH). *Pediatrics, 79*: 1–25 (1987).
83. Newman, W.P., III, Freedman, D.S., Voors, A.W., Gard, P.D., Srinivasan, S.R., Cresanta, J.L., et al. *N. Engl. J. Med., 314*: 138–144 (1986).
84. Oscai, L.B., in *Perspectives in Exercise Science and Sports Medicine*. Vol. 2, *Youth, Exercise, and Sport* (C.V. Gisolfi and D.R. Lamb, eds.). Benchmark Press, Indianapolis, pp. 273–292 (1989).
85. Pacelli, L.C., *Physician Sports Med., 17*(8): 16 (1989).
86. Paffenbarger, R.S., Hyde, R.T., Wing, A.L., and Hsieh, C., *N. Engl. J. Med., 314*: 605–613 (1986).
87. Parizkova, J., *Body Fat and Physical Fitness*. Martinus Nijhoff, The Hague (1977).
88. Pate R.R., and Ward, D.S., in *Advances in Sports Medicine and Fitness*. Vol. 3. (W.A. Grana, J.A. Lombardo, B.J. Sharkey, and J.A. Stone, eds.). Year Book, Chicago, pp. 37–55 (1990).
89. Perusse, L., Tremblay, A., LeBlanc, C., and Bouchard, C., *Am. J. Epidemiol., 129*: 1012–22 (1989).
90. Pfeiffer, R.D., and Francis, R.S. *Physician Sports Med., 14*(9): 134–143 (1986).
91. Plowman, S.A., *Pediatr. Exerc. Sci., 1*(4): 303–312 (1989).
92. Plowman, S.A., Liu, N.Y., and Wells, C.L. *Med. Sci. Sports Exerc., 23*: 23–29 (1991).
93. Powell, K.E., Thompson, P.D., Caspersen, D.J., and Kendrick, J.S. *Ann. Rev. Publ. Health, 8*: 253, 281–287 (1987).
94. President's Council on Physical Fitness and Sports. *Physical Fitness Research Digest*, Series 1, No. 1. Washington, D.C. (1971).
95. Rains, C.B., Weltman, A., Cahill, B.R., Janney, C.A., Tippett, S.R., and Katch, F.I. *Am J. Sports Med., 15*(5): 483–489 (1987).
96. Raithel, K.S., *Physician Sports Med., 16* (10): 146–154 (1988).
97. Reybrouck, T.M., in *Advances in Pediatric Sport Sciences*. Vol. 3. (O. Bar-Or, ed.). Human Kinetics, Champaign, Illinois, pp. 131–150 (1989).
98. Riopel, D.A. Boerth, R.C., Coates, T.J., Heunekens, C.H., Miller, W.W., and Weidman, W.H., *Circulation, 74*(5): 1189A–1191A (1986).
99. Rocchini, A.P., *Pediatr. Clin. North Am., 31*(6): 1259–1273 (1984).
100. Roche, A.F., Chumlea, W.C., and Thissen, D., *Assessing the Skeletal Maturity of the Hand-Wrist: Fels Method*. Thomas, Springfield, Illinois (1988).
101. Rogol, A.D., in *Competitive Sports for Children and Youth* (E.W. Brown and C.F. Branta, eds.). Human Kinetics, Champaign, Illinois, pp. 173–193 (1988).
102. Ross, J.G., and Pate, R.R., *J. Physical Ed. Rec. Dance, 58*(9): 51–56 (1987).

103. Rowland, T.W., *Pediatr. Exerc. Sci.*, *1*(4): 313–328 (1989).
104. Rowland, T.W., *Pediatr. Exerc. Sci.*, 1(4): 187–188 (1989).
105. Rowland, T.W., *Physician Sports Med.*, 14(2): 122–128 (1986).
106. Rowland, T.W., *Med. Sci. Sports Exerc.*, *17*(5): 493–497 (1985).
107. Rowland, T.W., and Green, G.M., *Med. Sci. Sports Exerc.*, 20(5): 474–478 (1988).
108. Roy, S., Caine, D., and Singer, K.M., *Am. J. Sports Med.*, *13*: 301–308 (1985).
109. Rutenfranz, J., *Med. Sci. Sports Exerc.*, *15*(6): 486–490 (1986).
110. Sady, S.P., in *Clinics in Sports Medicine* (F. Katch and P.F. Freedson, eds.). Saunders, Philadelphia, pp. 493–513 (1986).
111. Sale, D.G., in *Youth, Exercise, and Sport* (C.V. Gisolfi and D.R. Lamb, eds.). Benchmark Press, Indianapolis, pp. 165–216 (1989).
112. Sallis, J.F., Patterson, T.L., Buone, M.J. and Nader, P.R., *Am. J. Epidemiol.*, *127*: 933–941 (1988).
113. Saris, W.H.M., *Acta Paediatr. Scand.* *318*(Suppl.): 37–48 (1985).
114. Servido, F.J., Bartels, R.L., and Hamlin, R.L., *Med. Sci. Sports Exerc.* 17: 288 (abst.) (1985).
115. Sewall, L., and Micheli, L.J., *J. Pediatr. Orthop.*, *6*: 143–146 (1986).
116. Shephard, R.J., in *Advances in Pediatric Sport Sciences.* Vol I. (R.A. Boileau, ed.). Human Kinetics, Champaign, Illinois, pp. 1–28 (1984).
117. Shephard, R.J., *Physical Activity and Growth.* Year Book, Chicago, (1982).
118. Shephard, R.J., *Endurance Fitness.* University of Toronto Press, Toronto, (1977).
119. Shephard, R.J., Lavalleé, H., Rajic, M., Jéquier, J.C., Brisson, G., and Beaucage, C. in *Pediatric Work Physiology* (J. Borms and M. Hebbelnick, eds.). Karger, Basel, pp. 124–133 (1978).
120. Siegel, J.A., Camione, D.N., and Manfredi, T.G. *Med. Sci. Sports Exerc.* 20 (Suppl.): S53 (1988).
121. Smoak, C.G., Burke, G.L., Webber, L.S., Harsha, D.W., Srinivasan, S.R., and Berenson, G.S., *Am. J. Epidemiol.*, *125*: 364–372 (1987).
122. Stager, J.M., and Hatler, L.K. *Med. Sci. Sports Exerc.* 20(4): 369–373 (1988).
123. Strauzenberg, S.E., *J. Sports Med.*, *22*: 401–406 (1982).
124. Telford, R.D., McDonald, I.G., Ellis, L.B., Chennells, M.H. D., Sandstrom, E.R., and Fuller, P.J. *J. Sports Sci.* 6: 49–57 (1988).
125. Theintz, G.E., Howald, H., Allemann, Y., and Sizonenko, P.C., *Int. J. Sports Med.*, *10*: 87–91 (1989).
126. Trussel, J., *Hum. Biol.*, *52*: 711–720 (1980).
127. Vaccaro, P., and Mahan, A., *Sports Med.*, *4*: 352–363 (1987).
128. Von Döbeln, W., and Eriksson, B.O., *Acta Pediatr. Scand.* *61*: 653–660 (1972).
129. Vrijens, J., *Med. Sport*, *11*: 152–158 (1978).
130. Ward, D.S., and Bar-Or, O., *Med. Sci. Sports Exerc.*, *19*: 515 (1987).
131. Warren, M.P., *J. Clin. Endoctrinol. Metab.*, *51*: 1150–1156 (1980).

132. Washington, R.L., van Gundy, J.C., Cohen, C., Sondheimer, H.M., and Wolfe, R.R., *J. Pediatr.*, *112*: 223–233 (1988).
133. Webber, L.S., Cresanta, J.L., Voors, A.W., and Berenson, G.S., *J. Chronic Dis.*, *36*: 647–660 (1983).
134. Weiss, M.R., and Petlichkoff, L.M., *Pediatr. Exerc. Sci.*, *1*(3): 195–211 (1989).
135. Wells, C.L., in *American Academy of Physical Education Papers*, No. 19. (G.A. Stull and H.M. Eckert, eds.). Human Kinetics, Champaign, Illinois, pp. 114–126 (1986).
136. Wells, C.L., and Plowman, S.A., in *Competitive Sports for Children and Youth* (E.W. Brown and C.F. Branta, eds.). Human Kinetics, Champaign, Illinois, pp. 195–212 (1988).
137. Weltman, A., in *Advances in Pediatric Sport Sciences* (O. Bar-Or, ed.). Human Kinetics, Champaign, Illinois, pp. 101–129 (1989).
138. Weltman, A., Janney, C., Rains, C.B., Strand, K., Berg, B., Tippett, S., Wise, J., Cahill, B.R., and Katch, F.I., *Med. Sci. Sports Exerc.*, *18*(6): 629–638 (1986).
139. Zauner, C.W., Maksud, M.G., and Melichna, J., *Sports Med.*, *8*(1): 15–31 (1989).
140. Zwiren, L.D., *Pediatr. Exerc. Sci.*, *1*(1) 31–44 (1989).
141. Zwiren, L.D., in *American College of Sports Medicine: Resource Manual for Guidelines for Exercise Testing and Prescription*. Lea & Febiger, Philadelphia, pp. 309–314 (1988).

4

Exercise Testing and Training of the Middle Aged

Roy J. Shephard

University of Toronto
Toronto, Ontario, Canada

INTRODUCTION

This chapter will discuss features of exercise testing and prescription of particular relevance to the late middle-aged patient, whom we will arbitrarily define as having an age between 40 and 65 years. During this time, women pass through the menopause, and both sexes experience a major change of life roles. Children are becoming independent and taking their activity separately from the parents. Women may be returning to paid employment after a period as full-time homemaker. Men have often reached a plateau of achievement in their careers, and are beginning to seek other methods of self-actualization than working 16 h per day. Financial debts associated with education and house purchase have usually been repaid, and many couples note a substantial increase of disposible income, particularly in the latter half of late middle-age. Retirement is now seen as a less distant prospect, and people begin to recognize a need for interests and hobbies appropriate to a time of greater leisure.

At the same time, many patients become conscious of declining physical performance (Table 1). Some people become discouraged by slower swimming speeds, or an increased golfing handicap, and others note that domestic tasks once accomplished with ease are becoming more difficult. Chronic diseases have often made substantial pro-

Table 1   Age-Related Decline in Performance of Selected Events

Event	\multicolumn{6}{c}{Age (yrs)}

Event	40–44	45–49	50–54	58–59	60–64	65–69
100 m (s)	10.7	11.1	11.4	11.6	12.0	13.2
1500 m (min/s)	3:52	4:03	4:14	4:20	4:53	4:59
Marathon run (min/s)	131:19	140:12	145:17	146:35	167:46	173:03
Long jump (m)	7.34	6.68	6.23	6.03	5.38	4.68

Source: Based on data accummulated by Stones, M.L., and Kozma, A., *Exp. Aging Res.,*
7: 274 (1981).

gress relative to early adulthood. The typical patient has sustained a
10-kg increase of body mass, this representing a 15-kg accumulation of
body fat, and a 5-kg loss of lean tissue. Osteoporosis begins around
25–30 years of age (earlier in women than in men), and there is a major
acceleration of bone calcium loss in the 5-year perimenopausal period.
About 40% of many urban samples have smoked heavily for 30–50
years, with a cumulative deterioration of respiratory function. Perhaps
5–10% of the sample have become problem drinkers, in some cases
with an associated cardiomyopathy. Coronary atherosclerosis is still
typically silent, but in many patients the intravascular plaques are
beginning to reach the critical dimensions (>70% of the lumen) where
significant myocardial ischemia develops during vigorous exercise (46).

EVALUATION

In general, the principles of exercise evaluation are as in a young
adult, although such features as abnormal stress tests, body fat distribution, and bone density may need special consideration.

Stress Testing

A middle-aged adult can be tested on a treadmill; here, uphill walking
becomes the preferred mode of exercise, rather than running. If a cycle
ergometer is used, quadriceps weakness may begin to limit the attainment of an oxygen consumption plateau (56). Stepping is a third possible option, provided there has been no loss of stability of the knee
joints. Sport-specific tests are rarely necessary in the older adult; even
when there is participation in Masters' competition, most competitors
elect to contest a variety of sports.

　　Submaximal tests become progressively less satisfactory as a
means of predicting peak power output because aging leads to an

increasing interindividual variation in peak heart rates (2) (Fig. 1). A symptom-limited maximal test thus has increasing attraction as a method of assessing an individual's peak cardiorespiratory performance (11).

At one time, it was argued that a stress electrocardiogram was mandatory in any patient over the age of 40 years who wished to begin an exercise program (1,14). If the patient's intention is to begin some moderate walking, or to do a little more gardening (typical decisions in later middle age), a stress ECG seems an unnecessary expense. On the other hand, if there is a wish to undertake serious

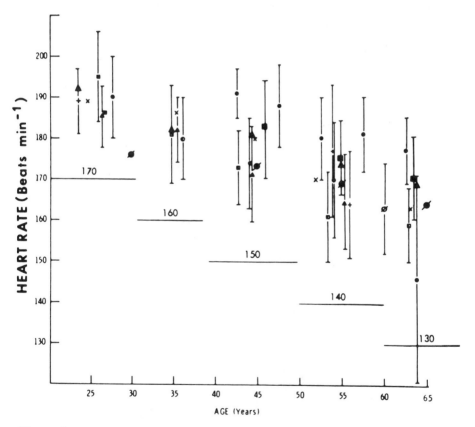

Figure 1 Decline of maximal heart rate with age. (Data from the world literature collected by S.M. Fox and W. Haskell, and reproduced by permission of the authors.) × Robinson (45a), ø Astrand et al. (3b), ⊡ Astrand (3a), ⊙ Bruce (11), ▲ Bink (5a), + Andersen (2a), ● Lester et al. (31a), ▲ Kasch et al. (28a), ■ Saltin & Grimby (46a), ♦ Hollmann (25a).

training (for example, in preparation for a marathon run or Masters' competition) (29,30,42), a careful evaluation of exercise responses is required. Particular features to note are (a) a poor peak performance, (b) the development of premature ventricular contractions (VPCs) and ST segmental depression (Fig. 2), (c) an excessive rise of blood pressure, (d) failure of blood pressure to show the anticipated rise, and (e) any unusual symptoms.

A poor peak performance is always an indication for caution, since it implies that a given exercise prescription will impose a greater stress upon the individual concerned, with a corresponding increase in the risks of an untoward event such as electrical failure of the heart and sudden death during exercise. Such patients usually show a poor cardiac ejection fraction, possibly due to incompetent or stenotic valves, prior undetected infarction or cardiomyopathy. Underlying

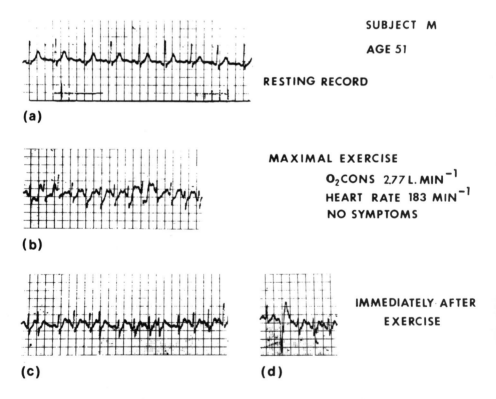

SUBJECT M

AGE 51

RESTING RECORD

(a)

MAXIMAL EXERCISE
O_2CONS 2.77 L. MIN^{-1}
HEART RATE 183 MIN^{-1}
NO SYMPTOMS

(b)

IMMEDIATELY AFTER EXERCISE

(c)   (d)

Figure 2 Exercise electrocardiogram signaling an adverse prognosis. The individual in question died a few weeks later while running up a flight of stairs to attend to an emergency.

pathologies can commonly be elucidated by echocardiographic investigation (20,55).

Occasional VPCs are observed in a person who has maintained a high level of cardiorespiratory training, with a corresponding augmentation of vagal tone and a slow resting heart rate. Such VPCs tend to become less frequent or disappear as the heart rate increases with exercise. In contrast, VPCs of ischemic etiology become more frequent as the intensity of exercise is increased (13,34,66). Adverse features of the ECG record are multiple VPCs (>3 in 10 s), runs, polyfocal VPCs, and the occurrence of VPCs early in the repolarization cycle (55). Many older adults show a slight ST segmental depression during vigorous exercise. True ischemic changes are horizontal or downsloping in type rather than the more commonly encountered J-point depression with subsequent upward slope. A 1-mm (0.1 mV) horizontal depression of the ST-segment is associated with a statistically increased risk of myocardial infarction (9,27), and it is commonly regarded as dangerous to allow a progressive exercise test to continue beyond a 2-mm ST depression. The difficulty in advising the individual patient is that whereas an abnormal ECG implies, on average, a two- to threefold increase in the risk of a heart attack over the next quinquennium (28), if the person is middle aged and symptom-free, some two-thirds of apparently positive test results are "false-positive" results (50) (Table 2). Cynics have suggested that relative to the stress ECG, the toss of a coin is a more effective way of distinguishing vulnerable patients! However, this may not be an entirely fair criticism, since a negative test result is correct 99% of the time, and many of the false-positive results can be clarified at some cost to the patient (anxiety, medical expense, and a finite risk from angiography) by such techniques as 2D echocardiography (64), computed tomographic scanning (47), and positron emission tomography (48).

It remains controversial whether such additional investigation is cost effective in the symptom-free middle-aged adult. The advice

Table 2 The High Incidence of "False-Positive" Tests with Routine Application of Exercise Electrocardiography to a Middle-Aged Population. True Incidence of Myocardial Ischemia 50 Cases per 1000.

Test result	Ischemia		Test errors (%)
	absent	present	
Positive	95	40	70.4
Negative	855	10	1.2

offered to the patient (moderate exercise, avoidance of prolonged isometric straining, and an improvement of overall lifestyle) is unlikely to be changed even if coronary narrowing is confirmed. The best plan is simply to set the intensity of the exercise prescription a little below the threshold where ECG abnormalities become marked. One exception is the patient who expresses a desire to engage in vigorous Masters' competition; here, it may be warranted to pursue a correct diagnosis, and if the vascular lesion is severe to consider angioplasty or coronary vascular bypass surgery.

Patients with a tendency to resting hypertension may show an even more abnormal pressure during exercise (Table 3). Moreover, while hypotensive medication may offer quite good control of the resting pressure, it is often relatively ineffective in controlling exercise pressures (19). The hypertension associated with exercise has particular importance, since it can lead to myocardial ischemia, cardiac failure, and (occasionally) vascular rupture. On the other hand, regular physical activity is likely to have a beneficial effect on both resting and exercise blood pressures (49,65). Some have argued that the impact of training on exercise pressures is much greater than that of hypotensive drugs (19). The optimum prescription is thus moderate exercise to a level of pressure that is well tolerated by the heart. Muscle-strengthening exercises may also help in controlling hypertension, since the rise of blood pressure during exercise is often linked to muscles that are contracting at an excessive fraction of their maximal voluntary force (33).

Failure of the blood pressure to show the anticipated rise with a further increment of work rate is an ominous sign of a failing circulation (26). It may reflect aortic valvular or vascular stenosis, or simply failure of a weakened and ischemic myocardium to respond to the challenge of increased afterload during vigorous exercise. Again, the

Table 3 Rise of Systolic Blood Pressure (kPa)[a] in Relation to Age and Work Rate (METs = ratio of exercise to resting oxygen consumption)

Age (yrs)	Rest		Exercise		
	(1 MET)	(4 METs)	(6 METs)	(8 METs)	(10 METs)
25	16.0	19.3	20.8	22.3	23.8
35	16.3	19.6	21.6	23.5	25.2
45	16.7	20.2	22.4	23.5	24.8
55	17.0	20.9	23.4	25.5	27.5

[a] (1 kPa = 7.5 Torr).
Source: Based on data of S. M. Fox, personal communication.

prescribed intensity of effort should be held below a level where this sign appears.

Significant symptoms are not common during routine stress testing. Sometimes, on close questioning, the patient with an apparently silent myocardial ischemia will admit to a little tightness in the chest, a sense of constriction in the throat, or a tingling sensation along the inner aspect of the left arm, whereas PVCs may be detected as a thump in the chest. If the patient learns to recognize such symptoms, this may be helpful in self-pacing and monitoring of exercise sessions.

Body Composition

Actuarial tables of "ideal weight" become harder to interpret in older adults (Fig. 3). There have been suggestions that the "ideal" figure assessed at the time of purchase of life insurance (usually as a young adult) is no longer relevant in middle age and later life. A lower mortality is apparently observed in those patients whose body mass has increased by some 10% over the working span (4,17,21,32,44,63). This advantage apparently still persists at least to some extent after elimination of effects attributable to current smoking habits (22) and preexistent disease, although it is less certain that the data have been adequately adjusted for former cigarette smoking. Possibly, there are significant health disadvantages in attempting to maintain the ideal body mass of a young adult through a combination of a sedentary lifestyle and rigid dieting.

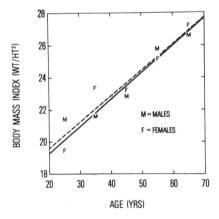

Figure 3 Changes of actuarial "ideal weight" with age. The body mass index associated with the lowest mortality is plotted against age. (From Andres, R., Bierman, E.L., and Hazzard, W.R., *Principles of Geriatric Medicine*. McGraw-Hill, New York, Fig. 29.2, p. 316 [1985]; used with permission.)

As adults become older, there is not only a tendency to an increase in the total body fat content (Table 4), but also an alteration in its pattern of distribution. A "central," masculine, pattern of accumulation over the abdomen is particularly associated with an increased risk of ischemic heart disease (6,7,10). In general, the proportion of deep to superficial fat rises (3,16), so that skin fold equations developed on young adults fail to predict either body density or total body fat accurately. Particularly in older women, the loss of calcium from the bones also leads to a substantial decrease in the density of lean tissue, so that the standard assumptions of hydrometry (a fat density of 0.9 g/ml and a lean tissue density of 1.1 g/ml) lead to an overestimation of body fat content (18,36,58).

Techniques of body composition assessment based on the lean tissue compartment (body impedance, total body water, and total body potassium measurements) are also complicated by age-related changes in the potassium and water content of the tissues, and the screening effect of an increased layer of superficial fat. Any assessment of body composition that does not use age-specific equations should thus be regarded with considerable suspicion (36,58).

Methods of measuring bone density (dual photon absorptiometry, whole body calcium counts following neutron activation) are now becoming more readily available (23,58,62), and should be considered in older adults who give a history of fractures with insignificant amounts of trauma.

Muscle Strength and Flexibility

Assessments of muscle strength in the older adult are hampered by a lack of normative data. Results are affected substantially by small

Table 4 Changes in "Excess Weight" and Skinfold Thicknesses with Aging

Age (yrs)	Men		Women	
	excess weight (kg)[a]	average skinfold (mm)[b]	excess weight (kg)[a]	average skinfold (mm)[b]
20–29	1.7 ± 8.7	11.3 ± 5.3	8.3 ± 5.3	16.2 ± 3.8
30–39	6.4 ± 8.5	16.1 ± 10.6	1.4 ± 5.3	13.5 ± 5.2
40–49	9.3 ± 9.5	14.0 ± 5.8	6.8 ± 8.4	17.3 ± 5.4
50–59	8.8 ± 7.7	15.2 ± 6.7	4.9 ± 7.2	18.2 ± 5.1
60–69	5.1 ± 7.3	15.4 ± 2.7	4.5 ± 9.5	22.5 ± 7.9

Mean ± SD of data for average Canadians living in metropolitan Toronto.

[a] Relative to actuarial "ideal weight" for height.

[b] Average of 8 skinfold readings.

alterations of joint angle and harnessing (in the case of isometric testing) and by speed, practice, and damping (in the case of isokinetic
measurements). All scores also depend strongly on motivation, and
thus the persuasive powers of the observer. The largest quantity of
normative information currently available relates to dynamometer
measurements of hand-grip force (Fig. 4), but even results for this simple observation depend heavily upon the design of the dynamometer,

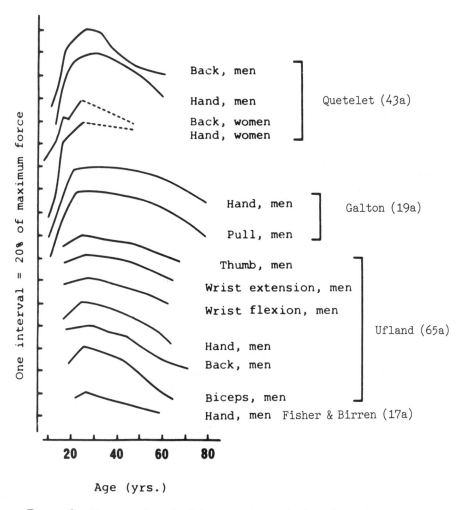

Figure 4   Changes of maximal isometric force of selected muscle groups with
aging. (Based in part on an analysis of Fisher, M.B., and Birren, J.E., *J. Appl.
Psychol.*, 31: 490–497 [1949].)

motivation of the subject, and opportunity for test practice; there may thus be only a limited correlation between hand-grip force and the strength of the muscles about the knee joint or in the back. For example, a person playing a game such as tennis regularly, or having a manual occupation is likely to have a selective preservation of hand-grip force.

The same problem of limited generality affects assessments of joint flexibility (59). The largest volume of normative data has been accumulated on "sit-and-reach" scores, and many individuals show a substantial decrease of score for this test over the span of adult life.

EXERCISE PRESCRIPTION

General considerations

The objectives of exercise prescription in an older adult are to suggest a safe intensity of physical activity, to motivate the individual to participate regularly in training sessions, and to sustain, if not restore, the function that has been lost since early adulthood.

Safety

Exercise training continues to be a very safe undertaking for the older adult—even in those who have sustained a myocardial infarction the average risk of a cardiac incident is only about 1 in 300,000 person-hours for a supervised exercise program, and 1 in 100,000 person-hours for an unsupervised program (24,57). Nevertheless, the immediate risk of a cardiac incident during the actual bout of physical activity is five to 50 times higher than that of continuing in a sedentary state (50,61,67). Moreover, although the absolute risk of exercise is lower for middle age than for the retirement years, the relative risk of increased physical activity is somewhat greater during middle age than in older people (Table 5). A possible explanation of this paradox is that some middle-aged men who have been sedentary for quite a number of years are reluctant to admit their lack of physical condition, and thus they are tempted to embark on bouts of very demanding physical activity with inadequate preparation. In contrast, the elderly adopt a very cautious approach to exercise.

The physician may encounter particular difficulty in regulating the prescription of the busy, overly competitive executive. Sometimes, such individuals will try to beat a superior opponent at a game of tennis or squash even when they have become extremely tired, or they will try to progress faster than a rival when given a sequential exercise training plan. A hectic schedule may also encourage them to exercise

Table 5 Relative Risks of Sudden Death During Nonstrenuous and Strenuous Exercises in Relation to Age

Age (years)	Nonstrenuous exercise[a]		Strenuous exercise[a]	
	M	R	M	R
20–39	26.0	2.5	6.1	10.0
40–49	5.2	3.6	1.2	13.1
50–69	3.4	2.5	1.2	5.3

[a] Number of exercise sessions ($\times 10^6$) for single death (M) and risk of sudden cardiovascular death in exercise relative to sedentary state (R).
Source: Based on data from Ref. 67.

without an adequate warm-up (a common cause of cardiac problems [5]), and they may decide that if a 30-min session of exercise has been prescribed for their health, even greater benefit will be obtained from a continuous 2-h session. Such individuals must be warned firmly against exceeding their prescription.

Older individuals may have previously encountered problems with their back or knees, and it is important to inquire about such possible disabilities before prescribing exercise. City jogging and violent ''dancercize'' classes are particularly likely to exacerbate musculoskeletal problems.

In older women with substantial osteoporosis, overvigorous muscle contractions may give rise to fractures, and in both sexes repeated pounding on a hard surface such as a concrete sidewalk or a tiled concrete floor in a dance studio can give rise to stress fractures, particularly of the metatarsal bones. A slowing of reflexes, with a weakening of tendons and muscles, also leads to a high incidence of musculotendinous tears and strains, particularly if an excessive weekly training distance is attempted (43).

Tolerance of heat and cold decrease with aging. Thus, the middle-aged adult must be more cautious than a younger person if the climate is unfavorable for a particular competition.

Motivation

Continued motivation of the participants is a major problem with most exercise programs for middle-aged adults. For instance, if a corporate fitness program is introduced at the worksite, only about a third of eligible employees are initially recruited to such a facility, and many of these are people who were previously active elsewhere (31). Moreover, there is a high drop-out rate; some 50% of initial recruits are lost to the exercise program after 6 months, and a steady rate of attrition continues thereafter, so that despite an influx of new employees, the 10-year experience is that only about 13% of employees are significantly involved in the program (54), many of these 13% being infrequent rather than frequent participants.

The usually cited reason for dropping out of an exercise program (Table 6) is lack of time (12,52). At first inspection, this seems a feeble excuse; most older adults have 3–4 h of free time per day, much of which is spent in watching television. However, there is an "opportunity cost" if such free time is assigned to an exercise program and any ancillary travel to and from the exercise facility (53). Participants intuitively make their calculation of opportunity foregone, and decide that the cost (which might be assessed at their average hourly wage) is too high relative to the benefits immediately anticipated from exercise participation.

The simplest approach to changing their unfavorable assessment is to lower the opportunity cost—particularly the travel component. Thus, if the exercise facility is nearby, or the physical activity is built into the normal day (such as walking to the subway, or cycling to work), the weekly time commitment of the participant is greatly reduced. The alternative approach is to increase the immediate dividends of exercise. The physiological and biochemical rewards of physical activity bear a relatively fixed relationship to the intensity and duration of exercise, but other types of reward (Table 7) may be increased by an up-grading of the exercise facility (a more pleasant decor,

Table 6 Reasons Cited for Dropping Out of Various Exercise Programs

Activity	% of Sample Stopping in Past Year	Obstacles
Jogging	12	Time, laziness
Swimming	5	Facilities, program, time
Tennis	7	Time, facilities, program
Cycling	3	Equipment
Home exercise	6	Laziness
Exercise classes	10	Time, facilities, program
Walking	2	Time, illness, injury

Source: Based on data of Canada Fitness Survey, 1981. (Fitness and Amateur Sport, 1983, Fitness and Lifestyle in Canada).

Table 7   Possible Rewards that Can Provide Positive Feedback in an Exercise Program

Rewards:	Symbolic	Badges, pins, T-shirts, awards, membership of club
	Material	Money, prizes, release time, assistance with dues
	Psychological	Encouragement from instructor, recognition of achievements by group or family, attention, friendship
Punishment:	Symbolic	Exclusion from group
	Material	Pain, injury, costs of tuition and clothing, time loss, physical effort and fatigue
	Psychological	Discouragement or ridicule (from instructor, group or family), failure to achieve goals, family complaints about absence, psychological fatigue due to program

Source: Based on an analysis by R. Danielson and K. Danielson, On-going motivation in employee fitness programming. in *Employee Fitness, the How To.* (L. Wanzel, ed.). Toronto, Ont: Ministry of Tourism and Recreation, 1979.

incidental music, better control of temperature and humidity, improved shower and locker facilities, greater opportunities for socialization), provision of positive feedback from the instructor (reporting of favorable test scores, presentation of award pins, T-shirts, and other symbols of achievement), and maximizing the gains of mood state by optimizing the intensity, duration, and volume of physical activity. It is also helpful to minimize negative feedback, and to eliminate (as far as possible) any practical barriers to exercise participation. A person who is in poor physical condition and who has become obese may be embarassed to exercise with those of the opposite sex, and the unrealistic demands of a fit instructor can also be discouraging. It is thus useful to arrange unisex beginners' classes for such individuals. At the other end of the spectrum, a person who has sustained an excellent level of physical condition for their age may become discouraged if an age-related exercise class offers so little physical challenge that it fails either to improve personal fitness or to induce a desired secretion of mood-elevating β-endorphins.

Sometimes, the barriers to participation can be very simple issues, such as the need to leave the worksite with other members of a car pool. Such difficulties can often be surmounted by developing flexible hours of work or flexible hours of program operation. The cost of facility membership is rarely a significant barrier in middle-age, but expectations of the purchase of expensive clothes, shoes, and equipment can discourage the participation of single parents.

Effectiveness

The considerations governing an appropriate and effective pattern of exercise are much as for a younger adult, although in terms of avoiding musculoskeletal and cardiac problems, it is usually desirable to reduce the intensity somewhat during middle age (commencing training, for example, at 60–70% rather than 70–80% of maximal oxygen intake). The duration of training sessions can be extended to compensate for their lower intensity. Quite low intensities of exercise can offer a satisfactory way of sustaining and even of slowly developing cardiorespiratory condition, provided that sessions are regularly repeated (15,60 [see Fig. 3, chapter 5]).

Muscle-strengthening exercises remain important during middle age, but particularly if the muscles are initially weak or there is a high resting blood pressure, it is important to avoid prolonged straining against a closed glottis.

In terms of controlling obesity, improving lipid profile, and extending lifespan, an effective regimen calls for a substantial weekly energy expenditure (Fig. 5), but this can be accomplished by such activities as walking and stair climbing (38,41). Benefit commences with an added leisure expenditure of about 2 MJ (500 kcal) per week, and a maximal response is seen with an expenditure of 8–9 MJ (2000 kcal) per week, the latter being equivalent to an hour or more of brisk walking per day.

Mode of Exercise

From a physiological point of view, any large muscle activity (fast walking or jogging, cycling, swimming, rowing, canoeing, or cross-country skiing) is effective in developing cardiorespiratory condition. Such activities can be combined with daily transportation needs (reducing opportunity, cost, above), or they can be undertaken in beautiful areas of the countryside (increasing the personal rewards). Unfortunately, such types of exercise often lack a social component (which is an important motivator for some people), and they do little to develop muscular strength. Indeed, long-distance jogging is sometimes associated with a loss of lean tissue from the upper half of the body.

Gymnastic and dance classes maximize the social rewards of

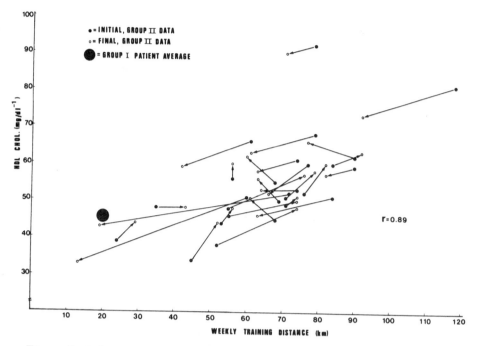

Figure 5 Influence of weekly jogging distance upon HDL cholesterol. Large circle represents patients involved in moderate jogging program. Lines represent individual patients who prepared themselves for marathon participation by a change in weekly jogging distance. (Kavanagh, T., Shephard, R.J., Lindley, L.J., and Pieper, M., *Arteriosclerosis*, 3: 249–259 [1983]; used with permission.)

physical activity, but the intensity of some forms of exercise can be rather light in terms of developing cardiorespiratory condition, unless movements are performed at a fast tempo. The speed of movement can be increased by an appropriate choice of music, but there is then a danger that twisting may provoke joint injuries.

Tennis and squash are very popular with middle-aged executives, and such games can provide a substantial cardiorespiratory stimulus if they are played against a vigorous opponent. The competitive nature of the pursuit is an important motivator for some business people, but it also leads to an increased secretion of catecholamines for a given intensity of effort (8) (Fig. 6), with a high incidence of PVCs (40), and thus an enhanced danger of a fatal cardiac arrhythmia.

Team sports offer substantial camaraderie, and appeal particularly to hourly workers. But as age advances, it becomes increasingly difficult to assemble a full team of players at an appropriately matched

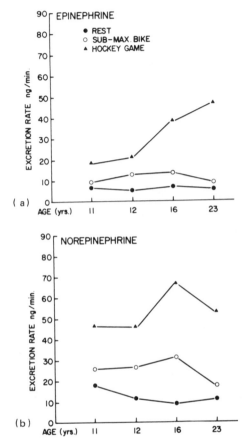

Figure 6 The influence of competition upon catecholamine secretion. Excretion of norepinephrine and epinephrine following hockey game and following equivalent intensity of cycle ergometer exercise. (From Ref. 8; used with permission.)

level of fitness and skill. Moreover, competition and excitement increase the output of catecholamines for a given intensity of exercise, and the body contact inherent in many team sports becomes increasingly hazardous for weakened bones.

The most effective approach to muscle building is a circuit training program (for instance, lifting weights about each of the major joints in turn). At each station on the circuit, a series of perhaps three sets of 10 repetitions is performed at 50–60% of the 1 repetition maximum for the movement in question. Some people can find motivation in an improvement of performance at the various stations, although unfortunately such gains tend to plateau as training continues (25).

Other recreational activities that require the lifting of heavy weights also develop muscle mass. In recommending such activities, care must be taken to avoid prolonged straining. However, it is interesting that three of 14 participants in the recent Canada/USSR Polar Ski Trek carried a 40-kg backpack some 2000 km across the icecap in difficult winter and early spring conditions, despite substantial resting and exercise-induced hypertension (46). Some patients seek to combine muscle building with aerobic exercise by carrying light weights while walking or jogging (35). This seems an unnecessary expense, and indeed the weights usually add little to the energy cost of movement. Simpler options are to swing the arms vigorously while walking with a briefcase or a bag of groceries, or to mow the lawn briskly with a handmower.

Flexibility is developed by taking the major joints gently through their full range of motion. Rowing and swimming are more effective than other types of aerobic exercise in this regard.

Any type of weight-bearing activity is effective in strengthening bones at the prime sites of osteoporotic fracture (the hip and the neck of the femur). Some authors have suggested that swimming also leads to an increase of bone density; this may reflect the pull of the active muscles upon the bones, but it is also possible that those patients who choose to swim engage in some form of weight-bearing activity.

If mood elevation is seen as an important objective of exercise, arousal can be obtained through any pattern of vigorous movement, but prolonged endurance exercise is needed to increase the secretion of endorphins. If the patient's problem seems an overhectic schedule, relaxation may be achieved most effectively by rhythmic, noncompetitive activity, performed alone or with a close friend, in a quiet, relaxing setting.

Spontaneous Choice

The spontaneous choice of the older adult concentrates upon walking and gardening as preferred forms of physical activity (37) (see Fig. 7).

Slow walking (2–3 km/h) will contribute little to health but is a pleasant form of relaxation. However, if the patient is encouraged to walk rapidly (up to 7–8 km/h), the exercise can become quite demanding—indeed, for most people, the energy demand associated with such a pattern of activity is more than the cost of running at the same speed (51). Walking has the additional advantage that the forces imposed upon the knees and back are only about a third as great as in running. Moreover, since one foot is always in contact with the ground, there is less danger of falls and slipping under winter conditions. Walking can be performed as a social activity (with the family or

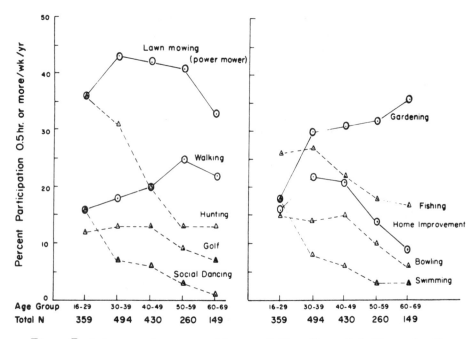

Figure 7 Influence of age upon leisure activities. (From Ref. 37; used with permission.)

close friends), and if the route is chosen appropriately, it can be combined with other pursuits (for instance, the study of nature or urban architecture), thus enhancing the quality of the activity.

Gardening is an activity of very variable intensity. For some people, it amounts to no more than a stroll through flower beds, sitting on a power mower, or holding the nozzle of a hose on a warm evening. However, planting and weeding give valuable exercise to the knees, hips and back, and digging in heavy soil provides a substantial stimulus to both cardiovascular and musculoskeletal systems. The intensity of digging depends on the hardness and wetness of the soil, the size of the shovel, and the pace of shoveling. Demand can be reduced to meet the effects of aging by use of a smaller shovel, a slower pace, and longer rest pauses. In countries such as Canada and the United States, it is important to recognize that gardening is a seasonal activity, and to allow a few days for muscles and joints to accept tasks that can be readily imposed at the end of the season. As with snow shoveling, there is some danger that heavy digging may provoke a heart attack. There is also some risk from pruning larger trees by handsaw, since heavy muscular exercise must then be performed with the hands held above the head. Caution is necessary when using ladders, particularly if reflexes and/or balance have deteriorated. In addition to physiological benefits, gardening offers quiet, relaxation, and a sense that something of permanence is being created—an appreciable reward, particularly for an older person.

While alternative modes of exercise can be considered, both walking and gardening have considerable potential for the older adult, and it may thus be appropriate for governments—and others interested in the promotion of fitness—to recognize this trend and to encourage it. Policy implications would include a diversion of funds from the building of hockey arenas to the construction of hiking trails, and the devlopment of gardening plots where older people could get both good exercise and sound nutrition by growing their own vegetables.

REFERENCES

1. American College of Sports Medicine, *Guidelines for Graded Exercise Testing and Prescription*. Lea & Febiger, Philadelphia (1986).
2. Andersen, K.L., Shephard, R.J., Denolin, H., Varnauskas, E., and Masironi, R., *Fundamentals of Exercise Testing*. World Health Organization, Geneva (1971).
2a. Andersen, K.L., Physical fitness—Studies of healthy men and women in Norway, in *International Research in Sport and Physical Education*. (E. Jokl and E. Simon, eds.) Charles C. Thomas, Springfield, Illinois (1964).
3. Ashwell, M., Cole, T.J., and Dixon, A.K., *Br. Med. J.* 290: 1691–1694 (1985).
3a. Åstrand, P.O. *Experimental Studies of physical working capacity in relation to age and sex*. Copenhagen: Monksgaard, 1952.
3b. Åstrand, I., Åstrand, P.O. and Rodahl, K. *J. Appl. Physiol.* 14:562–566 (1959).
4. Avons, P., Ducimitiere, P., and Rakatovao, R., *Lancet*, 1: 1104 (letter) (1983).
5. Barnard, R.J., Gardner, G.W., Diaco, N.V., MacAlpin, R.N., and Kattus, A.A., *J. Appl. Physiol.*, 34: 833–837 (1973).
5a. Bink, B. *Ergonomico* 5:25–28, 1962.
6. Bjorntorp, P., *Exerc. Sports Sci. Rev.*, 11: 159–180 (1983).
7. Blair, S.N., Ludwig, D.A., and Goodyear, N.N., *Hum. Biol.*, 60: 111–122 (1988).
8. Blimkie, C.J., Cunningham, D.A., and Leung, F.Y., in *Frontiers of Activity and Child Health* (H. Lavallée and R.J. Shephard, eds.). Editions du Pélican, Quebec City, pp. 313–322 (1977).
9. Bonow, R.O., Kent, K.M., Rosing, D.R., Lau, K.K., Lakatos, E., Borer, J.S., Bacharach, S.L., Green, M.V., and Epstein, S.E., *N. Engl. J. Med.*, 311: 1339–1345 (1984).
10. Bouchard, C., in *Metabolic Complications of Human Obesities* (J. Vague et al., eds.). Elsevier, Amsterdam, pp. 87–96 (1985).

11. Bruce, R.A., in *Principles of Geriatric Medicine* (R. Andres, E.L. Bierman, and W.R. Hazzard, eds.) McGraw-Hill, New York, pp. 87–103 (1985).

12. Canada Fitness Survey (1983). *Fitness and Lifestyle in Canada.* Fitness and Lifestyle Research Institute, Ottawa.

13. Chiang, B.N., Montoye, H.J., and Cunningham, D.A. *Am J. Epidemiol., 91*: 368–377 (1970).

14. Cooper, K.H., *J.A.M.A., 211*: 1663–1667 (1970).

15. Durnin, J.V.G.A., Brockway, J.M., and Whitcher, H.N. *J. Appl. Physiol., 15*: 161–165 (1960).

16. Durnin, J.V.G.A., and Womersley, J., *Br. J. Nutr., 32*: 77–97 (1974).

17. Dyer, A.R., Stamler, J., Berkson, D.M., and Lindberg, H.A., *J. Chron. Dis., 28*: 109–123 (1975).

17a. Fisher, M.B., and Birren, J.E., *J. Appl. Psychol. 31*:490–497 (1949).

18. Forsyth, R., Plyley, M.J., and Shephard, R.J., *Can. J. Appl. Sport Sci., 9*: 5P (1984).

19. Franz, I.W., *Can. J. Sport Sci.*, in press (1991).

19a. Galton (1884). Cited by Fisher and Birren (17a).

20. Gardin, J.M., Henry, W.L., Savage, D.D., and Epstein, S.E., *Am. J. Cardiol., 39*: 277 (1977).

21. Garn, S.M., Hawthorne, V.M., Pilkington, J.J., and Pesick, S.D. *Am. J. Clin. Nutr., 38*: 313–319 (1983).

22. Garrison, R.J., Feinleib, M., Castelli, W.P., and McNamara, P.M. *J.A.M.A., 249*: 2199–2203 (1983).

23. Harrison, J.E., McNeill, K.G., Hitchman, A.J., and Britt, B.A. *Invest. Radiol., 14*: 27–34 (1979).

24. Haskell, W.L., *Circulation, 57*: 920–924 (1978).

25. Hettinger, T., *Physiology of Strength.* Charles C. Thomas, Springfield, Illinois (1961).

25a. Hollmann, W. Changes for maximal and continuous effort in relation to age, in *International Research in Sport and Physical Education* (E. Jokl and E. Simon, eds.). Charles C. Thomas, Springfield, Illinois pp. 369–371 (1964).

26. Ivanova, L.A., Mazur, N.A., Smirnova, T.M., Sumarokov, A.B., Svet, E.A., Nazarenko, V.A., and Kotlyarov, V.V., in *Sudden Cardiac Death* (B.A. Lown and A.M. Vikhert, eds.). Washington, D.C.: National Heart and Lung Institute. NIH Publ. 81-2101, December, pp. 23–38 (1980).

27. Jennings, K., Reid, D.S., Hawkins, T., and Julian, D.J., *Br. Med. J., 288*: 185–187 (1984).

28. Kannel, W.B., and Brand, F.N., in *Principles of Geriatric Medicine* (R. Andres, E.L. Bierman, and W.R. Hazzard, eds.). McGraw-Hill, New York, pp. 104–119 (1985).

28a. Kasch, F.W., Phillips, W.H., Ross, W.D., Carter, J.E.L. and Boyer, J.L., *J. Appl. Physiol. 21*:1387–1388 (1966).

29. Kavanagh, T., and Shephard, R.J., *Ann. N.Y. Acad. Sci., 301*: 656–670 (1977).

29a. Kavanagh, T., Lindley, L.T., Shephard, T.J. and Campbell, R. *Ann. Sport Med. 4*:55–64 (1988).

30. Kavanagh, T., and Shephard, R.J., *Physician Sportsmed.* 18 (6):94–103 (1990).
31. Leatt, P., Hattin, H., West, C., and Shephard, R.J., *Can. J. Publ. Health,* 79: 19–25 (1988).
31a. Lester, F.M., Sheffield, L.T., Trammell, P. and Reeves, T.J., *Amer. Heart J.* 76:370–376 (1968).
32. Lew, E.A., and Garfinkel, L., *J. Chron. Dis.,* 32: 563–576 (1979).
33. Lind, A.R., and McNicol, G.W., *Can. Med. Assoc. J.,* 96: 706–712 (1967).
34. Madsen, E.B., and Gilpin, E., *J. Cardiac Rehabil.,* 3: 481–488 (1983).
35. Makalous, S.L., Energy expenditure during walking with *Physician Sportsmed.,* 16 (4): 139–148 (1988).
35a. McNeill, K.E., and Harrison, J.E. Partial body neutron activation-truncal, in *Non-invasive measurements of bone bass and their clinical application.* (S.H. Cohn, ed.) CRC Press, Boca Raton, Florida, pp. 165–190 (1981).
36. Mernagh, J.R., Harrison, J., Krondl, A., McNeill, K.G., and Shephard, R.J., *Nutr. Res.,* 6: 499–507 (1986).
37. Montoye, H.J., *Physical Activity and Health: an Epidemiological Study of an Entire Community.* Prentice Hall, Englewood Cliffs, New Jersey (1975).
38. Morris, J.N., Everitt, M.G., Pollard, R., Chave, S.P.W., and Semmence, A.M., *Lancet,* 2: 1207–1210 (1980).
39. Mueller, W.H., Joos, S.K., Hanis, C.L., Zavaleta, A.N., Eichner, J., and Schull, W.J., *Am J. Phys. Anthropol.,* 64: 389–399 (1984).
40. Northcote, R.J., Flannigan, C., and Ballantyne, D., *Br. Heart J.,* 55: 198–203 (1986).
41. Paffenbarger, R.S., Hyde, R.T., Wing, A.L., and Hsieh, C.C., *N. Engl. J. Med.,* 314: 605–613 (1986).
42. Pollock, M.L., Foster, C., Knapp, D., Rod, J., and Schmidt, D. *J. Appl. Physiol.,* 62: 725–731 (1987).
43. Pollock, M.L., Graves, J., Leggett, S., Braith, R., and Hagberg, J., *Med Sci. Sports Exerc.,* 21: S88 (1989).
43a. Quetelet, A. *Sur l'homme et le developpement de ses facultés.* Paris: Bachelier (1835).
44. Rhoades, G.G., and Kagan, A., *Lancet,* 1: 492–495 (1983).
45. Rissanen, V., *Adv. Cardiol.,* 18: 113–121 (1976).
45a. Robinson, S. *Arbeitsphysiologie* 4:251–323 (1938).
46. Rode, A. and Shephard, R.J., Some lessons from the Canadian/USSR Transpolar ski-trek. Basel: Karger (1992).
46a. Saltin, B. and Grimby, G. *Circulation* 38:1104–1115 (1968).
47. Scanlan, J.G., Gustafson, D.E., Chevalier, P.A., Robb, R.A., and Ritman, E.L., *Am. J. Cardiol.,* 46: 1263–1268 (1980).
48. Schelbert, H.R., Phelps, M.E., Hoffman, E., Huang, S.C., and Kuhl, D.E., *Am. J. Cardiol.,* 46: 1269–1277 (1980).
49. Seals, D., Hagberg, J., Hurley, B., Ehsani, A., and Holloszy, J., *J. Appl. Physiol.,* 57: 1024–1029 (1984).
50. Shephard, R.J. *Ischemic Heart Disease and Exercise.* Croom Helm, London (1981).

51. Shephard, R.J., *Br. J. Sports Med., 16*: 220–229 (1982).
52. Shephard, R.J., Fitness of a Nation: Lessons from the Canada Fitness Survey. Karger, Basel (1986).
53. Shephard, R.J., *Economic Benefits of Enhanced Fitness*. Human Kinetics, Champaign, Illinois (1986).
54. Shephard, R.J., in *Parke-Davis/AFB/TCOM Conference on the Economic Impact of Employee Health Promotion* (B. Kaman, ed.). Texas College of Osteopathic Medicine, Fort Worth (1990).
55. Shephard, R.J., in *Textbook of Clinical Sports Medicine* (C.B. Rians, ed.). Human Kinetics, Champaign, Illinois (1991).
56. Shephard, R.J., Allen, C., Benade, A.J.S., Davies, C.T.M., diPrampero, P.E., Hedman, R., Merriman, J.E., Myhre, K., and Simmons, R., *Bull. W.H.O., 38*: 757–764 (1968).
57. Shephard, R.J., Kavanagh, T., Tuck, J., and Kennedy, J., *J. Cardiopulm. Rehabil., 3*: 321–329 (1983).
58. Shephard, R.J., Kofsky, P.R., Harrison, J.E., McNeill, K.G., and Krondl, A., *Hum. Biol., 57*: 671–686 (1985).
59. Shephard, R.J., Montelpare, W., and Berridge, M., *Res. Quart., 61*:326–330 (1990).
60. Sidney, K.H., and Shephard, R.J., *Med. Sci. Sports, 10*: 125–131 (1978).
61. Siscovick, D.S., Laporte, R.E., and Newman, J.M., *Publ. Health Rep., 100*: 180–188 (1985).
62. Smith, E., Reddan, W., and Smith, P., *Med. Sci. Sports Exerc., 13*: 60–64 (1981).
63. Society of Actuaries, *Build Study, 1979*. Society of Actuaries and Association of Life Insurance Medical Directors of America, Chicago (1980).
64. Stack, R., and Kisslo, J., *Am. J. Cardiol., 46*: 1117–1124 (1980).
64a. Thomas, S.E., Cunningham, D.A., Rechnitzer, P.A., Donner, A.P., and Howard, J.H., *Med. Sci. Sports Exerc.* 17:667–672 (1985).
65. Tipton, C., *Exerc. Sports Sci. Rev., 12*: 245–306 (1984).
65a. Ufland, J.M. *Arbeitsphysiologie* 6:653–663 (1933).
66. Vedin, J.A., Wilhelmsson, C.D., Wilhelmsen, L., Bjure, J., and Ekstrom-Jodal, B., *Am. J. Cardiol., 30*: 25–30 (1972).
67. Vuori, I., Suurnakki, L., and Suurnakki, T., *Med. Sci. Sports Exerc., 14*: 114–115 (1982).

5

Exercise in Old Age (65-85)

Roy J. Shephard

University of Toronto
Toronto, Ontario, Canada

INTRODUCTION

In this chapter, we shall look specifically at patterns of exercise that are appropriate for the elderly individual. It will first be necessary to consider the definition of old age and to make an appropriate classification of the elderly. We shall then examine particular problems of exercise testing and prescription, the likely benefits of an enhanced physical activity, and safety precautions appropriate to this particular age group.

DEFINITION OF THE ELDERLY

Onset of Old Age

Influenced by considerations of safety and convenience of access, many research articles supposedly dealing with exercise for the elderly have focused upon people in the latter half of their working careers, with subjects ranging in age from 40 to 65 years. Such individuals are essentially late middle aged rather than elderly, and problems of exercise prescription peculiar to this group have already been discussed in Chapter 4.

One convenient milestone indicating passage into old age is normal retirement from work. This currently occurs at an age of 65 years in Canada and the United States, but is allowed a few years earlier in some European countries (120). In North America, "equal opportunity" and "human rights" legislations are tending to push back the age of mandatory retirement, but at the same time, automation is leading to redundancy and unemployment among many people previously regarded as late middle aged.

Gradations of Aging

Even when the age of onset has been agreed upon, the elderly cannot be regarded as a homogeneous group. Most people show a very substantial deterioration of physical capacity between the ages of 65 and 85 years. One method of allowing for this is to subdivide the elderly population on the basis of their calendar age. Three subcategories are then recognized: the young-old (65–75 years), the middle-old (75–85 years), and the very old (over 85 years).

However, such a basis of classification ignores the existence of very substantial differences of biological age between individuals who share an identical calendar age (24,49). There have been attempts to develop scales of biological age, using a variety of anthropometric, physiological, and psychological markers, but it has been far from clear how to combine data obtained from disparate disciplines, using varying techniques and scales of measurement. Too often, the biological age calculation has proven little more than a complicated way of determining calendar age (120).

Functional Classification

Neither calendar age nor biological age are entirely satisfactory as a basis for the classification of the elderly. Nevertheless, the differences between individuals are incontrovertible, and there is thus much to commend adoption of a simple functional classification, particularly when prescribing physical activity.

The *young-old* are then considered as a group who can live independently, with little or no restriction of their physical activity; the *middle-old* have some physical disability, and might require a little assistance with their daily activities; and the *very old* are those who have become almost totally disabled, requiring extensive support, often within an institution.

Prevalence of Disability

The Canada Health Survey (18a) found 26.5% of individuals over the age of 65 years had some major limitation of their habitual physical activity, and in 8.9% of senior citizens there was a total inability to undertake major physical activities; by the age of 80 years, a large proportion of subjects were limited by disturbances of either cardiac or mental function. Likewise, in the United States (72), 80% of older people have some type of chronic disability, with arthritis (44%) and heart disease (27%) being the commonest problems. Although only 11% of the population, the chronically disabled account for 30% of medical costs, 40% of acute hospital days, and 90% of nursing home care. At the age of 60 years, the active life expectancy of an American is 60% of a remaining 16.5 years, but by 85 years, the active expectancy is only 40% of a remaining 7.3 years (57).

The totally disabled are a small proportion of the elderly population, but they are responsible for a large part of these heavy and growing costs (119). On average, Canadian senior citizens live for 8–10 years in the middle-old category and a final year in the very old category before finally dying (121); together, these may be considered as the societal burden of the "frail elderly."

Distinguishing Disease from Aging

One important variable potentially limiting the physical activity of many old people is the onset of chronic disease (120,121); 85.6% of Canadians over the age of 65 years are said to have some type of chronic health problem (17a), and in the Canada Fitness Survey (18), "illness" was perceived as the major impediment to physical activity among the elderly. On the other hand, many of the chronic diseases that afflict senior citizens are relative rather than absolute contraindications to exercise. Given a suitably adapted exercise prescription, substantial gains of physical condition remain possible in such individuals.

There is often no clear dividing line between the effects of aging and those of disease. For example, it has generally been held that the elderly have difficulty in sustaining cardiac stroke volume as maximum aerobic effort is approached. However, Weisfeldt et al. (154) have argued that a decline of stroke volume at high work rates reflects undiagnosed cardiac disease. In their view, if silent myocardial ischemia is excluded by rigorous electrocardiogrpahy, echocardigraphy, and other techniques, then an old person can compensate for the inevitable decline of peak heart rate by application of the Frank-Starling mechanism and a compensatory increase of stroke volume, so that peak cardiac output remains unchanged.

This chapter will focus mainly upon the outwardly healthy elderly, recognizing that as age advances they constitute a diminishing fraction of the total population, and that the dividing line between health and illness becomes progressively obscured. The operational definition of "healthy" will be the absence of any well-defined symptoms, gross medical condition, or regular medication that would restrict the ability of the individual to participate effectively in a program of progressive conditioning exercise.

SPECIFIC PROBLEMS OF EXERCISE TESTING IN THE ELDERLY

General Considerations

It may be wise to consider first the need for exercise testing of the elderly. Often, the results are puzzling because of minor pathologies, and discovery of a seemingly dangerous but previously silent condition may lead to a prohibition of exercise that to this point has been enjoyed by the individual. Exercise testing will be desirable if a major increase of physical activity is contemplated (for example, preparation for some type of Masters' competition). It may also be helpful for personal motivation, to assess obscure symptoms, to help in diagnosis and prognosis, and to assess programs and the results of individual medical or surgical treatment, including rehabilitation. However, it is not mandatory when only a moderate increase of daily exercise such as light walking is contemplated; indeed, by suggesting that exercise is a dangerous habit, insistence upon rigorous testing may be counterproductive.

Most exercise programs tend to focus upon endurance activities, and the main focus of exercise testing in the elderly, as in younger age groups, thus remains the measurement or the estimation of maximum oxygen transport. It is also very helpful to have information on electrocardiographic and blood pressure responses to graded exercise, together with data on muscle function, body composition, and flexibility.

Maximum Oxygen Transport

Value of Test Data

Maximal oxygen intake is important in setting a safe upper limit for the person who wishes to undertake a vigorous endurance exercise program. Normally, an old person should hold sustained bouts of physical activity below the anaerobic threshold, about 70% of maximal oxygen intake. The maximal oxygen intake also indicates the likely fatigue threshold; over an 8-h day, fatigue is likely to develop if the average energy consumption amounts to more than about 40% of maximal oxygen intake (51,113). In the very old individual, maximal oxygen intake scores drop to such a low level that oxygen transport can become the main factor limiting independent living. The critical level for functional independence is generally a peak oxygen transport of about 12–14 ml/kg · min, although in some patients with chronic cardiac disease apparent maxima as low as 7–10 ml/kg · min have been reported (120,121).

Young-old

Choice of Test Equipment. The young-old are usually well able to undertake the laboratory tests of aerobic exercise adopted for younger individuals—treadmill walking, cycle ergometry, and stair climbing. However, due allowance must be made for the fact that many even of the young-old have not undertaken vigorous exercise recently. Relative to a young person, the senior citizen must thus be allowed more time for familiarisation with both the laboratory and the test equipment. For example, when walking on a treadmill, an older person adopts an awkward posture and tends to take small and hesitant steps, in part because of fear of falling. However, a more normal gait is restored with opportunity for practice of the test. Likewise, the older person often makes clumsy initial attempts to operate a cycle ergometer.

The knee joints may have become unstable with aging, and a light hand support is often welcomed by an older person, both for treadmill walking and for stepping. The use of such support alters the energy cost of movement, and the oxygen consumption must thus be measured directly rather than predicted from the supposed intensity of exercise, as is sometimes done when using the Bruce treadmill protocol or a simple step test. If a treadmill is not available, jogging in place has been suggested as a possible alternative method of exercising those who are reasonably fit (99); again, a measurement of oxygen consumption would be needed for such a test to have any precision. A final alternative for those with very unstable knees or a history of back problems is the use of a cycle ergometer, although maximal effort may then be limited by quadriceps weakness, and in some older men a varicocoele or prostatic problems are a further source of difficulty.

Direct Maximum Testing. As in a younger person, the most accurate method of determining maximal oxygen intake is to carry a progressive exercise test to voluntary exhaustion. A short bout of maximal effort is often tolerated surprisingly well by middle-aged and young-old patients (25a,128,142). The only changes of treadmill protocol that are necessary relative to a younger person are a longer period of warm-up, smaller increments of speed or slope per test stage, and a lower peak rate of working. If a stepping bench is chosen as the means of exercise, a step height of 35–40 cm rather than 45 cm may suffice to elicit maximum effort, and the use of the lower step may also be desirable because of a limited range of motion at the hip joint.

In healthy elderly volunteers, a traditional "plateau" of oxygen consumption can be demonstrated in as many as three-quarters of those undertaking a maximal stress test on the treadmill (128), although because the maximal oxygen intake decreases with age, the usually accepted precision of plateau demonstration (<2 ml/kg · min increment of oxygen consumption with an increment of power output) may require review in older patients. The proportion of plateau values has been rather low in some elderly samples (142), but the peak oxygen intake data for a given patient have nevertheless remained quite reproducible from one test day to another, showing a test/retest correlation as high as 0.90. Unfortunately, the ancillary criteria of maximal effort (peak heart rate, blood lactate concentration, and respiratory gas exchange ratio) become more fallible in an old person, so that in some individuals where a plateau reading cannot be elicited, the only option is to report the peak voluntary effort (Table 1).

If maximal exercise tests are conducted on a cycle ergometer, the peak performance of an elderly person is commonly halted by complaints of local weakness and fatigue in the quadriceps muscle rather than by the intended central circulatory limitation (120,121). The cycle ergometer values for directly measured or predicted peak oxygen intake thus tend to show a steeper age-related decline than the corresponding treadmill or step-test data (6).

Submaximal Exercise Tests. Because of fears about test safety, some authors have attempted to predict the maximum performance of older patients from data obtained during submaximum exercise. Unfortunately, such predictions (which are already imprecise in young adults) become progressively more unsatisfactory with aging (Table 2), since the maximum heart rate (an essential element in most prediction formulas) shows a large and very variable decrease with aging (3). The coefficient of variation for heart rate predictions of maximal oxygen intake in 65-year-old subjects may be 15–25%, sometimes with a superimposed systematic error (120,121). Attempts to estimate oxygen consumption from the rate of working are also unsatisfactory in the elderly. Treadmill walking is often mechanically inefficient owing to a

Table 1 Criteria of Maximal Effort Observed in Sample of 26 Men and 29 Women of Average Age 65 Years During Treadmill Testing

	Δ Plateau oxygen intake ≤1 ml/kg·min ≤2 ml/kg·min (%)	Δ Plateau ≤2 ml/kg/min (%)	Δ Plateau heart rate ≤5 beats/min (%)	Respiratory gas exchange ratio ≥1.15 (%)	Respiratory gas exchange ratio ≥1.00 (%)	Arterial blood lactate ≥8.8 mM/L (%)	Peak heart rate ≥160 beats/min (%)	Peak heart rate ≥165 beats/min (%)	Systolic blood pressure ≥200 Torr (26.7 kPa) (%)
Men									
Fair effort (n = 7)	14.2	42.8	28.6	0	85.7	25.0	42.8	14.2	57.1
Good effort (n = 19)	63.2	78.9	63.2	36.8	100.0	77.8	84.2	68.4	57.9
All male subjects (n = 26)	50.0	69.2	53.8	26.9	96.2	68.2	73.1	53.8	57.7
Women									
Fair effort (n = 9)	33.3	44.4	33.3	0	55.6	11.1	44.4	22.2	33.3
Good effort (n = 20)	55.0	75.0	75.0	20.0	80.0	50.0	60.0	35.0	35.0
All female subjects (n = 29)	48.2	65.5	62.1	13.8	72.4	37.9	55.2	31.0	34.5

Source: Based on data of Ref. 127. From Ref. 120; used with permission.

Table 2 Errors in the Prediction of Maximal Oxygen Intake in the Elderly
(for sample of average age 65 years, using the Åstrand nomogram)

Test method	Sex and N	Predicted $\dot{V}O_{2\,max}$ (L/min)STPD	Measured $\dot{V}O_{2\,max}$ (L/min) STPD	Discrepancy $\dot{V}O_{2\,max}$ (L/min) STPD	Percentage error
Cycle erg., 4 min/load {	13M	1.72 ±0.36	2.27 ±0.42	−0.56 ±0.33	−24.7 ±14.5
	17F	1.37 ±0.36	1.62 ±0.17	−0.25 ±0.26	−15.4 ±16.0
Treadmill 3 min/load {	26M	2.11 ±0.38	2.27 ±0.36	−0.16 ±0.35	−7.0 ±15.4
	29F	1.83 ±0.43	1.60 ±0.22	0.23 ±0.41	14.3 ±25.6

Source: Based on data of Ref. 127. From Ref. 120; used with permission.

short-paced, tentative pattern of stepping, and the energy cost of the activity may be further modified relative to anticipated values if the patient clutches the handrail while walking. Likewise, stair climbing is often performed awkwardly, while stiff joints and lack of recent familiarity with cycling give a mechanical efficiency for cycle ergometry that is less than the value of 23% normally assumed in young subjects (111,120). A final variable is medication; old people consume a wide range of prescribed and nonprescribed drugs. Some agents, such as β-blockers, impair the heart rate response to a given intensity of exercise, precluding the use of submaximum tests which are based upon heart rate readings. Possible alternatives are a determination of ventilatory threshold (152) or a rating of perceived exertion (13).

In middle-old patients, physicians are increasingly reluctant to require vigorous test exercise, as a large proportion of such populations show electrocardiographic abnormalities that would contraindicate vigorous exercise in a younger person (129). During the Canada Fitness Survey (18), for instance, 19% of subjects in the age 60–69 category saw themselves as unable to perform a simple submaximal step test, and a total of 55% of potential subjects in the same age category were "screened out" by the health professionals who were conducting the tests (18,118). Equally, if testing is conducted in the laboratory, effort tends to be halted because of symptoms or electrocardiographic findings that appear dangerous to the patient or the supervising physician. While a "symptom-limited" test probably remains useful for exercise prescription, it inevitably lacks scientific precision.

Possible alternatives to a laboratory physical assessment, which avoid the risk and the potential criticism that testing has provoked a cardiac catastrophe, are (a) to observe the range of normal daily activities (71), (b) to measure the normal rate of walking (8,17,26,27), or (c) to determine the heart rate which is developed at a moderate walking speed such as 1.3 m/s (9,27). The coefficient of correlation between walking speed and maximal oxygen intake is unfortunately quite weak, and certainly does not allow the observer to characterize the aerobic fitness of an individual patient. For example, Cunningham et al. (26) reported a correlation coefficient of only -0.25 when walking speeds were compared with maximal oxygen intakes over a broad age range from 19 to 66 years. The correlation with maximal oxygen intake was indeed only slightly greater than that with age itself (-0.13). Bassey et al. (9) noted that the walking speed was also influenced by the strength of the calf muscles. In subjects over the age of 65 years, correlation coefficients of 0.41 and 0.36 linked strength and walking speed in men and women respectively.

In very old individuals, physical limitations may preclude any type of testing that requires the patient to stand. Smith and Gilligan (137) proposed the adoption of a progressive step test that could be performed while the patient was seated in a straight-backed chair. Their test augmented metabolism progressively from an initial figure of 2.3 to a final value of 3.9 METs (ratios to basal metabolic rate). The mechanical efficiency is inevitably very variable for seated exercise, being affected among other things by habitual posture and thigh length. In order to draw precise conclusions from such a test, direct measurements of oxygen consumption are needed. Unfortunately, limited dentition makes it very difficult for old people to use a mouthpiece, and hollowed cheeks may also limit the effectiveness of gas collection if a face mask is substituted. Nevertheless, the peak MET value that a patient can reach gives some indication of both the potential to initiate an exercise program and the subsequent prognosis.

A second possible method of evaluating the aerobic fitness of the very old is to assess their ability to perform specific activities of daily living (71). This approach lacks scientific precision, since the tasks that are accomplished depend greatly upon the determination of the individual concerned; however, an inventory of this sort may at least allow a ranking of aerobic fitness and provide some indication of activities that the individual is likely to undertake.

Electrocardiographic Changes

Clinicians commonly set great diagnostic and prognostic store by the electrocardiographic response to exercise. As patients become older, an ever-increasing proportion of the total sample show exercise-

induced abnormalities of ECG waveform and rhythm (90a,129), including ST segmental depression (Fig. 1) and premature ventricular contractions. However, as in younger patients, questions remain about
the reliability and the validity of such information (112), and if a silent
ischemic abnormality is detected, the subsequent management of the
individual is much more controversial than at a younger age.

It has been argued that because of an increased prevalence of
clinically significant myocardial ischemia, the number of false-positive

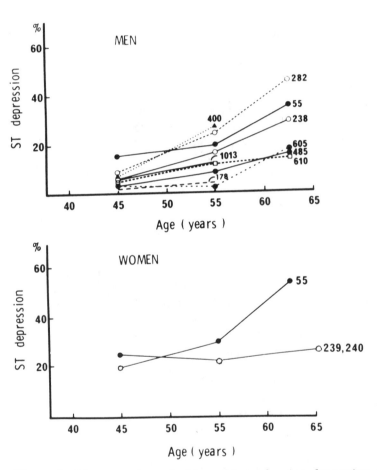

Figure 1 The percentage of older subjects showing depression of the ST-
segment of the electrocardiogram during or following maximal or near-
maximal exercise. For details of references corresponding to individual lines,
see source. (From Ref. 120; used with permission.)

results should be lower in the elderly than in a younger person. At first inspection, Bayes' theorem would certainly support such a hypothesis. However, other complicating factors are a high incidence of resting ECG abnormalities and an overall physical weakness that prevents many of the frail elderly from reaching a diagnostically adequate level of cardiovascular stress. Moreover, many older people take diuretics on a regular basis, and the resultant potassium excretion can influence both ECG appearances and vulnerability to an abnormal cardiac rhythm. The use of other medications, such as β-blockers and calcium channel antagonists, also influences the extent of ST depression by altering exercise heart rate and/or by modifying myocardial contractility. For these various reasons, a fair number of the apparently abnormal records seen in older people are still false-positive responses (129). In general, an abnormal ECG is more likely to be a true-positive result if it is associated with other cardiovascular risk factors, abnormalities of heart rhythm, a low peak heart rate, failure of the blood pressure to show the anticipated rise, chest pain, and a low peak power output or maximal oxygen intake. False-positive tests can generally be clarified by further laboratory investigation, but at substantial cost to the patient or insuring agency.

A proportion of exercise-induced ECG changes undoubtedly reflect the onset of significant myocardial ischemia, with implications of an adverse prognosis. The questions that thus arise are (a) is it safe for individuals with positive exercise ECG findings to undertake regular bouts of physical exercise, (b) should continuous electrocardiographic monitoring be provided during such exercise, and (c) can the threshold for the appearance of such abnormalities be used as a guide to an appropriate intensity of prescribed exercise?

Safety

The safety of appropriately prescribed exercise is increasingly recognized for younger patients, even when they have established cardiovascular disease. A survey of 167 supervised cardiac rehabilitation programs in the United States (143) provided data on 51,303 patients covering a total of 2,351,916 person-hours of prescribed exercise. Results were very similar to our own personal experience, where some 5000 "postcoronary" patients have been exercised regularly for up to 20 years (125). Van Camp et al. (143) noted a total of 21 incidents of cardiac arrest and eight myocardial infarctions across the 167 programs; the incidence rates were 1 per 111,996 patient-hours of exercise for cardiac arrest, 1 per 293.990 patient-hours for myocardial infarction, and 1 per 783,972 patient-hours for a fatality (Table 3). The risks were

Table 3 The Incidence of Cardiovascular Complications During Cardiac Rehabilitation Programs in Relation to Program Size

Program size (PH)	No. of reports	Patients	PH	Cardiac arrests (10^6 PH)	Fatal (10^6 PH)	Total MI (10^6 PH)
<5000	51	8582	115,152	8.7	0	0
5000–24.999	94	30335	1,135,157	8.8	0.9	4.4
>25,000	22	12386	1,101,607	9.1	1.8	2.7
Total	167	51303	2,351,916	8.9	1.3	3.4

PH = Patient hours.
Source: Based on data of Ref. 143.

apparently similar for both large- and small-scale programs, and were uninfluenced by the availability of continuous electrocardiographic monitoring.

While we presently lack such large-scale statistics for the elderly person who has not sustained an infarct, it is unlikely that they are at greater risk than the postcoronary patients, provided that they undertake a similar pattern of moderate, progressive activity appropriate to their initial physical condition. Exercise is thus a very safe recommendation to make to an older person—indeed, Vuori and associates (151) have suggested that because the elderly are less likely to undertake vigorous feats for which they are ill prepared, the relative risk of death from either "nonstrenuous" or "strenuous" exercise is lower in the 50- to 69-year-old group than in younger age categories (Table 4). Moreover, if account is taken of all 24 h of the day, a modest increase of physical activity remains a less dangerous recommendation than prolonged sitting or bed rest (133). Certainly, it would seem inappropriate to restrict the activity of middle-old or very old patients on the basis of asymptomatic electrocardiographic abnormalities. Why persuade an 80-year-old man who enjoys a weekly game of golf that it would be "safer" to give up this habit? What social good would be served, even if the patient lived 5 years longer, but spent 4 of those years paralyzed by a severe stroke, and unable to recognize his golfing friends?

Continuous Monitoring

Motivation to regular and progressive physical activity is a substantial problem in elderly patients. Given also the demonstrated safety of exercise, it is counterproductive to suggest that physical activity

Table 4   Influence of Age upon the Risk of Sudden Cardiovascular Death
During Exercise

	Age (years)					
	20–39		40–49		59–69	
Type of exercise	D	RR	D	RR	D	RR
Walking	0	0	37.9	0.2	11.7	0.5
Jogging	14.3	9.3	4.5	4.7	6.7	0.7
Nordic skiing	10.0	9.3	1.3	9.0	0.6	6.1
Ballgames	11.9		3.8		6.2	
Nonstrenuous exercise	26.0	2.5	5.2	3.6	3.4	2.5
Strenuous exercise	6.1	10.0	1.2	13.1	1.2	5.3

Abbreviations: D, number of deaths per 10^6 exercise sessions; RR, relative risk for the
given age group (observed deaths/expected deaths for same time interval).
Source: Based on data of Ref. 151.

requires detailed, minute-by-minute electronic surveillance; such monitoring (45) immediately suggests that exercise is an abnormal and
dangerous process rather than a feature of normal life.

Several studies have suggested that ambulatory electrocardiographic monitoring is an unnecessary luxury, even for patients with a
history of previous myocardial infarction. DeBusk et al. (130) arranged
home exercise programs for cardiac patients up to the age of 70 years;
the only personal monitoring came from heart rate monitors and
twice-weekly telephonic transmission of the ECG signal to the
supervising clinic. None of the patients who were under observation
developed any cardiovascular complications over a 26-week period of
vigorous exercise, although it must be admitted that a number of
patients with high-risk conditions such as congestive failure and
unstable angina were excluded from their trial.

Prescription Ceiling

In prescribing exercise for an elderly person, it seems prudent to set an
exercise "ceiling" at an intensity a little below that which provokes
symptoms (angina, abnormalities of pulse rhythm), signs (such as a
fall in blood pressure), or major electrocardiographic abnormalities.

On the other hand, ECG abnormalities give only a statistical indication of cardiovascular risk, even when they are considered in con-

junction with adverse symptoms and signs. The most commonly discussed finding (a deep, >0.2 mV, horizontal or downsloping depression of the ST-segment) is associated with about a twofold increase in the risk of exercise-induced cardiac incidents (114,115). Moreover, the safe ceiling of energy expenditure varies widely with the circumstances of exercise, including the type of activity that has been prescribed (the ceiling is lower for activities that involve vigorous contraction of relatively small muscles, an awkward posture, straining, or movements of the arms above the head), the general condition of the individual (the ceiling is lower if there is a history of recent illness or intercurrent emotional stress), and environmental conditions (for example, the ceiling is lower if the participant faces emotional excitement from competition or exposure to extreme heat or cold).

Blood Pressure Responses

Normally, exercise is associated with a progressive rise of systolic blood pressure, in an attempt to sustain the perfusion of muscles that are contracting at a large fraction of their maximal force (60,75,106). The cardiovascular response is most obvious during isometric straining against a closed glottis; in such circumstances large increases of blood pressure can develop within a minute. However, a slower increase of systolic pressure is also seen over 10–15 min of vigorous endurance activity. The resultant increase of cardiac afterload is one factor contributing to a decrease of stroke volume when older people are performing heavy physical work (Fig 2). If the myocardium has been weakened by the formation of scar tissue and chronic fibrotic degeneration, or left ventricular contractility is impaired by a relative myocardial ischemia, there may be not only a decrease of stroke volume, but also difficulty in sustaining blood pressure at high work rates.

Failure of the systemic blood pressure to show the normally anticipated rise over a progressive exercise test is an ominous warning that effort should be halted urgently (2). A meta-analysis (42) has further shown that an abnormally low blood pressure response to exercise indicates a poor prognosis following myocardial infarction.

Postural hypotension immediately following vigorous activity is a third problem, particularly if there is some initial tendency to hypotension (28,76). Factors predisposing to a decrease of blood pressure after exercise include "drop" attacks from arthritic compression of a vertebral artery (94), a substantial rise of core temperature, prolonged swimming, lack of an adequate warm-down, and standing in hot and

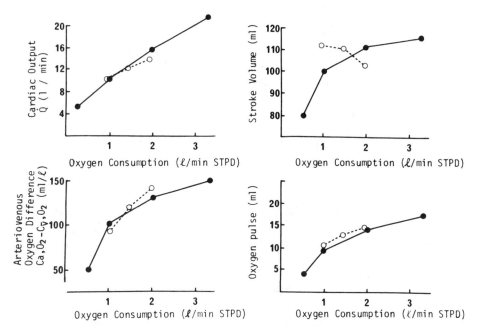

Figure 2 A comparison of exercise responses between young adults (solid line, average age 25 years) and elderly subjects (interrupted line, average age 65 years). (Graphs drawn from data of Ref. 91; first published in Ref. 112. Used with permission.)

humid shower areas (112). Consciousness may be lost, with an associated risk of physical injury, and the decrease of coronary perfusion may precipitate cardiac arrhythmia and sudden death. The few reported fatalities in cardiac exercise programs have tended to arise in shower areas following the exercise session (86,112).

If there is a history of fainting, it may be worth undertaking a tilt-tolerance test. A person with good cardiovascular reflexes typically shows a small increase of systemic blood pressure in response to sudden assumption of the upright position. In examining the blood pressure responses of the frail elderly, it is important to obtain full details of any continuing medication, as many commonly prescribed drugs modify the blood pressure during and following exercise.

Muscle Function

In principle, standard laboratory approaches can be applied to the assessment of isometric, isokinetic, and isotonic muscle function (113) in young-old and middle-old patients, but such procedures are of doubtful value in the very-old. In practice, observations on senior citizens have commonly been limited to measurements of peak isometric force on a few key muscle groups (120), although isokinetic data are now becoming available (36,43) (Table 5). The hand-grip dynamometer score, although important in a functional context, does not provide a good indication of overall body strength; moreover, results are lower if overall weakness precludes measurements in a standing position (141).

It is important that testing be preceeded by enquiry regarding musculoskeletal disorders affecting the joints under investigation. There must also be an adequate warm-up, to avoid causing musculoskeletal injuries during testing. Finally, prolonged straining against a closed glottis is to be avoided because of the associated rise of systemic blood pressure. Relative to young subjects, longer periods of practice may be needed to reach stable scores, not only during the dynamometric or a tensiometric determination of maximum isometric force, but also in determinations of isokinetic strength (using a device such as the Cybex II or the Kin-Com isokinetic tester), and during measurements of isotonic strength (using, for instance, an incremental dynamic lifting task).

Under field conditions, explosive strength could theoretically be evaluated by a squatting jump (Table 6), a standing broad jump, or a jump-and-reach test, although unstable knees, poor coordination, impaired balance, and lack of recent practice of the skill frequently lead to scores that are unrepresentatively low relative to actual strength. A combination of muscle strength and endurance can be assessed from such items as timed push-ups and sit-ups (118), but such tests are hard upon an aging vertebral column, and may give rise to an undesirably large rises of systemic blood pressure.

Table 5 Isokinetic Torque About Knee Joint at Rotation Speeds of 180 and 240°/s (data for three groups of older males)

Average age (years)	Knee flexion		Knee extension	
	180°/s (Nm)	240°/s (Nm)	180°/s (Nm)	240°/s (Nm)
57.1	47.9	47.9	66.0	65.3
63.1	45.0	34.9	68.1	57.4
74.0	34.6	28.1	51.1	42.4

Source: Adapted from Ref. 43; used with permission.

Table 6 Force and Power Developed During Squatting Jump in Men of
Various Ages

Age (years)	N	Body mass (kg)	Average Force (N)	Average power W/leg/kg
18–28	35	80	618	23
29–40	16	79	508	17
41–49	18	77	435	14
54–65	4	76	320	19
71–73	11	74	315	7

Source: Based on data of Bosco, C., and Komi, P.V., *Eur. J. Appl., Physiol.*, 43: 209–219 (1980).

The observed scores for most laboratory and field tests of strength depend heavily upon the motivation of the subject, and more encouragement may be need to elicit maximal effort in an old person than in someone who is younger. Pain may also limit effort about an arthritic joint. Rapid spinal movements are probably unwise in those with a history of back problems, and in the frail elderly with signs of osteoporosis such as a "dowager's hump," there is also some risk that overvigorous muscular efforts could cause a fracture.

DeVries (31) has suggested that problems of motivation and physical injury can be avoided by relating submaximal force development to the corresponding level of electromyographic activity; a fit person is able to develop a large force with less electromyographic activity. Functional capacity may also provide some guide to muscle performance in the middle-old and the very old. The relationship of triceps surae strength to walking pace (9) has already been noted. A survey of the activities of daily living may be informative (Table 7). One particularly important item is the ability of the quadriceps to lift the body mass from a chair or a toilet seat (120,121).

Table 7 Percentage of U.S. Adults of Various Ages Who Have Difficulty in
Doing Heavy Housework

Sample	Age				
	65–69	70–74	75–79	80–84	85 % over
Men	9.8	13.0	14.6	18.9	33.3
Women	21.8	27.3	33.2	41.7	54.2

Source: U.S. National Center for Health Statistics, Advanced data report 133 (1987).

Body Composition

One simple assessment of body composition is based upon the patient's weight-for-height relative to actuarial tables. Another approach is to determine the thickness of skin folds, or to carry out hydrostatic weighing. Finally, there are various more sophisticated laboratory methods for the determination of lean tissue and bone density (123).

Actuarial Tables

While actuarial tables of "weight for height" or ratios of body mass to height^2 have some usefulness as a method of assessing obesity in younger sedentary individuals, there are several sources of difficulty in applying such norms to the elderly patient:

1. Special weighing devices are needed for subjects who have difficulty in standing (22). Alternatively, body mass can be estimated from calf (C) and arm circumference (AC), knee height (K), and subscapular skinfold thickness (SS) (22):

    For men, M = 0.98C + 1.16K + 1.73AC + 0.37SS(cm) − 81.69

    For women, M = 1.27C + 0.87K + 0.98AC + 0.40SS(cm) − 62.35

2. The setting of an "ideal weight" is complicated by a decrease of stature due to kyphosis and vertebral collapse; overall stature may need to be estimated from knee height K:

    For men, H = 2.20K(cm) − 0.04A(yr) + 64.19

    For women, H = 1.83K(cm) − 0.24A(yr) + 84.88

3. The "ideal weight" indicated in such tables applies to survival from the age when insurance was purchased, commonly as a young adult; however, it cannot necessarily be used to interpret the prognosis of individuals who are first weighed as senior citizens; indeed, the "optimum" body mass seems to rise slightly as a person becomes older (4).
4. Progressive muscle wasting and mineral loss from bones may give a normal total body mass in relation to standing height; a substantial accumulation of body fat has been masked by loss of muscle protein and bone calcium.

Skinfold Measurements

A second simple approach to body composition is to determine the thickness of representative double folds of skin and subcutaneous fat. Again, there are some specific problems when applying this technique to middle-old and very old individuals. The patient may be reluctant to shed the layers of overlying clothing necessary for the examination, and in any event undressing is a time-consuming operation at this age. Measurement errors tend to arise because the skin moves independently of subcutaneous fat if it is lifted from the body. Moreover, the overlying skin is thinner and more compressible than in a younger person, and the ratio of deep to superficial fat tends to be greater than in a younger individual (134); a given skinfold reading thus implies a greater amount of body fat in an older person.

All of these issues point to the need for age-specific formulas if an attempt is to be made to predict body density or total body fat from skinfold readings. The alternative preferred by many investigators is to interpret the skinfold data in their own right, but again age-specific norms are required (Table 8). Particular attention has recently been directed to the relative amounts of fat over the chest and the hips; if the ratio is high (the so-called masculine pattern of fat distribution), then the risk of ischemic heart disease is increased.

Underwater Weighing

For a long period, underwater weighing was regarded as providing the "gold standard" of body composition determinations at all ages (123). The body mass was partitioned between two arbitrary compartments ("fat" and "fat-free tissue"), and by assuming a fixed density for each of the two compartments, the percentage of body fat was estimated. However, the progressive loss of bone mineral greatly reduces the density of "lean" tissue in the elderly, thus limiting the validity of this approach (89).

Table 8 Age-related Increase of Skinfold Thicknesses at Selected Sites

Body site	Men	Women
Chin	+39%	+67%
Subscapular	31	77
Triceps	12	26
Suprailiac	8	59
Waist	62	101
Suprapubic	111	68
Chest	49	106
Knee	37	90
Average, all sites	25	51

Data from seven surveys of elderly adults compared with values for young adults approaching the "ideal" body mass, expressed as a percentage increase.
Source: From Ref. 120; used with permission.

Technically, it remains quite possible to undertake underwater weighing in the young-old, but there are increasing practical difficulties when dealing with middle-old and very old patients. Many old people are nervous about total immersion; there may be a history of blackouts, or hypotensive episodes on emerging from the water, and there is also a danger of slipping on wet decks, particularly if balance is impaired (120).

Because aging leads to an increased probability of chronic chest disease, and a variable deterioration of lung function, it is no longer possible to assume the residual gas volume, or to predict it from vital capacity, as is sometimes done in younger individuals. Chronic chest disease slows expulsion of air from the lungs if a forced expiration is performed when the individual is underwater, and a combination of uneven gas distribution and frank bronchospasm may delay the equilibration of helium or oxygen when estimating residual gas volume. The use of a closed-circuit breathing apparatus may also be complicated by poorly fitting dentures, and thus mouthpiece leakage. One helpful possibility is to measure the residual gas volume with the head out of the water (34).

Determinations of Lean Tissue

Methods of lean tissue determination based upon body potassium measurements (89) require access to a whole body counter, but have the important advantage that minimal cooperation is required from the patient. Difficulties of interpretation arise in senior citizens because the potassium content of lean tissue is lower than in younger adults (149), whereas the natural ^{40}K radiation emanating from the muscles may be screened from the scintillation counter by an increased thickness of the subcutaneous fat layer.

Likewise, estimates of lean tissue mass which are based upon the dilution of deuterated or tritiated water are complicated by the need for assumptions about the water content of the tissues, which changes substantially with aging (123).

Other Techniques

A variety of other methods of determining body composition are currently being introduced (123). Whole body impedance can be determined relatively simply, but if body fat content is to be predicted, some major assumptions must be made regarding the electrical conductivity of lean tissue and the geometry of the body parts.

These assumptions may not be valid for an older person because of differences in the amount and distribution of body water (68,144) and the thickness of fascial sheaths.

Flexibility

Flexibility assessment is usually only a minor part of a fitness evaluation in a younger individual. However, it become an increasingly important determinant of function as age increases.

One difficulty in assessing flexibility is that it is relatively specific to a given articulation (126). There are general effects of aging upon collagen (147), but the range of movement becomes increasingly joint specific in older people, as general changes and the impact of inherited local anatomical peculiarities are compounded by the effects of local arthritic change.

For those patients who are able to sit upon the floor, the standard sit-and-reach test (40,153) provides a stable and reproducible measure of spinal flexibility (Table 9). The range of movement at other joints can be assessed by a simple goniometer, but the results are inherently unreliable (126), since the observed range of motion depends largely on success in aligning the goniometer with the axis of rotation of the joint.

Balance

Balance is quite important to the function of the middle-old and the very old. Determinations in the laboratory can be based on stabilometer scores (113), or more precisely upon movements of the center of

Table 9 Scores for Sit-and-Reach Test of Flexibility at Various Ages

Age (years)	Men (cm)	Women (cm)
20–29	30.3	32.7
30–39	28.8	31.8
40–49	24.9	29.9
50–59	24.6	29.5
60+	22.1	27.6

Note: score of 25 cm implies the ability to touch the floor with the tips of the fingers while the knees are fully extended.
Source: Based on data of Canada Fitness Survey of 1981 (Fitness and Lifestyle Research Institute, 1983: Fitness and Lifestyle in Canada. Ottawa, Ontario).

gravity as observed by a force plate. In the field, approximate data can be obtained by timing the ability to stand on one leg with and without the eyes closed.

EXERCISE PRESCRIPTION FOR THE ELDERLY

We will now consider certain general principles of exercise prescription in the elderly, will discuss the issues of an appropriate intensity, frequency, and duration of activity in relation to the anticipated training response, will make an optimum exercise recommendation for the several categories of older patient, and will consider methods of sustaining motivation.

Principles of Exercise Prescription

Occasional Masters' class athletes may still want to stress themselves to the limit of their potential (93), but it is not the purpose of this book to discuss the training of such individuals. The majority of older people wish to participate in much milder forms of physical activity which are perceived as more appropraite to their age group (93a). In essence, they seek an exercise prescription that will maintain a reasonable level of physical condition and improve their general health.

Until recently, it was assumed that exercise had to be relatively intense either to restore function or to assure health benefit. However, this dogma is now coming under increasing scrutiny, particularly with respect to the elderly. Physicians are realising that in a very sedentary senior citizen, both functional capacity and health can be improved by quite modest increases of regular physical activity; moreover, gains of endurance performance may outstrip the observed gains of maximal oxygen intake (85). However, maximization of the ultimate training response depends upon the individual's continuing compliance with the exercise prescription, and upon a regular upward adjustment of the required training program by the supervising physician; as in younger individuals, a large part of the conditioning response is dissipated by 2–3 weeks of detraining or bed rest (25,90).

Intensity

It was for long held that at all ages, endurance training required regular 30- to 60-min sessions of large muscle exercise such as jogging, cycling, or vigorous swimming, pursued on at least alternate days at an initial intensity of 60–70% of maximal oxygen intake. It was further assumed that to maximize the gains of physical condition, there should be a progression of training intensity from 60–70% to 60–80% of maximal oxygen intake as soon as the condition of the patient permitted. The empirical data supporting this type of prescription is discussed in Chapter 1.

Another important determinant of the training response is the initial fitness of the individual relative to the intensity and frequency of the prescribed activity. In older individuals, some training occurs in response to relatively low intensities of effort. Thomas et al. (142) suggested that intensity and frequency of exercise explained only 10% of the training-induced gains of performance in the elderly.

Sidney and Shephard (130a) compared various self-selected patterns of training in sample of young-old volunteers with an average age of 65 years (Fig. 3). The largest increase of maximal oxygen intake (a dramatic 33% over 7 weeks) was seen in subjects who averaged 3.3 training sessions/week at an intensity rising from 60 to 80% of their maximal oxygen intake. However, ˙a slower increment of aerobic power (a useful 10% over 14 weeks) was seen in subjects who exercised frequently, but failed to progress beyond an intensity equivalent to 60% of maximal oxygen intake. The improvement of cardiovascular endurance in response to low-intensity training, was subsequently confirmed by Badenhop et al. (5); they found equal gains of maximal

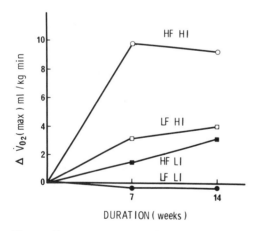

Figure 3 Influence of frequency (high versus low) and intensity of exercise (high versus low) upon the increase of predicted aerobic power of 65 year old adults participating in a 14 week training program. (From Sidney, K., and Shephard, R.J., *Med. Sci. Sports, 10*: 125–131 (1978); used with permission.)

oxygen intake with training at 30–45% and 60–75% of the maximum heart rate reserve. Likewise, Seals et al. (109) found some response to 6 months of training at 40% of the heart rate reserve, although further gains of physical condition developed when the intensity of training was increased to 75–80% of the heart rate reserve. Such observations have considerable practical importance for feeble middle-old and very-old patients, who initially may find great difficulty in exercising beyond 30–45% of their heart rate reserve.

Several recent reports have examined the influence of high- versus low-intensity training following myocardial infarction. In the first few months of rehabilitation, there seems little advantage to the adoption of a vigorous regimen (12,101). On the other hand, if training is continued for a year a more, intensive activity seems to induce a continuing increase of maximal oxygen intake (112), with an associated increase of stroke volume, whereas lighter exercise merely improves peripheral circulatory function (37,101). There is no evidence that regular exercise causes osteoarthritis (69,97,98), but an overvigorous program can aggravate preexisting disease. For instance, the impact stress on the knee joint is three to six times higher during jogging than during walking, even at an equivalent oxygen consumption (100). Further, the chances of a cardiovascular emergency (low with all patterns of physical activity [112] are likely to be particularly low if training is restricted to moderate rather than strenuous exercise) (151).

Finally, it should be emphasized that any specific benefit of intensive training is focused upon myocardial performance. In contrast, the consumption of fat is likely to be greater with prolonged bouts of moderate exercise than with shorter periods of very intensive effort, since fat cannot be metabolized under anaerobic conditions (113). Thus, if an objective of an exercise prescription is to reduce the amount of body fat, a program calling for moderate activity may be more effective than an intensive training plan.

Frequency and Duration of Effort

Recent investigations have stressed that the beneficial effects of exercise upon longevity are most likely to be realised if a critical volume of training is undertaken regularly every week. For example, the longevity of Harvard alumni (95) was increased with an added leisure energy expenditure of 2.2 MJ or more per week (500 kcal/week), and benefit was apparently maximized with an added weekly expenditure of 8.8 MJ (2000 kcal). It has further been shown that little benefit is obtained from irregular or seasonal bursts of activity (80); indeed, attempts to sustain a given exercise bout beyond the current capacity of the individual may provoke a heart attack (112).

Most of the training research which has been completed to date has focused upon young and middle-aged adults rather than the elderly. The beneficial impact of regular exercise upon the cardiovascular system (73) seems to be less marked in senior citizens than in younger people, possibly because the more vulnerable individuals have already died (95,96,102); for example, the gain of longevity decreases from about 2.5 years at age 35–39 years to 0.4 years at age 75–79 years (95). The optimum investment of training time in the various categories of elderly patient thus has yet to be defined. However, prolonged exercise sessions are impractical for the frail middle-old and very old. In order to undertake any substantial volume of training in such groups, it becomes necessary to break the prescribed activity into several sessions per day.

Recovery processes, such as the replenishment of glycogen stores and the repair of microtraumas proceed more slowly in the elderly, taking as long as 2 days to complete. The optimal frequency of exercise for older people might thus be three formal sessions per week, with provision for light walking on intervening days.

The optimum duration of cardiovascular training per session can be related to the prescribed intensity of effort in METs, using a formula of the type (7):

$$\text{duration (min)} = 218/\text{MET} - 60$$

For example, if an intensity of 2 METs is selected, then the optimum recommendation for an improvement of cardiovascular function would be to undertake 49 min of exercise per day. When physical activity is first renewed, a frail elderly person would lack the strength needed to continue a bout of conditioning for 49 min; the best plan might thus be to break the exercise prescription into several feasible segments of effort, with alternating periods of rest and light activity. Some authors have found a good response to a circuit training plan, where 1- to 2-min periods of light activity are interspersed between 5-min bouts at five or six different tasks (156).

If optimization of the serum lipid profile is seen as an important objective of training (84,157), data from middle-aged adults suggests the need for an energy expenditure equivalent to the walking or jogging of at least 18–20 km per week (35,59,155). In a senior citizen, such an amount of activity would best be distributed over at least three sessions per week.

Others aspects of training such as the strengthening of muscles (46) or the increase of joint flexibility may require relatively brief periods of definitive activity per session, whereas some objectives (such as increased social contacts) may be satisfied by program attendance without active participation.

Anticipated Response

On theoretical grounds, it might be anticipated that training would be less easily accomplished in a frail elderly person than in a younger adult. Functional adaptations to most types of stress are reduced with aging, and slower rates of protein synthesis could reduce the likelihood of morphological adaptations such as hypertrophy of cardiac or skeletal muscle. On the other hand, the physiological gap between the sedentary person and the active individual or continuing athlete remains much as in a younger individual (120), implying that while the old person may move more slowly from a sedentary to a trained state, the ultimate potential of the conditioning response is not greatly altered by aging.

It is difficult to make more formal comparisons of trainability between young and older individuals because the low initial fitness level of many old people in itself enhances their potential to develop a training response (56). The ideal experiment takes people of different ages but at same level of physical condition relative to their age-matched peers; if this is done, 65-year-old people seem to show at least the same percentage gains of fitness as younger individuals (31,5,31,47,130a), although in the short term (14 weeks), their absolute response is less than in a younger sample. Certainly training cannot restore tissue that has been destroyed by disease, but it can maximize residual function.

IDEAL PROGRAM

The form of the ideal exercise prescription must plainly be tailored carefully to both the physical and the medical condition of the individual patient. In essence, the search is for a recommendation that is not only safe, but also effective and sufficiently motivating to give a good chance of sustained compliance.

Effectiveness

An effective prescription aims to check the commonly observed age-related deterioration of cardiovascular function and muscular strength, to maintain flexibility, and to counter osteoporosis, while serving social and mood-elevating functions.

Cardiovascular Function

Cardiovascular function is improved by any training program that involves a substantial fraction of the body musculature—for example, regular walking, cross-country skiing, or vigorous swimming. If the patient is unable to stand, a considerable cardiovascular stimulus can still be developed using the muscles of the arms and shoulder girdle (124). For instance several arm and wheelchair ergometers are now available (124), and McNamara et al. (87) have described chair exercises to mimic both cycling and rowing.

Many elderly patients have undertaken almost no activity for many years, and in such individuals, some cardiovascular stimulus initially results from heart rates in the range 110–120 beats/min, although gains of condition quickly plateau unless the intensity of exercise is increased as fitness improves. Some patients have difficulty in palpating their heart rates accurately. Other practical guidelines to an appropriate intensity of effort are a level of activity that is perceived as "somewhat hard," that induces some sweating, and that induces some breathlessness while allowing conversation to continue. Initially, individual exercise bouts may be for periods of 10–15 min, but as condition improves the patient should be encouraged to extend the duration of each session to 30–60 min, using an intensity-related equation of the type discussed above.

Muscle Function

At any given fraction of the patient's maximum voluntary force, isometric exercise gives a similar rise of systemic blood pressure in young and older adults (106). Many early exercise prescriptions neglected to develop or even to sustain muscular strength because of fears of provoking an excessive rise of blood pressure. However, an exclusive cardiovascular focus (for example, exclusive walking or slow jogging) is undesirable, and can actually lead to a weakening of muscles, particularly in the upper half of the body.

Both cardiac patients and the young-old can undertake the full range of isotonic, isometric, and circuit exercises that younger adults use to develop muscle function, provided that individual muscular contractions are not held for more than a few seconds, and an adequate recovery interval is allowed between contractions (39,62). For a middle-old or very old person with limited mobility, muscle condition can still be improved by tensing one muscle group against another, or pressing periodically against the back of a chair or a bed board. Weights such as books can also be secured to a short plank which is balanced on the ankles; raising of this weight then provides a valuable stimulus to the leg muscles.

Flexibility

Era (38) has argued that when prescribing exercise for the elderly, attention should be paid to balance, coordination, agility, joint flexibility, and reaction speed. The leisure activities of the average senior citizen are unlikely to take all of the major joints through their full range of motion, and the patient should thus be encouraged to exercise all major joints on a regular basis. The mobility of most joints can be improved by a combination of flexibility exercises and dance-type movements (74).

If individual joints have become painful or unstable, weight-supported activities in a heated swimming pool provide a useful component of training (66,70,116). Particularly where movements are becoming restricted, it may also be helpful to engage in gentle stretching at the extremes of motion, using either the body weight or a partner as the driving force for such stretching. However, sudden, jerky movements could cause injury, and are to be avoided.

Osteoporosis

The precise pattern of exercise needed to reduce the risk of osteoporosis is still under investigation (107). The loss of bone mineral in astronauts during actual and simulated space missions suggests that one important element conserving bone density is normal gravitational stimulation, although Smith et al. (135) claimed that 80-year-old subjects gained some protection from chair exercises at 1.5–3.0 METs.

Walking provides a good stimulus to bones of the lower limbs, the hips, and the spine, but weights must be held in the hands if the arms are also to receive adequate stimulation. Likewise, it is probable that swimming and water-supported gymnastics will not provide an appropriate stimulus to strengthen the bones.

Mood Elevation

An elevation of mood may arise from the secretion of endorphins and other hormones (48), but elderly subjects are unlikely to take the prolonged and intense exercise necessary to induce such a response.

A further factor improving mood is the arousal associated with increased proprioceptive stimulation. The associated intensity of activity is a much more practicable goal for all categories of seniors;

indeed, some proprioceptive stimulation could be realized by a patient even while sitting in bed.

Other factors elevating the mood state of the exerciser are the increased opportunities for social contacts provided by some types of group exercise, and the pleasant esthetic experience of, for example, a walk in the country.

Irrespective of mechanisms, the end result is a lessening of anxiety and depression (52).

Overall Recommendation

An appropriate program for the senior citizen will include a fairly lengthy warm-up, endurance work involving a variety of the large muscle groups, weight-bearing activity (if possible), some strengthening of major muscles by resisted activity, and an extended (10–15 min) cool-down period.

Motivation

Perhaps the most difficult part of any exercise program is continuing motivation of the participants. Even in young adults, the drop-out rate is very discouraging (117). Typically, as many as 50% of those initially recruited have left exercise programs after 6 months. In old people, poor memory and necessary interruptions of training by intercurrent illness give even poorer prospects. Unfortunately, gains of fitness cannot be stored (25,90), and benefit is thus realized only if the prescribed activity is repeated on a regular basis several times per week.

Factors in the retention of initial enthusiasm for exercise include a careful matching of the prescription to the goals, aptitudes, interests, and skill levels of the individual patient.

Goals

The primary goals of an older exerciser are usually an improvement of health, and (particularly in women) an increase of social contacts (130). The search of the younger person for activities that involve speed, danger, and demanding competition against others or self is much reduced. Emphasis should thus be placed upon linkages between the prescribed activities and health, preferably within the framework of a total health promotional "package." Feedback should be provided to participants in terms of gains in health-related components of fitness such as increased cardiovascular endurance or a reduction of body fat. Care should also be taken to allow adequate time for social interaction within the structure of any formal exercise classes without compromising training objectives.

Aptitudes

Habit has a strong influence upon behavior (44), and it can be helpful to build the exercise prescription around the past aptitudes and experience of the patient, using sporting equipment that may be hidden in the corner of an attic. However, much depends on the personality of the individual; in some instances, the poor current performance of a previously mastered skill can have a negative impact upon motivation.

Interests

It is vital that prescribed activities be matched with the interests of the patient—a solitary jogging prescription is unlikely to be accepted if the person concerned hates jogging, and is looking for social contacts; for such a person, pool or gymnasium exercise and folk games will be much more appropriate (145). On the other hand, an introverted person may react negatively to the somewhat artificial jollity of an exercise class (82), while showing a positive response to a graded walking prescription.

Skill and Fitness Levels

The person who drops out of an exercise program is typically obese and a heavy smoker (82,180). This reflects in part the lesser interest of such individuals in all aspects of health, but a further factor is that the gap between the skills and fitness levels of the participant and the expectations of the instructor has become too wide. Attempts to meet fitness and health demands are thus unsuccessful, with a negative impact upon both body image and motivation to continued participation (130).

It is sometimes helpful if exercise classes are taught by an older instructor, since such individuals tend to have more empathy for the problems of the elderly. Specific classes for the obese and those with low skill levels are further mechanisms of reducing embarrassment and setting goals that the patient perceives as attainable.

Other Motivational Tools

Regular positive feedback is most important to motivation. The form of feedback may be physiological (demonstration of an improvement in exercise test scores), psychological (words of encouragement), or symbolic (provision of T-shirts or pins for specific achievements within the capacity of participants). It may also be helpful to have the patient draw up a decision balance sheet, or to contract for the attainment of specific fitness goals (33).

Obstacles to exercise participation should be minimized—failing memory could be countered by telephone reminders and/or provision of transport to activity classes, and limited socioeconomic resources should be recognized by minimum-cost programs that avoid demands for the purchase of expensive clothing and equipment.

Finally, as much as possible of the prescribed exercise should be built into the normal activities of daily living; for example, the patient should be encouraged to walk rather than to drive to the store when buying a newspaper, and to use hand rather than power tools around the home and garden.

BENEFITS OF EXERCISE

Many of the accepted benefits of an active lifestyle apparently have a differential impact with aging. For example, the cross-sectional statistics of Hammond and Garfinkel (47a) show that the actuarial risk arising from a 20% excess of body mass drops from 225% of the standard value in men aged 40–49 years to 119% of standard at an age of 70–79 years; this may reflect not only an approach to the "square" part of the mortality curve (41), but also an increased influence of a loss of lean tissue upon total body mass and thus "ideal" weight. The same cross-sectional data suggest an increasingly adverse effect of physical inactivity (from 180% of standard mortality in sedentary men aged 40–49 years, and 131% in men aged 50–59 years, to 285% in men aged 70–79 years).

However, cross-sectional comparisons can be misleading. For example, those who report that they are still taking heavy exercise at the age of 70–79 years are presumably both a health-conscious and a healthy subsegment of the general population. On the other hand, longitudinal studies show progressively less impact of regular physical activity upon life expectancy in older cohorts of patients (95,102). Likewise, any encouragement that exercise gives to the adoption of a more general healthy lifestyle (for example, the cessation of smoking or a reduced consumption of saturated fat) could have progressively less effect on older patients, since many of those with inherited susceptibility to such risk factors have already died by the years of retirement.

Particular benefits of exercise in the elderly include (a) the maintenance of function, independence, and life quality; (b) the halting of osteoporotic changes; (c) social gains; and (d) relief of depression.

Independence

Regular physical activity has a positive impact upon a number of the common factors that contribute to a loss of independence in the elderly.

An active lifestyle averts an increase of body mass, but otherwise does not materially inhibit the progressive age-related deterioration of oxygen transport (the loss is 0.4–0.5 ml/kg · min per year in continuing athletes, only marginally less than in sedentary subjects [122]). However, regular exercise does move the individual from a sedentary to an active aging curve (55,122). An optimal training regimen can increase the maximum oxygen intake of a sedentary 65-year-old adult by as much as 10 ml/kg · min (128), and this is equivalent to a 20-year gain in what has been termed "functional aerobic age" (16). Thus, if the person had remained inactive, the maximum oxygen intake would have dropped to the critical threshold for independence (around 12–14 ml/kg · min) by the age of 80 years, but renewed physical activity may delay this situation to the age of 90 or even 100 years (Fig 4).

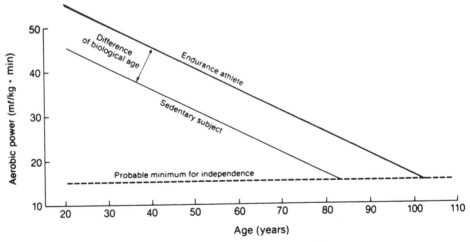

Figure 4   To illustrate the potential gain from an aerobic training program. In a sedentary subject, the maximal oxygen intake drops to the minimal value required for independent living (12–14 ml/kg/min) soon after the age of 80 years. However, involvement in an endurance training program moves the individual in the direction shown by the arrow, to the aging line for an endurance athlete. It now takes 10–20 years longer for the aerobic power to drop to the threshold required for independent living. (From Shephard, R.J., *Exercise Physiology*. B.C. Decker, Burlington, (1987); used with permission.)

Independence can also be threatened by a loss of muscular strength; for example, a senior may be unable to lift the body mass from a chair or a toilet seat. Again, there is no evidence that regular exercise can halt the progressive, age-related loss of lean tissue, but nevertheless training can increase strength by 10–15% (29,120). The active person thus follows a different aging curve from the person who is sedentary, and at any given calendar age the active patient remains much further from the limiting value of muscle strength and power needed for independence (81).

A third problem of advancing years is loss of movement at key joints. Flexibility becomes insufficient to allow such daily activities as climbing into a bath or dressing. Again, exercise does not reverse the aging process in ligamentous collagen, but if the main articulations are taken regularly through their full range of motion, the critical level of function for independent living may be conserved to a much greater age. Exercise cannot restore damaged articular surfaces, but a strengthening of the major muscles around an arthritic hip, knee, or ankle can substantially improve the stability of these joints, enabling continued performance of the vital activities of independent living.

A final important cause of loss of independence is a progressive deterioration of cognition. It is difficult to measure mental function quantitatively, but there is some evidence that the mental ability of an older person can be conserved by involvement in a regular physical activity program (14,104,127,139), probably by increasing cerebral arousal, and perhaps also by increasing cerebral perfusion.

Osteoporosis

Senescence is associated with a progressive loss of both mineral content and matrix from the bones (19,105), with a corresponding increase in the risk of fractures (50). There is now increasing evidence that regular, weight-bearing activity can check this process (1,15,20,67, 132,136).

Social Gains

For a variety of reasons that include a deterioration of the special senses, death of friends and relations, and increasing poverty, the social world of the middle-old and very old often becomes increasingly circumscribed (127). An exercise class provides a valuable occasion for friendly contact with other people, and can thus be very helpful in reversing this process of social disengagement.

Relief of Depression

Depression is a common accompaniment of aging. There are obvious physical, social, and economic reasons why the life of a senior citizen can be hard.

Many patients will explain that the reason they exercise regularly is in order to feel better. Experimental demonstration of the improved mood is more difficult, although some reports have claimed a lessening of anxiety and a relief of depression following adoption of a regular exercise program, particularly where patients were initially anxious or depressed (131,140). Possible mechanisms include greater arousal, new interests and social contacts, an improved body image, and a greater feeling of self-efficacy.

SAFETY OF EXERCISE

A discussion of the safety of exercise for the elderly inevitably raises potential dangers of physical injury, environmental hazards, infection, and death, which must be weighed against any gains of life expectancy and quality-adjusted life expectancy.

Despite the various potential benefits discussed above, most old people are cautious about exercising. With a few exceptions, they err by taking an inadequate dose of physical activity. The role of the physician should thus be to encourage rather than to discourage physical activity. Such a recommendation is clinically justifiable, since the risks for a 24-h period are lower for an active than for an inactive person (although there may be some transient increase of risk while the exercise is being performed [112,133]).

Because the patient is inherently cautious, exercise for the elderly is very safe. The main emphasis of any prescription must be to do just a little more than was accomplished safely in the preceeding week; if the new program can be accomplished without symptoms, then there is little need for detailed clinical surveillance. Nevertheless, a few simple precautions should be observed. The prescribed intensity of exercise should normally leave the patient with no more than a pleasant tiredness on the following day. Activities should be held below a level provoking deep ST segmental depression, frequent premature ventricular contractions, or a decline in systemic blood pressure. Moderation of the prescription is advisable during extremes of hot and cold weather; in both situations, the optimum arrangement is to move the exercise class to an air-conditioned facility. An excessive rise of blood pressure should be avoided by prohibiting the prolonged lifting of heavy weights and straining against a closed glottis. The impact stress on the knees and the vertebral column should be reduced by substituting walking for jogging. Violent twisting movements of the spine should be avoided, and situations predisposing to a fall should also be avoided, particularly in the frail elderly with disturbances of balance or a history of "drop attacks."

Injury

Even in young adults, well-conceived epidemiological surveys of injuries incurred in the various classes of sport and exercise are only beginning to appear. There is no great difficulty in accumulating sport-specific injury totals, but very little is known about the corresponding number of participants or the average period for which they were active. Nevertheless, many forms of vigorous physical activity have a substantial annual injury rate (111), including substantial numbers of preventable injuries; Koplan et al. (65) noted that as many as a third of participants in a 10-km race had been injured during the previous year.

Leg, ankle, and back injuries apparently occur with some frequency among elderly exercisers (10). About a half of Masters' competitors are injured in a typical year (58), with one participant in six needing to withdraw from competition for 4 weeks or more. One study of older individuals attending an outpatient sports medicine clinic suggested that in elderly subjects the majority of problems were due to overuse (Table 10), and only in 4% of consultations was surgical treatment required (83).

Violent muscular efforts and sudden twisting movements seem particularly undesirable, and straight leg lifts, traditional knee bends, and hyperextension of the back have also been criticized as increasing the likelihood of injury (78). Old people generally recognize their limitations, and relative to the young, they are less likely to engage in excessive competition; nevertheless, safety can be increased by age-specific leagues, simple modifications of the rules, and skillful "officiating" which slows the pace of a team game when necessary. With activities such as jogging the incidence of stress injuries rises sharply once a certain weekly distance—perhaps 40–50 km/week in a young adult—is exceeded (103). The influence of calendar or biological age on this injury threshold is unknown, but it seems likely that the tolerated distance will decrease with aging. On the other hand, most older people have less inclination to indulge in excessive and obsessional activity, and for this reason fewer old people may sustain injury (83).

Table 10 Type of Injuries Incurred by Older (mean age 57 years) and Younger (mean age 30 years) Patients Attending a Sports Injury Clinic

	Percent of Sample	
Diagnosis	older	younger
Tendinitis	25.3%	26.2%
Patellofemoral pain	10.9	22.6
Ligament sprain	7.9	12.6
Muscle sprain	7.0	9.0
Metatarsalgia	6.9	2.8
Osteoarthritis	6.6	1.7
Plantar fasciitis	6.6	2.5
Meniscal injury	5.4	1.4
Degenerative disc disease	4.8	1.5
Stress fracture	4.2	11.2
Morton's neuroma	3.2	0.5
Inflammatory arthritis	2.6	1.1
Vascular/compartment	1.5	0.3
Bursitis	1.0	2.2
Multiple diagnoses	2.3	1.3
Unknown	3.8	3.1
Total	100.0	100.0

Source: Matheson, G.O., MacIntyre, J.G., Taunton, J.E., Clement, D.B., and Lloyd-Smith, R., *Med. Sci. Sports Exerc.*, 21: 379–385 (1989).

A number of factors increase the risk of a mechanical injury in an elderly person. Poor vision, disturbed balance (23), unstable knee and hip joints, reduced foot-lift, postural hypotension, and drop attacks all increase the likelihood of slips and falls (94). Moreover, osteoporosis increases the likelihood of a fracture if a fall is sustained (11,88). Care must thus be taken to provide nonslip flooring, free of obstacles which could trip up the unwary. When playing competitive games, a reduction in the field and the acuity of vision plus some impairment of hearing increase the risk of collision with an opponent and/or moving or stationary obstacles (111). Careful design of an exercise facility can minimize such risks, although as age increases it may be wise to avoid forms of activity where there is a substantial risk of colliding with an opponent, a racquet, or a ball. Impairments of balance, attacks of unconsciousness, and hypotension on leaving the water may all increase the risks of swimming; handrails and nonslip flooring can reduce risks, and elderly subjects should avoid swimming alone. Pursuits such as cycling and downhill skiing also become inappropriate if balance is disturbed.

Environmental Hazards

Aging is associated with difficulty in adapting to all forms of stress, including extremes of both heat and cold.

In the heat, problems of a low general level of fitness and poor cardiovascular function (138) are compounded by a greater rate of body heat production (because of a lesser mechanical efficiency, more of the total energy expenditure appears as heat, and less as usable work). There is also a decreased secretion of sweat at any intensity of effort, (63), while accumulated heat is less readily eliminated because of an increased thickness of subcutaneous fat and poorer vascular regulation (64). Even moderate activity can cause fatalities in the frail elderly who are exposed to extremes of continental heat (92,108). Methods of combating heat and other environmental hazards are discussed in Chapter 1.

The elderly also have an increased vulnerability to the various general, local cutaneous, and local respiratory problems of a cold environment, including hypothermia, chilblains, frostbite, and exercise-induced bronchospasm. Because of poor general condition, it is not possible to work hard enough to avoid hypothermia under cold conditions. An excessive drop in core temperature also reflects difficulty in regulating blood flow distribution. Limited intramuscular stores of glycogen and an impaired shivering response further restrict the maximum rate of heat production. There may also be an impaired function of the cutaneous thermoreceptors, an inappropriate setting to the hypothalmamic thermostat (23a), a lesser capacity for cutaneous vasoconstriction (151a), treatment with vasodilator drugs that increase the rate of heat loss (9a), and in some instances lack of money to purchase adequate protective clothing.

One important factor predisposing the elderly to the peripheral effects of cold is a poor circulation. Loss of cutaneous sensitivity and lack of adequate clothing may again contribute to the development of lesions.

The frail elderly are also more vulnerable to the other environmental hazards discussed in Chapter 1. They are unwise to engage in underwater exploration, as even a brief loss of consciousness underwater is likely to be fatal. Care is need to avoid hypotensive episodes following normal swimming or pool exercises, and pools should be fitted with adequate handrails and nonslip decks (116). The moderate hypoxia of mountain resorts (3000–4000 m altitude) may be sufficient to provoke an attack of myocardial ischemia in the frail elderly. Finally, such individuals are particularly vulnerable if they attempt to exercise out-of-doors during bouts of severe air pollution.

Infections

There is increasing evidence that very strenuous bouts of physical activity may impair the function of the immune system, at least briefly (161,146); however, the elderly are unlikely to undertake exercise of this intensity. On the other hand, regular training may increase the resistance of the immune system to a single bout of vigorous exercise, and by increasing natural killer cell activity, it may protect against age-related deterioration of cell structure (79).

A combination of insipient diabetes, a poor blood supply to the skin, and a slow rate of healing increases the risk of serious staphylococcal infections of the skin, ulcers, and slow-healing abrasions. An older person must thus be very careful to avoid superficial injuries, to ensure cleansing and drying of the skin after exercising, and to monitor the healing of any minor skin injuries that are incurred.

Risk of Death, and Quality-adjusted Life Expectancy

When a middle-old or very old patient asks a physician for advice about exercising, the common reply is, "Be careful." However, such advice largely ignores both the limited life expectancy of an old person and the impact of being careful upon the quality of the remaining years of life. If there are no close relatives, and the prognosis for the ultracareful individual is nine years of partial dependency followed by a year of total dependency, then there is much to commend a more carefree attitude to life. Such a philosophy would recognize that on occasion exercise can apparently provoke death (112), while ameliorating overall prognosis; it would also note that an increase in the range of physical pursuits commonly enhances life quality, in part by maintaining the physical condition needed for independent living, and it would place more emphasis upon the quality than upon the length of life (53).

It is perhaps dangerous to draw conclusions from cross-sectional data, since results may be influenced by cohort effects; nevertheless, the figures of Vuori et al. (151) suggest that the relative risk of provoking sudden death by vigorous exercise is actually lower in a person aged 50–69 years than in a younger individual. Certainly, the dangers of exercise prescription for the elderly have been greatly overrated, and some authors have even suggested that it is the chair or bed-bound senior citizen who needs regular medical surveillance rather than the person who is prepared to increase their physical activity. A moderate, progressive exercise program is a safe and desirable recommendation, even for the person of advanced age.

REFERENCES

1. Aloia, J.F., Cohn, S.H., Ostuni, J.A., Cane, R., and Ellis, K. *Ann. Intern. Med.*, *89*: 356–358 (1978).
2. American College of Sports Medicine, *Guidelines for Graded Exercise Testing and Prescription*. Lea & Febiger, Philadelphia, (1986).
3. Andersen, K.L., Shephard, R.J., Denolin, H., Varnauskas, E. and Masironi, R., *Fundamentals of Exercise Testing*. World Health Organization, Geneva (1971).
4. Andres, R., in *Principles of Geriatric Medicine* (R. Andres, E.L. Bierman, and W.R. Hazzard, eds.) McGraw-Hill, New York; pp. 311–318 (1985).
5. Badenhop, D.J., Cleary, P.A., Schaal, S.F., Fox, E.L., and Bartels, R.L., *Med. Sci. Sports Exerc.*, *15*: 496–502 (1983).
6. Bailey, D.A., Shephard, R.J., and Mirwald, R.L., *Can J. Appl. Sport Sci.*, *1*: 67–78 (1976).
7. Barry, H.C., *Geriatrics, 34*: 155–162 (1986).
8. Bassey, E.J., Fentem, P.H., MacDonald, I.C., and Scriven, P.M., *Clin. Sci. Mol. Med.*, *51*: 609–612 (1976).
9. Bassey, E.J., Bendall, M.J., and Pearson, M., *Clin. Sci.*, *74*: 85–89 (1988).
9a. Besdine, R.W. and Harris, T.B., ALteration in body temperature (hypothermia and hyperthermia). *Principles of Geriatric Medicine*. R. Andres, E.L. Bierman, and W.R. Hazzard, eds. McGraw Hill, New York pp. 209–217 (1985).
10. Billings, R.A., Burry. H.C., and Jones, R., *Rheumatol. Rehabilit., (Lond.)*, *16*: 236–240 (1977).
11. Block, J.E. and Genant, H.K., in *Physical Activity, Aging and Sports* (R. Harris and S. Harris, eds.). Center for Studies of Aging, Albany, pp. 295–299 (1989).
12. Blumenthal, J.A., Rejeski, W.J., Walsh-Riddle, M., Emery, C.F., Miller, H., Roark, S., Ribisl, P.M., Morris, P.B., Brubacker, P., and Williams, R.S., *Am. J. Cardiol.*, *61*: 26–30 (1988).
13. Borg, G., in *Frontiers of Fitness* (R.J. Shephard, ed.). Thomas, Springfield, Illinois, pp. 280–294 (1971).
14. Bortz, W.M., *J.A.M.A.*, *248*: 1203–1208 (1982).
15. Brewer, V., Meyer, B.M., Keele, M.S., Upton, S.J., and Hagan, R.D., *Med. Sci. Sports Exerc.*, *15*: 445–449 (1983).
16. Bruce, R.A., in *Principles of Geriatric Medicine* (R. Andres, E.L. Bierman, and W.R. Hazzard, eds.). McGraw-Hill, New York, pp. 87–105.

17. Butland, R.J.A., Pang, J., Gross, E.R., Woodcock, A.A., and Geddes, D.M., *Br. Med. J., 284*: 1607–1608 (1982).

17a. Canada Health Survey. Ottawa: Health & Welfare Canada, 1982.

18. Canada Fitness Survey, *Fitness and Lifestyle in Canada.* Canadian Fitness and Lifestyle Research Institute, Ottawa (1983).

18a. Canada Health Survey. Ottawa: Health & Welfare Canada, 1982.

19. Chestnut, C.H., in *Principles of Geriatric Medicine* (R. Andres, E.L. Bierman, and W.R. Hazzard, eds.). McGraw-Hill, New York, pp. 801–812 (1985).

20. Chow, R.K., Harrison, J.E., Sturtridge, W., Josse, R., Murray, T.M., Bayley, A., Dornan, J., and Hammond, T., *Clin. Invest. Med., 10*: 59–63 (1987).

21. Chumlea, W.C., Roche, A.F., and Steinbaugh, M.L., *J. Am. Geriatr, Soc., 33*: 116–120 (1985).

22. Chumlea, W.C., Roche, A., and Mukherjee, D., *Nutritional Assessment of the Elderly Through Anthropometry.* Ross Laboratories, Columbus, Ohio (1987).

23. Claussen, C.-F., and Claussen, E., in *Physical Activity, Aging, and Sports* (R. Harris and S. Harris, eds.) Center for Study of Aging, Albany (1989).

23a. Collins, K.K., Dore, C., Exton-Smith, A.N., Fox, R.H., MacDonald, I.C., and Woodward, P.M. *Brit. Med. J.* (i) 353–356 (1977).

24. Comfort, A., *Lancet, 2*: 411–414 (1969).

25. Convertino, V., Hung, J., Goldwater, D. et al., *Circulation, 65*: 134–140 (1982).

25a. Cumming, G.R., and Borysyk, L.M., *Med. Sci. Sports, 4*: 18–22 (1972).

26. Cunningham, D.A., Rechnitzer, P.A., Pearce, M.E., and Donner, A.P., *J. Gerontol., 37*: 560–564 (1982).

27. Cunningham, D.A., Rechnitzer, P.A., and Donner, A.P., *Can. J. Aging, 5*: 19–26

28. Dambrink, J.H.A., and Wieling, W., *Clin. Sci., 72*: 335–341 (1987).

29. Davies, C.T.M., and White, M.J., *Gerontology, 1 29*: 19–25 (1983).

30. DeBusk, R.F., Houston, N., Haskell, W.L., Fry, G., and Parker, M., *Am. J. Cardiol., 44*: 1223–1229 (1979).

31. DeVries, H.A., *J. Gerontol., 25*: 325–336 (1970).

32. DeVries, H.A., *Physiology of Exercise.* 4th Ed. W.C. Brown, Dubuque, Iowa (1986).

33. Dishman, R., *Exercise Adherence: Its Impact on Public Health.* Human Kinetics, Champaign, Illinois (1987).

34. Donnelly, J.E., and Sintek, S.S., in *Perspectives in Kinanthropometry* (J.A.P. Day, ed.). Human Kinetics, Champaign, Illinois (1986).

35. Drygas, W., Jegler, A. and Kunski, H., *Int. J. Sports Med., 9*: 275–278 (1988).

36. Dummer, G.M., Clarke, D.H., Vaccaro, P., Vander Velden, L., Goldfarb, A.H., and Sockler, J.M., *Res. Quart., 56*: 97–110 (1985).

37. Ehsani, A.A., Martin, W.H., Heath, G.W., and Coyle, E.F., *Am J. Cardiol., 50*: 246–254 (1982).

38. Era, P., *Scand. J. Soc. Med.*, *39* (Suppl.): 1–77 (1987).
39. Franklin, B.A., Hellerstein, H.K., Gordon, S. and Timmis, G.C., *J. Cardiopulm. Rehabil.*, *6*: 62–79 (1986).
40. Frekany, G., and Leslie, D., *Gerontologist*, *15*: 182–183 (1975).
41. Fries, J.F., *N. Engl. J. Med.*, *303*: 130–135 (1980).
42. Froelicher, V.F., Perdue, S., Pewen, W., and Risch., M., *Am. J. Med.*, *83*: 1045–1054 (1987).
43. Gandee, R., Hollering, B., Kikukawa, N., Rogers, S., Narraway, A., Newman, I., and Haude, R., in *Physical Activity, Aging and Sports* (R. Harris and S. Harris, eds.). Albany, Center for Study of Aging, pp. 369–373 (1989).
44. Godin, G., Valois, P., Shephard, R.J., and Desharnais, R., *J. Behav. Med.*, *10*: 145–158 (1987).
45. Gorden, N.F., Levinrad, L.I., Faitelson, H.L. et al. *S. Afr. Med. J.*, *64*: 169–172 (1983).
46. Grimby, G., Anianson, A., Danneskold-Samsoe, B., and Saltin, B. *Med. Sci. Sports*, *12*: 95 (1980).
47. Haber, P., Honiger, B., Klicpera, M. et al., *Eur. Heart J.*, *5*: Suppl. E 37–39 (1984).
47a. Hammond, E.C., and Garfinkel, L., *Arch. Env. Health 19*: 167–182 (1969).
48. Harber, V.J., and Sutton, J., Sports Med., 1: 154–171 (1984).
49. Heikkinen, E., in *Recent Advances in Gerontology* (H. Orimo, K. Shimada, M. Iriki, and D. Maeda, eds.). Excerpta Medica, Amsterdam, pp. 501–503 (1979).
50. Horowitz, M., Wishart, J.M., Bochner, M., Need, A.G., Chatterton, B.E., and Nordin, B.E.C., *Br. Med. J.*, *297*: 1314–1315, 1988 (1988).
51. Hughes, A.L., and Goldman, R.F., *J. Appl. Physiol.*, *29*: 570–572 (1970).
52. Ingebretsen, R., *Scand. J. Soc. Med.*, *29*: 153–159 (1982).
53. Kaplan, R.M., and Criqui, M.H., Plenum Press, New York (1985).
54. Karvonen, M.J., Kentala, E., and Mustala, O., *Ann. Med. Exp. Fenn.*, *35*: 307–315 (1957).
55. Kasch, F. & Kulberg, J., *Scand. J. Sports Sci.*, *3*: 59–62 (1981).
56. Kasch, F., Wallace, J.P., and Van Camp, S.P., *J. Cardiopulm. Rehabil.*, *5*: 308–312 (1985).
57. Katz, S., Branch, L.G., Branson, M.H. et al., *N. Engl. J. Med.*, *309*: 1218–1224 (1983).
58. Kavanagh, T. & Shephard, R.J. Ann. N.Y. Acad. Sci., *301*: 455–465 (1977).
59. Kavanagh, T., Shephard, R.J., Lindley, L.T., and Pieper, M., *Arteriosclerosis*, *3*: 249–259 (1983).
60. Kay, C., and Shephard, R.J., *Int. Z. Angew. Physiol.*, *27*: 311–328 (1969).
61. Keast, D., Cameron, K., and Morton, A.R., *Sports Med.*, *5*: 248–267 (1988).
62. Keber, R.E., Miller, R.A., and Najjar, S.M., *Chest, 67*: 388–394 (1975).
63. Kenney, W.L., and Fowler, S.R., *J. Appl. Physiol.*, *65*: 1082–1086 (1988).

64. Kenney, W.L., and Hodgson, J.L. *Sports Med., 4*: 446–456 (1987).
65. Koplan, J.P., Powell, K.E., Sikes, R.K. et al., *J.A.M.A., 248*: 3118–3121 (1982).
66. Koszuta, L.E. , *Phys. Sportsmed., 17*(4): 203–206 (1989).
67. Krølner, J.P., Toft, B., Nielsen, S.P., and Tondevold, E., *Clin. Sci., 64*: 541–546 (1983).
68. Kushner, R.F., and Schoeller, D.A., *Am. J. Clin. Nutr., 44*: 417–424 (1986).
69. Lane, N.E., Bloch, D.A., Jones, H.H. et al., *J.A.M.A., 255*: 1147–1151 (1986).
70. Lawrence, G., *Aquafitness for Women*. Personal Library, Toronto (1981).
71. Lee, T.H., Shammash, J.B., Ribeiro, J.P., Hartley, L.H., Sherwood, J., and Goldman, L., *Am. Heart J., 115*: 203–204 (1988).
72. Lenfant, C., and Wittneberg, C.K., *Physical Activity, Aging and Sports* (R. Harris and S. Harris, eds.). Albany, : Center for Study of Aging, Albany (1989).
73. Leon, A., *Med. Clin. N. Am., 69*: 3–20 (1985).
74. Levarlet-Joye, H. and Simon, M., *J. Sports Med. Phys. Fitness, 23*: 8–13 (1983).
75. Lind, A.R., and McNicol, J.W., *Can. Med. Assoc. J., 96*: 706–712 (1967).
76. Lipsitz, L.A., Wei, J.Y., and Rowe, J.W., *Quart. J. Med., 55*: 45–54 (1985).
77. Lohman, T.G., Slaughter, M.H., Boileau, R.A., Bunt, J., and Lussier, L., *Hum. Biol., 56*: 667–679 (1984).
78. MacCallum, M., in *The Coming of Age of Aging* (R.C. Goode & D.J. Payne, eds.). Ontario Heart Foundation, Toronto, pp. 83–111 (1980).
79. MacKinnon, L.T., *Sports Med., 7: 141–149 (1989)*.
80. Magnus, K., Matroos, A., and Strackee, J., *Am J. Epidemiol., 110: 724–733 (1979)*.
81. Makrides, L., Heigenhauser, G.J., McCartney, N., and Jones, N.L., *Clin. Sci., 69*: 197–205, 1985 (1985).
82. Massie, J., and Shephard, R.J., *Med. Sci. Sports 3*: 110–117 (1971).
83. Matheson, G.O., MacIntyre, J.G., Taunton, J.E., Clement, D.B., and Lloyd-Smith, R., *Med Sci. Sports Exerc., 21*: 379–385 (1989).
84. Matter, S., Stanford, B.A., and Weltman, A., *J. Gerontol., 35*: 332–336 (1980).
85. Mazzeo, R.S., Brooks, G.A., and Horvath, S.M., *J. Appl. Physiol., 57*: 1369–1374 (1984).
86. McDonough, J., and Bruce, R.A., in *Proceedings of the National Conference on Exercise in the Prevention, in the Evaluation and in the Treatment of Heart Disease. J.S. Carol. Med. Assoc., 65* (Suppl. 1): 26–33 (1969).
87. McNamara, P.S., Otto, R.M., and Smith, T.K., *Med. Sci. Sports Exerc., 17*: 266 (Abstr.) (1985).
88. Melton, L.J., in *Biological and Behavioral Aspects of Falls in the Elderly Proc.* Natl. Inst. Aging, Bethesda, Maryland Sept. 17–18 (1984).

89. Mernagh, J.R., Harrison, J.E., Krondl, A., McNeill, K.G., and Shephard, R.J., *Nutr. Res.*, *6*: 499–507 (1986).
90. Miyashita, M., Haga, S., and Mizuta, T., *J. Sports Med. Phys. Fitness, 18*: 131–137 (1978).
90a. Montoye, H.J., *Physical activity and health: an epidemiological study of an entire community*. Prentice Hall, Englewood Cliffs, New Jersey (1975).
91. Niinimaa, V., and Shephard, R.J., *J. Gerontol., 33*: 362–367 (1978).
92. Oeschli, F.W., and Buechley, R.W., *Environ. Res., 3*: 277–284 (1970).
93. Oja, P., Kukkonen-Harjula, R., Nieminen, R., Vuori, I., and Passanen, M., *Int. J. Sports Med., 9*: 45–51 (1988).
93a. Ostrow, A.C., and Dzewaltowski, D.A., *Res. Quart. 57*: 167–169 (1986).
94. Overstall, P.W., Exton-Smith, A.N., Imms, F.J., and Johnson, A.L., *Br. Med. J., 1*: 261–264 (1977).
95. Paffenbarger, R.S., Hyde, R.T., Wing, A.L., and Hsieh, C.C., *N. Engl. J. Med., 314*: 605–613 (1986).
96. Palmore, E.D., in *Physical Activity, Aging and Sports* (R. Harris and S. Harris, eds.). Center for Study of Aging, Albany pp. 151–156 (1989).
97. Panush, R.S., and Brown, D.G., *Sports Med., 4*: 54–64 (1987).
98. Panush, R.S., Schmidt, C., Caldwell, J.R. et al., *J.A.M.A., 255*: 1147–1151 (1986).
99. Papazoglou, N.M., Kolokouri-Dervou, E.S., Viaros, P.A., Vassilou, S.V., and Korkodilos, G.A., *Am. J. Cardiol., 61*: 1146–1147 (1988).
100. Pascale, M., and Grana, W.A., *Physician Sportsmed., 17*(3): 157–166 (1989).
101. Paterson, D.H., Shephard, R.J., Cunningham, D., Jones, N.L., and Andrew, G., *J. Appl. Physiol., 47*: 482–489 (1979).
102. Pekkanen, J., Marti, B., Nissinen, A., Tuomilehto, J., Punsar, S., and Karvonen, M.J., *Lancet, 1*: 1473–1477 (1987).
103. Pollock, M.L., Gettman, L.R., Milesis, C.A. et al., *Med. Sci. Sports, 9*: 31–36 (1977).
104. Powell, R.R., *J. Gerontol., 29*: 157–161 (1974).
105. Raab, D.M., and Smith, E.L., in *Topics Geriatr. Med., 1*(1): 31–39 (1985).
106. Sagiv, M., and Grodjinovsky, A., in *Physical Activity, Aging and Sports* (R. Harris and S. Harris, eds.). Center for Study of Aging, Albany, pp. 51–55 (1989).
107. Schoutens, A., Laurent, E., and Poortmans, J.R., *Sports Med., 7*: 71–81 (1989).
108. Schuman, S.H., *Environ. Res., 5*: 59–75 (1972).
109. Seals, D.R., Hagberg, J.M., Hurley, B.F. et al., *J. Appl. Physiol., 57*: 1024–1029 (1984).
110. Shephard, R.J., *Int. Z. Angew. Physiol., 28*: 38–48 (1968).
111. Shephard, R.J., *Endurance Fitness*. 2nd Ed. University of Toronto Press, Toronto (1977).
112. Shephard, R.J., *Ischemic Heart Disease and Exercise*. Croom Helm, London (1981).

113. Shephard, R.J., *Physiology and Biochemistry of Exercise*. Praeger, New York (1982).
114. Shephard, R.J., *Eur. J. Cardiol.*, *11*: 147–157 (1980).
115. Shephard, R.J., *J. Cardovasc. Pulm. Med.*, *12*: 29–32 (1984).
116. Shephard, R.J., *CAHPER J.*, *50*(6): 2–5, 20 (1985).
117. Shephard, R.J., *Sports Med.*, *2*: 348–366 (1985).
118. Shephard, R.J., *Fitness of a Nation. Lessons from the Canada Fitness Survey*. Karger, Basel (1986).
119. Shephard, R.J., *Economic Benefits of Enhanced Fitness*. Human Kinetics, Champaign, Illinois (1986).
120. Shephard, R.J., *Physical Activity and Aging*. 2nd Ed. Croom Helm, London (1987).
121. Shephard, R.J., in *International Perspectives on Adapted Physical Activity* (M. Berridge and G. Ward, eds.). Human Kinetics, Champaign, Illinois, pp. 235–242 (1987).
122. Shephard, R.J., in *The Academy Papers* (H. Eckert and W. Spirduso, eds.). Human Kinetics, Champaign, Illinois (1988).
123. Shephard, R.J., *Body Composition*. Cambridge University Press, London (1989).
124. Shephard, R.J., *Fitness Assessment and Programming for Disabled Populations. Research and Practice*. Human Kinetics, Champaign, Illinois (1989).
125. Shephard, R.J., Kavanagh, T., Tuck, J., and Kennedy, J., *J. Cardiac Rehab.*, *3*: 321–329 (1983).
126. Shephard, R.J., Montelpare, W., and Berridge, M., *Res. Quart.*, (1989).
127. Shephard, R.J., and Leith, L., in *Cognitive Change and Aging*. (M.L. Howe, ed.)., Springer, New York (1989).
128. Sidney, K.H., and Shephard, R.J., *J. Appl. Physiol.*, *43*: 280–287 (1977).
129. Sidney, K.H., and Shephard, R.J., *Br. Heart J.*, *39*: 1114–1120 (1977).
130. Sidney, K.H., and Shephard, R.J., *Med. Sci. Sports*, *8*: 246–252 (1977).
130a. Sidney, K.H., and Shephared, R.J., *Med. Sci. Sports 10*: 125–131 (1978).
131. Sidney K.H., Niinimaa, V., and Shephard, R.J., *J. Sports Sci.*, *1*: 194–210 (1983).
132. Sidney, K.H., Shephard, R.J., and Harrison, J., *Am J. Clin. Nutr.*, *30*: 326–333 (1977).
133. Siscovick, D.S., Laporte, R.E., and Newman, J.M., *Publ. Health Rep.*, *100*: 180–188 (1985).
134. Skerlj, B., Brozek, J., and Hunt, F.E., *Am J. Phys. Anthropol.*, *11*: 577–600 (1953).
135. Smith, E.L., Reddan, W., and Smith, P.E., *Med. Sci. Sports Exerc.*, *13*: 60–64 (1981).
136. Smith, E.L., Smith, P.E., Ensign, C.J., and Shea, M.M., *Calcif. Tiss. Int.*, *36*: s129–s138 (1984).
137. Smith, E.L., and Gilligan, C., *Phys. Sportsmed.*, *11*(8): 91–101 (1983).
138. Soltysiak, J., Golec, L., and Sokolowski, E., *Acta Physiol. Pol. 22*: 639–648 (1971).

139. Stamford, B.A., Hambacker, W., and Fallica, A., *Res. Quart.*, 45:34–41 (1974).
140. Taylor, C.B., Sallis, J.F., and Needle, R., *Publ. Health Rep.*, 100: 195–202 (1985).
141. Teraoka, T., *Kobe J. Med.*, 25: 1–17 (1979).
142. Thomas, S., Cunningham, D.A., Rechnitzer, P.A., Donner, A.P., and Howard, J.H., *Can. J. Sport Sci.*, 12: 144–151 (1987).
143. Van Camp, S.P., and Peterson, R.A., *J.A.M.A. 256*: 1160–1163 (1986).
144. Van Loan, M., and Mayclin, P., *Hum. Biol.*, 59: 299–309 (1987).
145. Van Rensel, B., Renson, R., and deMeyer, H., *Int. Rev. Sports Soc.*, 18: 103–114 (1983).
146. Verde, T., Thomas, S.G., and Shephard, R.J., *Med. Sci. Sports Exerc.* 21: S 110 (1989).
147. Viidik, A., *Biomed. Eng.*, 2: 64–67 (1967).
148. Viitsaalo, J.T., Era, P., Leskinen, A.L., and Heikkinen, E., *Ergonomics*, 28: 1653–74 (1985).
149. Von Kriegel, W., and Airsherl, W., *Acta Endocrinol.*, 46: 47–64 (1964).
150. Vuori, I., in *Guide to Fitness After Fifty* (Harris, R. and Frankel, W., eds.). Plenum Press, New York (1977).
151. Vuori, I., Suurnakki, L., and Suurnakki, T., *Med. Sci. Sports Exerc.*, 14: 114–115 (1982).
151a. Wagner, J.A., Robinson, S., and Marino, R.P. *J. Appl. Physiol. 37*: 562–565 (1974).
152. Wasserman, K., Beaver, W.L., and Whipp, B.J., *Med. Sci. Sports Exerc.*, 18: 344–52 (1986).
153. Wells, K.F., and Dillon, E.K., *Res. Quart.*, 23: 115–118 (1952).
154. Weisfeldt, M.L., Gerstenblith, M.L., and Lakatta, E.G., in *Principles of Geriatric Medicine* (R. Andres, E.L. Bierman, and W.R. Hazzard, eds.). McGraw-Hill, New York, pp. 248–279 (1985).
155. Williams, P.T., Wood, P.D., Haskell, W.L., and Vranizan, K., *J.A.M.A.* 247: 2672–2679 (1982).
156. Wolfel, E.E., and Hossack, K.F., *J. Cardiopulm. Rehabil.*, 9: 40–45 (1989).
157. Yano, K. Reed, D.M., Curb, J.D., Hankin, J.H., and Albers, J.J., *Arteriosclerosis*, 6: 422–433 (1986).
158. Yoshikiwa, M., Okano, K., Nakai, R., Tomori, T., and Takneawa, M., *Asian Med. J.*, 21: 359–378 (1978).

6

General Principles of Exercise Testing and Training in a Cardiac Population

Deborah Morley

Temple University School of Medicine
Philadelphia, Pennsylvania

Henry S. Miller, Jr.

Bowman Gray School of Medicine, Wake Forest University
Winston-Salem, North Carolina

INTRODUCTION

In this chapter, we will discuss principles of exercise testing and training in a cardiac population. The principles we will outline apply both to the population of patients with known coronary artery disease as well as to those who are at high risk for coronary artery disease.

The objectives of available therapy for atherosclerotic coronary artery disease include preserving viable myocardium, control of angina, arrhythmias, and other symptoms, and improving survival. The now widespread use of intracoronary and intravenous thrombolytic therapy which dissolves occlusive thrombi in the coronary arteries has been instrumental in limiting myocardial damage in acute infarctions. The advent of percutaneous transluminal coronary angioplasty (PTCA) as a method of reducing coronary artery obstruction has provided another therapeutic option for restoring blood flow to the heart muscle and decreasing myocardial ischemia. The development of new pharmacological agents, particularly angiotensin converting enzyme (ACE) inhibitors and antiarrhythmics, are significantly improving the clinical status of patients with heart failure or other complications of coronary heart disease. Coronary artery bypass graft (CABG) surgery is still a useful way to augment myocardial blood flow to ischemic myocardium before and after an infarct. Advances in nuclear cardiology and echocardiography are also providing more accurate diagnostic and prognostic information. Finally, physicians and other health care professionals are emphasizing preventive medicine by modification of lifestyle risk factors for coronary atherosclerosis and its complications.

Technological advances in medicine have enabled us to identify atherosclerosis much earlier in its clinical course. This is particularly true for the peripheral arteries (i.e., carotid, abdominal aorta, ileofemoral, etc.) where high-resolution ultrasound is now capable of detecting small plaques. Early detection of small plaques in peripheral vessels is important because the risk of concomitant coronary artery disease is high for individuals with peripheral vascular disease. We are learning more about atherogenesis and the contribution of genetic and environmental factors each day. Thus, not only are more people surviving cardiac events, but we are also able to identify more persons with early atherosclerotic disease or who have a high risk of coronary artery disease.

Treatments for nonatherosclerotic forms of heart disease have also improved. More and more individuals are having valvular and congenital lesions repaired, allowing near-normal activity. Previously, these cardiac defects may have resulted in profound disability or death. New medications for reducing left ventricular work, controlling arrhythmias, and cardiac transplantation have improved survival and the functional capacity of cardiomyopathic patients. Thus, the number of patients surviving with a wide range of cardiovascular problems has dramatically increased. All of these individuals can benefit from exercise evaluation and conditioning with regular exercise.

One important point to make in this overview of exercise testing and training is that the *general principles* of cardiac exercise testing and training are the same no matter what the patient population. Since an exercise prescription establishes a safe, individualized exercise program, specifically defining intensity, duration, frequency, and mode of activity, these parameters are simply adjusted to meet specific patient needs.

PURPOSES OF EXERCISE TESTING

In patients with known cardiac disease, exercise testing is performed to determine the patient's functional capacity. For persons with symptoms of or high risk for cardiac disease, the exercise test is done to obtain diagnostic information. A diagnostic exercise test documents the adequacy of myocardial blood flow with or without therapy. It is frequently performed to assist the physician in the selection of medical, interventional, or surgical options and to evaluate the adequacy of therapy to control angina, arrhythmias, or blood pressure during physical activity. In patients in whom a diagnosis of coronary artery, valvular, or myocardial disease has been already made, the test is used to determine a safe and effective level of exercise for the individual patient.

Functional capacity defines the amount of work a subject can do before showing signs or symptoms of ischemia, arrhythmias, or other cardiac dysfunction. Functional testing should be done while the patient is taking medications as usual. Since blood pressure and heart rate at maximal exercise are often used to determine a patient's exercise prescription, the values used must represent the effect of medications or patients will not be able to adhere to prescriptions when exercising. Functional exercise testing is also employed widely for the evaluation of new drug efficacy. A good functional exercise test, especially with oxygen uptake, is also important in timing the need for cardiac interventions; e.g., valve replacement, coronary bypass surgery, or cardiac transplantation. The remainder of our discussion will focus on functional exercise testing for the cardiac patient.

EXERCISE TESTING

Pretest History

Prior to an exercise test, the testing personnel should have available as much information about the patient as possible. At a minimum, the medical history and physical findings documenting cardiac diagnosis, medication being taken, and a resting electrocardiogram must be available. Other information such as previous exercise tests, results of cardiac catheterization, echocardiogram, or other diagnostic tests are helpful to the physician in planning and interpreting the test. At the time of the test (or before if information is available), the test staff should review the names and dosages of all the patient's medications and determine whether there are any pulmonary, orthopedic, or other problems that might limit the subject's ability to exercise.

Selection of Protocol and Mode

It is preferable to conduct exercise testing of cardiac patients on a treadmill. This weight-bearing exercise utilizes the large muscles of the body in a way that is familiar and usually accomplishes enough work to adequately test the function of the heart. However, if the patient is unable to walk, non-weight-bearing aerobic exercise modalities (i.e., biking, rowing, or an arm ergometer) are suitable. When doing serial exercise testing, the same modality should always be used because the ischemic threshold can vary with the type of exercise, particularly when the patient has dynamic coronary stenoses (1). Arm crank ergometers should be used only for cardiac patients who are paraplegic or otherwise unable to exercise. Keyser et al. (2) have demonstrated that when compared to arm egometry, treadmill testing was more specific for ischemia. Even varying the crank speed within a given workload provided different ischemic and hemodynamic responses to exercise.

Monitoring

During the exercise test, ECG and blood pressure monitoring should be done. The capacity for 12-lead electrocardiograms and continuous oscilloscope monitoring of the patient should be available. It is recommended that a full 12-lead ECG be run once during each exercise level. The ECG is used to obtain accurate heart rates, record dysrhythmias, and detect ST-segment and T-wave changes as evidence of ischemia. Similarly, blood pressure should be monitored at least once per stage or at least every 3 min. If the heart is able to meet the increasing demands of exercise, the systolic blood pressure should rise as exercise demand increases. Careful monitoring of the blood pressure is of equal, if not more, importance than the ECG in the evaluation of patients with valvular or cardiomyopathic heart disease.

In addition to these measures, it is helpful to monitor the patient's degree of perceived exertion. Numerous scales are available which ask the patient to match a verbal descriptor of how hard they are working and/or how they feel to the corresponding number. Borg's scale of perceived exertion (Table 1) is probably the best known (2a). Monitoring the patient's perception of their activity during exercise allows them to monitor their activity at home. The way a patient feels at a given level of exercise can be correlated to their heart rate and any signs or symptoms they may have while working on the job, at home, or during recreational activities. Similar charts and scales are available for patients to monitor the severity of any angina they experience (Table 2) as well as for dyspnea (Table 3). Evaluating local muscle fatigue in a similar way should be done when modalities such as the bicycle are employed for exercise testing. The use of ratings of perceived exertion (RPE) and other measures of dyspnea are very important for exercise prescription in heart failure and transplant patients.

Table 1 Borg's Scale of Perceived Exertion

RPE	Verbal anchor
6	
7	Very, very light
8	
9	Very light
10	
11	Fairly light
12	
13	Somewhat hard
14	
15	Hard
16	
17	Very hard
18	
19	
20	Very, very hard

Table 2 Angina Scale

1+	Light, barely noticeable
2+	Moderate, bothersome
3+	Severe, very uncomfortable
4+	Most severe pain ever experienced in the past

Table 3 Dyspnea Scale

1. Mild, noticeable to patient—not to observer
2. Some difficulty—noticeable to observer
3. Moderate difficulty—but can continue
4. Severe difficulty—patient cannot continue

Measurement of Oxygen Uptake

The functional capacity of the patient should also be estimated or measured in terms of the amount of oxygen consumed (VO_2). Specifically, this is termed the MET (metabolic equivalent term) capacity: 1 MET translates into the amount of oxygen necessary for one to maintain one's body at rest, estimated at 3.5 ml of O_2/kg of body weight/min;

i.e., 10 METs = 35 ml of O_2/kg/min. As the patient's heart and body work increases to meet the challenge of exercise, the number of METs necessary to support this work increases. Most standard cardiac protocols have estimated MET levels calculated from oxygen uptake measurements drawn from large-scale population studies. These protocols can be used to estimate the MET capacity for cardiac patients when O_2 uptake equipment is not available. Because of the influences that medications, training, and clinical problems may have on pulse rate and blood pressure, it is often best to estimate the patient's functional capacity in terms of METs. You can counsel patients with regard to their ability to perform work or leisure activities based on the numerous charts which associate various work/leisure activities with the required energy in terms of METs. As a general rule, the maximum MET capacity (estimated or measured) of a patient on a symptom-limited exercise test should be twice the estimated MET capacity for the work performed by the individual.

Test Endpoints

In cardiac exercise testing, the test should be terminated when the patient reaches his or her symptom-limited maximum. Termination may be due to general fatigue, ischemic ECG changes, an increase in arrhythmias, or changes in conduction with exercise or symptomatic changes of angina and dyspnea. All may indicate that the heart is no longer able to meet the demands of the exercise safely. The reader should consult the *American College of Sports Medicine Exercise Testing Guidelines* (3) for a detailed list of the criteria for test termination in a cardiac population.

Graded exercise testing can also be used for persons with other forms of heart disease and medical problems. Exercise testing has to be individualized for each patient, depending on the exercise restriction, but there is little change in the way the test is conducted or monitored. In patients with valvular, congenital, or cardiomyopathic heart disease, exercise testing is extremely useful for establishing the functional capacity of the individual. This information is helpful either for advising the adolescent with congenital disease as to activities in which it is safe for them to participate, or for telling a patient with cardiomyopathy whether they can safely achieve the physical capacity necessary for a given job.

In all forms of heart disease discussed, exercise may cause a reduction in left ventricular contractility, resulting in a drop or plateau in the blood pressure as exercise increases. The test should be terminated with any significant fall in systolic blood pressure. Symptoms that may limit exercise in noncoronary heart disease patients include dyspnea, weakness, sudden fatigue, dizziness, syncope, and arrhythmias. Frequent premature ventricular beats, premature atrial beats, and tachy/dysrhythmias are commonly noted in patients with valvular and cardiomyopathic disease. In this situation, exercise testing is helpful to ascertain the specific activity level or heart rate at which the rhythm problems occur and whether they increase with exercise.

In older individuals, valvular heart disease and cardiomyopathy may be associated with obstructive coronary artery disease. Again, exercise testing may help sort out the underlying causes of patient symptoms. However, ECG changes at rest in this population, such as with left ventricular hypertrophy, often make interpretation of the exercise ECG for ischemic changes difficult. However, the symptoms that develop and the level of exercise are helpful to the physician when making decision regarding the timing and nature of treatment. Exercise radionuclide studies to more accurately assess the presence of myocardial ischemia in a population where chest pain may not necessarily occur is also very useful for evaluating a patient's functional capacity and directing the treatment course.

The exercise test protocol chosen for cardiac patients should begin at a low level (approximately 2–3 METs) and progress slowly by 1 MET every stage. The length of each exercise stage should be 2–3 min, allowing the patient to achieve some degree of steady state. This is particularly important in testing cardiac patients because the exact level at which angina or ECG changes of ischemia begin may be difficult to determine when larger jumps in workload are used. When the patients are carefully monitored, endpoints can be determined. It is critical for the safety of the patient that the physician exercising the patient has this information. Cardiac protocols for treadmill testing and bicycle ergometry are shown in Table 4 and 5, respectively.

Interpretation of Exercise Test

The primary purpose of functional exercise testing in the coronary heart disease population is to determine at what, if any, level the myocardium becomes ischemic (i.e., myocardial oxygen supply no longer meets its demand). As such, the exercise test is usually interpreted as positive (there is ECG and/or symptomatic evidence of ischemia) or negative (there is no evidence of ischemia) for coronary ischemia at the exercise level attained. While ST-segment changes on the ECG may be the primary evidence of myocardial ischemia, the presence of angina,

Table 4 Cardiac Protocol for Treadmill GXT

Speed	% Grade	Min	Estimated Min
1.7	0	2–3	1.7
1.7	5	2–3	3.5
2.0	10	2–3	5.2
2.5	10	2–3	6.4
2.5	12.5	2–3	8.5
3.0	12.5	2–3	8.5
3.0	15	2–3	9.5
3.4	15	2–3	10.6
4.0	15	2–3	12.3
4.2	17.5	2–3	13.4

Table 5 Cardiac Protocol for Bicycle Ergometry

Workload	Min	Estimated METs
150	2–3	2.5
300	2–3	3.7
450	2–3	4.9
600	2–3	6.1
750	2–3	7.3
900	2–3	8.6
1050	2–3	9.8
1200	2–3	11.0
1350	2–3	12.2
1500	2–3	13.5

failure of blood pressure to rise, or arrythmias may be equally helpful in the detection of heart disease. In other cardiac patients such as those with heart failure, the primary objective of exercise testing is to determine the level of exercise that may cause left ventricular (LV) deterioration, to determine the efficacy of medical therapy, or to gauge the timing of transplantation. In any event, *the objective of exercise testing should be established prior to doing the test*. The exercise prescription developed for a given patient is formulated so that the patient can exercise at an intensity that is safe, effective, and does not cause significant myocardial ischemia or the other signs of exercise intolerance. The reader is referred to any standard cardiology or exercise testing text for a further discussion of the interpretation of exercise tests.

The symptom-limited functional graded exercise test provides information crucial to appropriate exercise prescription. The resting heart rate (HR) before exercise and the HR at their symptom-limited maximum exercise level are used to calculate the exercise heart rate range using the Karvonen formula (4). The heart rates at the desired exercise intensity can be correlated with signs, symptoms, and ratings of perceived exertion to make the activity safe and effective. For many noncoronary populations, the MET capacity and subjective ratings of exertion are relied upon heavily for exercise prescription, so care should be taken in collecting this data.

PROGNOSTIC VALUES OF EXERCISE TESTING

The cardiac patient is assessed very carefully for those complications that significantly affect morbidity and mortality. Information obtained from an exercise test performed following the event is very helpful. The findings of residual ischemia of the left ventricle, left ventricular dysfunction, or sustained ventricular arrhythmias, particularly when associated with one of the other complications, carries an increased risk of death during the 6–12 months following myocardial infarction (5–25%). Functional exercise testing, when conducted prior to hospital discharge at 7–9 days and particularly at 3 weeks following myocardial infarction, provides good information with respect to the occurrence of ischemic events and left ventricular function. Much of the research available predicting the risk from exercise testing results has been collected in cardiac populations at the time of low–level exercise testing done before hospital discharge. However, more recent reports indicate that a symptom-limited exercise test at 3 weeks post–myocardial infarction (NI) or bypass or valve surgery is more prognostic of future events than a low-level predischarge exercise test if the level achieved is less than 4 METs.

ST-segment depression is the ECG marker of coronary ischemia. When definite ST-segment depression of greater than 2 mm occurs during an exercise test, there is a 36% chance of a recurrent coronary event and a 6–10% risk for sudden cardiac death in the first year after myocardial infarction. These data are from a summary of five studies that looked at discharge treadmill test of 838 post-MI patients done 10–14 days after MI (5). Angina associated with ischemic ST-segment changes increased the risk of morbidity and mortality even more. Angina pectoris alone predicted an 11% risk for recurrent ischemic events in 1 year (5). ST-segment elevations seen on exercise testing in patients with residual aneurysm or abnormal LV wall motion have been associated with an increased risk for recurrent events in the first year after MI when seen on discharge exercise testing (6). When these signs and symptoms of ischemia are noted, the patient should be referred for appropriate therapy. Options usually include PTCA or CABG of the obstructed coronary artery with or without medications to control myocardial ischemia.

Blood pressure (BP) response to exercise is an important predictor of future risk. A drop in systolic BP when the total workload is less than 9 METs is associated with increased cardiac death in the first year post-MI. A failure of the blood pressure to rise above 130 torr with activity, especially when associated with ischemic ST-segment changes, also indicates a poorer prognosis. In interpreting BP responses to exercise, one is cautioned to take into consideration the effect the patient's medications may have on test results. One investigator (5) has noted a 60% rate of cardiac events, reinfarctions, and sudden death in patients with an abnormal blood pressure response to exercise. This inability of the BP to increase with increasing exercise, particularly when it falls at an exercise level of 7 METs or less, is usually associated with severe left ventricular functional impairment. In the presence of coronary artery disease, this carries a very high mortality rate.

Interestingly, common arrhythmias such as premature ventricular beats, even with couplets and triplets, on exercise testing do not increase the risk for cardiac events (5,6). In the evaluation of combined complications of an infarction, one study demonstrated that ventricular tachycardia that could be reproduced by programmed stimulation and which was associated with ischemic ST-segment changes provided almost a 100% accurate prediction of a poorer prognosis in the first year after infarction (7).

Other factors noted at treadmill testing also contribute to predictions of a patient's prognosis. These include an inability to attain an exercise level of 4 METs or maintain this level for 3 min (5); a prolonged QT interval, and a total treadmill time of less than 9 min on a modified Bruce protocol. Other factors which usually indicate a poorer prognosis include frequent arrhythmias and an impaired left ventricular function to a significant degree. Clearly, exercise testing has been of great value in cardiac patients both for determination of prognosis as well as exercise prescription and indications for the appropriate treatment.

Recent reports conclude that little prognostic information is obtained from early low-level exercise tests in patients with uncomplicated non-Q-wave infarction. Testing has been found to be very helpful in patients with non–Q-wave infarction and clinical complications (8). Abnormal exercise ECG findings have been shown to be predictive of future cardiac events in patients tested within 1 month of angioplasty (9).

EXERCISE PRESCRIPTION

In order to provide cardiac patients with a safe, beneficial exercise level which is commensurate with their cardiac ability, each patient should be give an exercise prescription based on the results of the patient's symptom-limited graded exercise test. An exercise prescription is like a prescription for medication and is individualized. In this case, the patient is given an intensity, frequency, mode, and duration of exercise. If the patient adheres to the exercise prescription, the benefits of exercise training discussed earlier should be achieved. The importance and value of an appropriate warm-up before and cool-down after exercise should be discussed with patients, and cannot be overemphasized.

Intensity

The exercise intensity for most cardiac patients is based on their symptom-limited maximum HR compared to their resting HR. A HR range is determined from this information based on the method of Karvonen. To determine the patient's heart rate at the upper limit of his or her range, the following formula is used:

$$0.85 \times (symptom - limited\ maximum\ HR - resting\ HR)$$

The lower limit of the HR range is determined by multiplying the difference between these two HRs by 0.65. If the patient exercises at a pace at which the HR is maintained between this upper and lower limit, they can feel confident that they are not exercising at a level which will cause cardiovascular problems. Moreover, by staying within the HR range, they will achieve aerobic training benefits. Research has shown that training benefits are not improved by exercising at a HR higher than the 85% range in normals and patients with coronary disease. Levels below 60% in subjects that have been inactive can be used for initial stages of the exercise program. Allow the subject to begin exercising at a comfortable level and then gradually increase the intensity. We do not currently have such guidelines for patients with nonischemic forms of cardiac disease, but intensities used should be dependent on the capacity and needs of specific patients. It is common with cardiac patients who have not been exercising or who have recently had myocardial infarction, bypass surgery, or unstable angina to be given an initial (1–2 months) prescription of 40–60%, perhaps with a longer duration of activity. Other modifications will be discussed later in chapters dealing with special cardiac populations.

Mode

The mode of activity should be aerobic. Aerobic activity is defined as activity for which the oxygen demands of the exercise can be met by the body's mechanisms for metabolizing substrates with oxygen. Aerobic activities employ use of the large muscles of the body and entail rhythmic and continuous movement. Walking, jogging, bicycling, swimming, and rowing are all examples of aerobic activities. Because it is a weight-bearing activity and is thus advantageous for weight loss, cardiac patients should be encouraged to walk. Jogging has the same advantage; however, the risk of orthopedic injury, particularly in the elderly, makes it a less desirable activity for cardiac patients. In the event that a patient cannot exercise by walking or if their personal preference is for another activity, any of the aerobic modalities may be employed to achieve the benefits of exercise training. Examples ae cycling, rowing, or swimming. Weight training with low resistance and other specific exercise programs can also be designed for aerobic training.

Frequency

In order to achieve a training benefit, an individual should exercise at least three times per week. As long as a cardiac patient is capable of monitoring his or her own HR and understands the importance of adhering to the HR range, there is no harm in exercising four to seven days/week. Daily or weekly activities such as mowing the grass, raking leaves, gardening, or vacuuming floors when 30–60 min are required to complete the task and the HR response is appropriate may count as an exercise session.

Duration

Ideally, the aerobic portion of the exercise should be maintained for 30 min per exercise session. This duration is the minimum required to achieve a training effect. Many cardiac patients are not able to sustain activity for this length of time, but they should be encouraged to work toward this goal. Intermittent short periods of activity of 5–10 min alternating with rest periods can be very beneficial. In this way, the patient can gradually increase the length of activity periods and shorten rest periods. Eventually the goals of continuous exercise for 30–40 min or 10–15 min, two to three times/day at a higher intensity will be achieved. Both methods will improve conditioning.

Modifications of Exercise Prescription in Non-Coronary Heart Disease Patients

The exercise prescription is individualized and based on the symptom-limited maximum exercise test for patients with acquired or congenital forms of heart disease, as in the case of those with coronary heart disease. With patients who demonstrate myocardial functional deficit, as with cardiomyopathy, exercise intensity and duration will usually need to be reduced. As an example, a patient may be started with a prescription for 20–40% of capacity for 5–10 min with activity interspersed with rest periods. Care should be taken to ensure that the patient does not exercise in a dehydrated or hypovolemic state or when the environmental humidity and temperature are high (e.g., more than 78°F). Added to the limited cardiac output of these patients, such conditions would exacerbate the potential for syncopal episodes. Patients with coexistent ischemic heart disease requiring nitroglycerin for angina may develop a symptomatic decrease in blood pressure coupled with their limited cardiac output. Arrhythmias are also commonly associated with cardiomyopathy and valvular disease and may worsen with exercise or produce a fall in blood pressure. Be sure the symptoms and signs are maximally controlled medically prior to beginning an exercise program.

Exercise in patients following cardiac transplantation is now common and is discussed in Chapter 8. If testing and prescription are individualized and the patient's condition is medically stable, significant benefits of training will occur in markedly debilitated patients. Changes will be confined primarily to peripheral adaptations. Exercise prescription and training of patients with chronic heart failure and cardiomyopathy is an emerging field. Clinicians are now recognizing the potential benefits of activity for these groups, contraindicating previous dogma recommending forced rest for this subset of patients. This topic addressed in Chapter 12.

EXERCISE TRAINING

Supervised Versus Unsupervised Training

When recommending exercise as therapy to improve functional capacity in cardiac patients, one is always confronted with the issue of whether or not a patient's rehabilitation program should be supervised. This question is frequently answered on the basis of program availability. Cardiac rehabilitation programs are now widespread and in many areas of the country they are reasonably available to more and more patients. Little controlled research has been done in the area of supervised versus unsupervised rehabilitation in cardiac patients, but some recommendations can be made.

In general, patients with a poorer prognosis as demonstrated on treadmill testing as well as those with previous infarctions, three-vessel disease, or poor left ventricular function should participate in a supervised program when possible (10). Other conditions which are felt to mandate supervised activity include an abnormal blood pressure response to exercise, indicative of left ventricular dysfunction, and angina or ECG evidence of myocardial ischemia at a functional capacity of less than 7 METs. Arrhythmias or conduction defects, a functional capacity of less than 5 METs, a history of syncope, pacemakers which do not allow appropriate heart rate increases with exercise, uncontrolled hypertension with exercise, and patients with other physical problems that require special equipment for aerobic exercise to be performed should be supervised (11). Frequently, patients who are deconditioned owing to long-term inactivity, as with bed rest due to illness, can progress from a supervised to unsupervised program after initial instruction and training.

In the absence of the above criteria, the decision as to whether or not supervised exercise is recommended depends very much on the patient. For example, patients who are "Type A" personalities or are very hard-driven emotionally tend to exercise at an intensity that is greater than that prescribed for them (12). These noncompliant patients need supervision to ensure that they do not develop cardiac complications by exercising excessively. Conversely, patients who are depressed or lack motivation and thus would benefit from frequent encouragement should be advised to exercise in a supervised environment. Any patient for whom unsupervised exercise is allowed should be trained to accurately monitor his or her pulse rate before, during, and after exercise. They should also clearly understand the signs and symptoms of cardiovascular and pulmonary problems requiring medical attention before beginning unsupervised activity. To achieve these goals, it is often best to ask cardiac patients to exercise with a supervised program for several sessions to allow assessment of the exercise prescription and to initiate dietary or psychological therapy as needed. The environment of a supervised program can provide support for risk factor modification. Discussing the rehabilitation goals for each individual will provide the patient with the information necessary to adequately monitor their physical activity, dietary needs, and other therapy necessary to return to a safe, useful, and productive lifestyle.

SUMMARY

Coronary heart disease affects millions of people and claims the lives of several hundred thousand each year. Better recognition and control of the factors leading to coronary atherosclerosis, along with improved therapy of the acute and chronic problems, are enabling many people who develop coronary heart disease to live very productive lives for many years. Exercise is thought to reduce the risk of heart disease by positively affecting the factors that induce the disease. Exercise training helps maximize the efficiency of the uninjured myocardium and reduces the risk of recurrent ischemic events in coronary heart disease patients. Knowledge about the relationship of exercise to heart disease is only beginning to be acquired; much is yet to be learned. In any event, whether causal or not, exercise has a positive impact on the lives of cardiac patients. Therefore, physicians caring for patients with cardiovascular disease should provide them with a safe and effective exercise prescription and program.

SAFETY OF EXERCISE TESTING AND TRAINING PROGRAMS IN SUBJECTS WITH MEDICAL PROBLEMS

This chapter and the chapters that follow will address the specific concerns of the patient population with cardiovascular and associated diseases. The general principles of exercise testing and training discussed are applicable to the patients following myocardial infarction, with and without angina, coronary artery bypass graft surgery, precutaneous transcoronary angioplasty, and in the high-risk population.

The risks of an appropriate well-monitored exercise test in this high-risk population has been shown to be extremely low. Resuscitation of the subjects who have had events in this monitored environment is usually 85–90% in most laboratories (100% in ours). In approximately 72,000 maximum exercise test in 34,300 middle-aged adults with a low prevalence for coronary heart disease, only six major cardiac events occurred. All were resuscitated with one person dying 1 week later (13). In our experience in a hospital-based exercise testing laboratory where the patient population either has a high probability of having cardiovascular or other medical disease problems, the event rate is similar: about one major cardiac event in 11,000.

Perhaps a better substantiation of the safety of testing and exercise in a cardiac population are noted in articles by Haskell (14) and later by Van Camp and Peterson (15). Haskell surveyed 30 cardiac rehabilitation programs in the mid to late 1970s and received information on 13,570 participants who accumulated about 1,634,000 h of exercise. Fifty cardiac events occurred, and 42 were resuscitated. In this group, seven patients had myocardial infarctions, five of whom survived. The rate for nonfatal events was one out of 34,700 and the fatal event rate one out of 116,400 patient-h of exercise. Van Camp and Peterson (15) surveyed data from 167 programs some 8 years later in which 51,300 patients exercised 2,351,916 hours. Twenty patients had cardiac arrest, 18 were resuscitated, with eight sustaining a myocardial infarction. The event incidence was one arrest per 112,000 patient-h, one myocardial infarction per 294,000 patient-h, and a fatality occurring every 784,000 patient-hrs. The event rate and occurrence did not differ in patients attending large or small programs nor were they related to the intensity of electrocardiographic monitoring. From these studies and knowing that all patients have cardiovascular disease, one can conclude that the likelihood of problems developing while attending a cardiac rehabilitation exercise programs is extremely low.

Hossack and Hartwig (16) evaluated the participants in the Multiple Exercise Center of the CAPRI Program (cardiopulmonary rehabilitation) in Seattle where out of 2464 patients, 25 had cardiac arrest and all were resuscitated. The patients who experienced cardiac arrest had an above-average exercise tolerance on exercise test and were usually exercising above their prescribed heart rate. Of the 17 patients who had cardiac catheterization, 12 had high-grade occlusive disease in the left anterior descending coronary artery, and the other five patients had complete occlusion of this coronary artery. Hossack and Hartwig (16) concluded that carefully watching the patients for excessive exercise, particularly in those who were more fit and tended to exceed their prescribed heart rates, would have markedly reduced this risk.

In assessing the benefits and risks of exercise training in the chronic coronary artery disease patient population, Thompson (17) noted that the incidence of cardiac events, even though extremely low, was higher during the time the patient was exercising than when they were not. However, the overall mortality in the patients who did exercise was significantly lower than those who were inactive. Cobb and Weaver (18) in their evaluation of cardiac rehabilitation participants in Seattle noted that even though cardiac arrest was usually unrelated to exertion, there was an increased risk of sudden events in patients with coronary heart disease associated with strenuous exercise. Those who had cardiac arrest following a maximum exercise test or maximum exertion had ventricular fibrillation and usually responded to prompt electrical shock. The events were usually not related to an acute myocardial infarction. These authors referred to the Framingham Study in which community members followed over 20 years were noted to have a lower incidence of sudden death if their daily exercise and physical fitness were good. Even in this population, there was a significant association of sudden death occurring in the setting of physical activity.

Considering the fact that the patients discussed in most of these studies had coronary disease, the risk of sudden death or of major cardiac events with exercise is quite low in the carefully controlled setting as is practiced in prescribed exercise programs. In a meta-analysis of the results of numerous exercise versus control studies in patients with cardiovascular disease, Oldridge et al. (19) noted that being in an exercise program significantly reduced the cardiovascular as well as overall mortality. In the analysis of O'Connor et al. (20) in a large number of patients, it was noted that the effect of exercise on cardiovascular and all cause death rate improved significantly over a 3 year period. However, these positive effects do not preclude the fact that careful evaluation of the subjects by exercise testing and emphasizing the importance of exercising within a safe heart rate range and work level is very important. The fact that these patients have a significantly higher risk for cardiac events because of their disease and the mortality is significantly less in physically active patients are compelling reasons to have them participate in an exercise program.

REFERENCES

1. Pupita, G., Kaski, J.C., Galassi, A.R., Vejor, M., Crea, F., and Maserj, A., *Am Heart J.*, 118: 539–545 (1989).
2. Keyser, R.E., Andres, R.F., Warken, D., Greninger, L.O., and Morse, D.E., *J. Cardiopulm. Rehabil.*, 9: 145–154 (1989).

2a. Borg, G., *Med. Sci. Sports Exerc.* 14: 377 (1982).
 3. American College of Sports Medicine, *Guidelines for Exercise Testing and Prescription*. Lea & Febiger, Philadelphia (1986).
 4. Karvonen, M., Kentala, K., Musta, O. *Ann. Med. Exp. Biol. Fenn.*, 35: 307 (1957).
 5. Weiner, D., in *Exercise and the Heart* (N.A. Wenger, ed.). Davis, Philadelphia, pp. 95–105 (1985).
 6. Hamm, L.F., Stull, G.A., and Crow, R.S., *Prog. Cardiovasc. Dis.*, 28(6): 463–476.
 7. Denniss, A.R., Baailens, J., Cody, D.V., Richards, D.A., Russel, P.A., Young, A.A., Ross, D.L., and Uther, J.B., *Am. J. Cardiol.*, 56: 213–220 (1985).
 8. Krone, R.J., Dwyer, E.M., Greenberg, H., Miller, J.P. and Gillepsie, J.A., *J. Am. Coll. Cardio.*, 14: 31–37 (1989).
 9. Deligonul, U. Vandormael, M.G., Shah, Y., Galan, K., Kern, M.J., Chaitman, B.R., *Am. Heart J.*, 117: 509, (1989).
10. Haskell, W., in *Clinics in Sports Medicine* (B.A. Franklin and M. Rubenfire, eds.). Saunders, Philadelphia, pp. 455–471.
11. Miller, H.S., in *Exercise and the Heart* (N.A. Wenger, ed.). Davis, Philadelphia, pp. 193–201 (1985).
12. Rejeski, W.J., Morley, D., and Miller, H. *J. Cardiac Rehabil.*, 3: 339–346 (1983).
13. Gibbons, L., Blair, S.N., Kohl., H.W., and Cooper, K., *Circulation*, 80(4): 846–852 (1989).
14. Haskell, W.L., *Circulation*, 57(5): 920–924 (1978).
15. Van Camp, S.P., and Peterson, R.A., *J.A.M.A.*, 256(9): 1160–1163 (1986).
16. Hossack, K.F., and Hartwig, R., *J. Cardiac Rehabil.*, 2(5): 402–408 (1982).
17. Thompson, P.D., *J.A.M.A.*, 259 (10): 1537–1540 (1988).
18. Cobb, L.A., and Weaver, W.D., *J.A.C.C.* 7(1): 215–219 (1986).
19. Oldridge, N.B., Guyatt, G.H., Fischer, M.E., and Rimm, A.A., *J.A.M.A.*, 260(7): 945–948 (1988).
20. O'Connor, G.T., Buring, J.E., Yusuf, S., Goldhaber, S.Z., Olmstead, E.M., Pfaffenbarger, R.S., and Hennekens, C.H., *Circulation*, 80: 234–244 (1989).

7

The Prevention and Treatment of Coronary Disease: The Case for Exercise

Henry S. Miller, Jr.

Bowman Gray School of Medicine, Wake Forest University
Winston-Salem, North Carolina

Ralph S. Paffenbarger, Jr.
Stanford University School of Medicine
Stanford, California

INTRODUCTION

Prior to the 1940s, the majority of the world population was employed in occupations requiring a moderate to high degree of physical activity, and there was little written about the relationship of physical activity and the development of cardiovascular diseases. With industrialization, automation minimized the manual labor involved in jobs of moderate and high exercise levels. Since that time, there has been a gradual and progressive elimination of any significant physical activity related to most of the occupations in the industrialized world. Therefore, to be physically active one has to add sports and games or other leisure time activities to obtain the amount of exercise that our ancestors attained with their gainful employment.

In the early 1950s, Morris and his coworkers (1) pointed out that there was a relationship between physical activity and coronary disease. In studies of London busmen, they contrasted the activity of the drivers with that of the "conductors," who repeatedly traversed the stairs between the upper and lower deck of the London bus. They found coronary disease incidence less in the more active conductors. Morris et al. later studied the health records of almost 18,000 British civil servants (2,3) whose sedentary desk jobs deprived them of any significant physical activity while working. Again, they showed that those who had been vigorous in performing their yard work, hiking, running, and playing games had a coronary heart disease incidence of one-half that of the workers who were less active. Paffenbarger and his coworkers (4,5) evaluated and followed over 6000 San Francisco longshoremen for over 22 years (early 1950s to early 1970s). They showed that the heavy physical activity of the cargo handlers during those decades, with an average energy expenditure of 8500 kcal or more per week, had a significantly lower risk of fatal coronary heart disease than men with less physically demanding jobs, such as hoist operators, foremen, and clerks. In a 7-year follow-up of participants in the Multiple Risk Factor Intervention Trial (MRFIT), Leon and his coinvestigators (6) observed a decrease in the relative risk of coronary heart disease as the degree of physical activity increased in this population. The subjects were divided into tertiles according to their level of leisure time physical activity calculated in kilocalories per day, with the lowest group being approximately half as active as the middle group and the high group more than twice as active as the middle group. Paffenbarger et al. (7,8) assessed the physical activity index in kilocalories per week based on habitual walking, stair climbing, leisure time sports play, and similar activities in almost 17,000 Harvard alumni over 10–16 years. In the 40% that had an index of 2000 kcal or more per week, the relative risk of developing coronary heart disease during the year follow-up was approximately 39% lower than the same risk in men who had an index of less than 2000 kcal.

In a review of these and other similar studies, several interesting facts are noted. First, in contrast to the Harvard alumni, the MRFIT study showed little or no benefit in mortality from exercise beyond a moderate level, even though there was a very significant benefit of moderate- over low-level exercise. Compared to the Harvard graduates, the MRFIT population differed: The subjects were primarily middle-aged men at presumed high risk for coronary disease and their overall participation in vigorous physical activity was far less than that noted in the Harvard alumni.

Second, in contrast to the other groups, the cardiovascular disease risk was lowered in the London civil servants surveyed by Morris et al. (2,3) only when their physical activity included vigorous sports play in contrast to all leisure moderate-level activities in the other groups. These differences among the studies may be related to the personal characteristics of the study populations, the classification of exercise activities, and perhaps even the diagnostic criteria used for determining the presence or absence of cardiovascular disease. However, in these and other studies, moderate-level or higher physical activity is related to decreased mortality and prolonged cardiovascular health.

More recent studies have looked at the levels of physical fitness and the risk of cardiovascular disease, primarily by measuring cardiovascular fitness parameters during exercise testing. This method of population study based on a single test measurement to evaluate fitness and compare the results to is much easier than trying to assess the degree of leisure and work activity by various mechanisms. The evaluation of the subjects in the MRFIT Study (6) show that treadmill times and percentage of subjects achieving target heart rates were significantly high when their leisure time activity assessment was greater. More importantly, coronary heart disease risk was less in those individuals as compared to those with the least exercise tolerance on treadmill testing.

Other studies should be noted as correlating measurements of physical fitness to coronary heart disease and all cause mortality. In one, Lie and coworkers (9) evaluated the fitness by submaximal ergometer testing and followed approximately 2000 middle-aged male industrial government workers in Oslo for 7 years. They noted that the more fit participants had lower resting heart rates, blood pressure, and serum lipids, higher maximum heart rates and blood pressure during exercise, smoked less than the less fit individuals, and approximately one-fifth the incidence of fatal coronary heart disease.

Ekelund et al. (10) evaluated the 4276 middle-aged men in the Lipid Research Clinic Study by the heart rate determined at the second stage of a submaximal test and maximum time on the treadmill test. The subjects were divided into four groups and followed over an average of 8.5 years. The coronary heart disease mortality in the most fit quartile was six times less than that in the least fit.

Slatterly and coworkers (11) evaluated 2400 railway workers by recording the exercise heart rates at various stages of a treadmill fitness test. It was noted that the group with the slowest heart rate at each level had about one-third the number of deaths due to coronary heart disease as did those with the fastest heart rate response. All these studies were adjusted for age and in the Lipid Research Clinic Study for cigarette smoking, blood pressure levels, lipoprotein profiles, etc., and the physical fitness determinations proved to be an independent predictor.

More recently, 10,250 middle-aged men were divided into five levels of fitness based on maximum treadmill performance when evaluated at the Cooper Clinic in Dallas (12). They were followed for 8 years for all-cause mortality with the death rate in the most fit group being 70% less than that in the least fit group. An increasing mortality gradient was noted from the most to least fit with the middle group showing 45% less mortality than the lowest risk group. These trends persisted even when factoring out cigarette smoking, elevated blood pressure, elevated cholesterol, elevated glucose, and family history of heart disease. More recently, Blair and his associates (12) have reanalyzed this data and added other subjects, again showing that there is a gradient in the reduction of mortality as related to fitness levels. This correlates with previous studies noting that even low moderate exercise is better than none if the effect of fitness on mortality is judged important. Maximum protection against heart disease may be at a moderate level of exercise with the more aggressive training techniques allowing one to be more competitive but perhaps not increasing life expectancy or reducing the frequency of coronary heart disease.

From these and many other studies, one can surmise that being physically active and maintaining a high level of physical fitness lessens the mortality due to coronary disease. For the patient with known cardiovascular disease in a rehabilitation program in which physical activity and risk factor control are the methods of intervention and secondary prevention, the evidence of mortality reduction from any one study is encouraging but not statistically significant. However, two recent publications have carefully looked at several studies utilizing therapeutic physical activity training programs in the patients with known heart disease. These selected studies differed in the length of time the subjects were in the training programs and the time in which they started to exercise following the cardiac event. However, all studies compared the patients in the exercise program to controls as to improvement in physical performance, the influence on risk factors, and, more importantly, the influence on all-cause and cardiovascular mortality and recurrence of myocardial infarction. In the first review, Oldridge and his colleagues (13) surveyed a number of Scandinavian and European studies and one study from the United States, all of which had excellent controls and well-documented data. They found a significant reduction in all-cause and cardiovascular disease mortality in those subjects who were in the exercise training programs. Of interest, there was no significant group differences in the recurrence of myocardial infarction, but the mortality associated with the recurrent myocardial infarction was dramatically reduced in those patients in the physical exercise programs. Later, O'Connor et al. (14) reviewed some of the same studies reviewed by Oldridge (13) and added others based on slightly different inclusion criteria. Importantly, they reported the influence of the physical activity programs on mortality at 1, 2, and 3 years regardless of the patients' duration in an exercise program. They noted that the greatest reduction on all-cause and cardiovascular mortality and sudden death was in the first year. But even after 3 years, there was approximately a 20% decrease in all three. Again, there was little effect on recurrence of myocardial infarction, but mortality from the recurrent myocardial infarction was quite low in the exercise group. In only one study was smoking control assessed, as no other risk factors were addressed. These studies were designed specifically to evaluate the influence of exercise on mortality and myocardial infarction recurrence rate following a cardiac event. Both studies used meta-analysis to analyze the multistudy data. Each individual study reviewed had positive trends, but usually because of the number of subjects the influence of exercise on mortality was not statistically significant. Combining the number of subjects in each study allowed several thousand subjects to be analyzed and made the statistical difference significant. There are many skeptics who find it difficult to accept this, but whether analyzed individually or collectively, all studies follow the same trend, noting that the exercise group had a reduction in mortality.

As the evidence builds supporting the premise that serum lipid reduction can control atherosclerotic plaque progression and, at times, regression of plaque size, one has to conclude that a well-designed multidisciplinary cardiac rehabilitation program should be extremely beneficial to the patient who has had a major coronary event.

This very brief review of the relation of physical activity and fitness levels on mortality in the cardiovascular disease patients is an introduction to the chapters that follow. It will be noted that patients with coronary artery disease treated medically for symptomatic and asymptomatic disease, and/or by interventional therapy, i.e., coronary artery bypass graft surgery, balloon angioplasty, etc., can benefit from exercise therapy. The more critically ill patients with congestive heart failure and those treated by cardiac transplant can also benefit from the effectiveness and safety of a rehabilitation program. Patients with congenital and valvular heart disease can be functionally improved. Exercise is the base around which rehabilitation and prevention programs can be developed to positively return the patient to an as near normal lifestyle as possible in a safe effective way. It also creates an environment in which all other risk factors for coronary disease can be evaluated, treated, and hopefully controlled.

REFERENCES

1. Morris, J.N., Heady, J.A., Raffle, P.A.B., Roberts, C.G., and Parks, *Lancet*, 2: 1053–1057, 1111–1120 (1953).
2. Morris, J.N., Kagan, A., Pattison, D.C., Gardner, M., and Raffle, P.A.B., *Lancet*, 2: 552–559 (1966).
3. Morris, J.N., *Uses of Epidemiology*. 3rd Ed. Churchill Livingstone, Edinburgh, pp. 159–186 (1975).
4. Paffenbarger, R.S., Jr., Laughlin, M.E., Gima, A.S., and Black, R.A., *N. Engl. J. Med.*, 282: 1109–1114 (1970).
5. Paffenbarger, R.S., Jr., and Hale, W.E., *N. Engl. J. Med.*, 292: 545–550 (1975).
6. Leon, A.S., Connett, J., Jacobs, D.R., Jr., and Rauramaa, R., *J.A.M.A.*, 258: 2388–2395 (1987).
7. Paffenbarger, R.S., Jr., Wing, A.L., and Hyde, R.T., *Am. J. Epidemiol.*, 108: 161–175 (1978).
8. Paffenbarger, R.S., Jr., Hyde, R.T., Wing, A.L., and Hsieh, C.-C., *N. Engl. J. Med.*, 314: 605–613, 315: 399–401 (1986).
9. Lie, H., Mundal, R., and Erikssen, J., *Eur. Heart J.*, 6: 147–157 (1985).
10. Ekelund, L.G., Haskell, W.L., Johnson, J.L., Whaley, F.S., Criqui, M.H., and Sheps, D.S., *N. Engl. J. Med.*, 319: 1379–1384 (1988).
11. Slatterly, M.L., Jacobs, D.R., Jr., and Nichaman, M.Z., *Circulation*, 79: 304–311 (1989).
12. Blair, S.N., Kohl, H.W., Paffenbarger, R.S., Clark, D.G., Cooper, K.H., and Gibbons, L.W., *J.A.M.A.*, 262: 2395–2401 (1989).
13. Oldridge, N.B., Guyatt, G.H., Fischer, M.E., and Rimm, A.A., *J.A.M.A.*, 260: 945–950 (1988).
14. O'Connor, G.T., Buring, J.E., Yusuf, S., Goldhaber, S.Z., Olmstead, E.M., Paffenbarger, R.S., Jr., and Hennekens, C.H., *Circulation*, 80: 234–244 (1989).

8

Exercise and Therapy of the Cardiac Transplant Patient

Terence Kavanagh

University of Toronto
Toronto, Ontario, Canada

INTRODUCTION

The typical heart transplant recipient is a 45-year-old male who, as a result of severe ischemic heart disease or cardiomyopathy, has developed New York Heart Association Class IV cardiac failure (1). He has experienced varying periods of preoperative invalidism, suffers from generalized muscle weakness, has not worked steadily for some time, and is depressed and fearful. It is hard to imagine a more appropriate candidate for exercise rehabilitation. Of course, the first positive step toward full recovery is the transplant procedure itself, with its rapid alleviation of disabling cardiac symptoms and its increasingly optimistic long-term outlook (5- and 10-year survival rates of 85 and 75%, respectively). However, successful exploitation of the new heart requires a program to improve physical fitness, restore self-confidence, and hasten return to full-time employment. Since the patient is committed to a life-long regimen of medical supervision, there is ample opportunity for the rehabilitation team to become involved in the ongoing medical care, particularly in the first postsurgical year.

PHYSIOLOGICAL RESPONSES TO EXERCISE
AFTER HEART TRANSPLANTATION

Although the rehabilitation goals and the method of achieving these are the same for cardiac transplant recipients as they are for coronary artery bypass graft and postmyocardial infarction patients, the fact that we are dealing with a transplanted denervated heart requires special consideration.

The resting rate of the donor heart is high (approximately 100 beats min^{-1}) both during waking and sleeping hours; this is due to the intrinsic rate of its sinoatrial node, now free from the customary vagal inhibition (2–6). The minor 24-h fluctuations in resting rate which do occur are a result of variations in the levels of circulating catecholamines (7).

Given a normal peripheral demand for blood flow, the denervated heart's relative tachycardia implies a small stroke volume at rest. Thus, even in the absence of further increase in heart rate, the Frank Starling mechanism has the potential to induce a substantial increase of cardiac output during exercise. In practice, the response of the transplanted heart to both postural and light exercise appears to be mediated by an increase in venous return with a consequent increase in stroke volume. During more vigorous activity, any further augmentation in cardiac output depends on circulating catecholamine-induced chronotropic and inotropic response (3,8,9). This explains the attenuated heart rate response to an incremental exercise test, sluggish in the first few minutes and then rising more steeply as serum levels of catecholamines rise, and even continuing to rise after cessation of effort and during the first few minutes of recovery when catecholamine levels are presumably still high and accumulating (10). Recovery rates are also delayed because of the slow clearance of circulating catecholamines, which may exert their chronotropic action for up to 10 min in recovery (11,12) (Fig. 1). Support for this interpretation of the denervated heart's response to effort come from animal and human studies which show that they are abolished by the administration of a β-blocker (8,13–16). Peak heart rates, on the other hand, are approximately 20–25% lower than those seen in age-matched controls (Table 1) owing to the absence of direct sympathetic innervation of the sinoatrial node (17–20).

Interpretation of changes in blood pressure responses after transplantation is difficult because both cardiac and peripheral vascular components are involved, and one cannot easily differentiate between the various potential mechanisms (Table 2). Resting hypertension is a

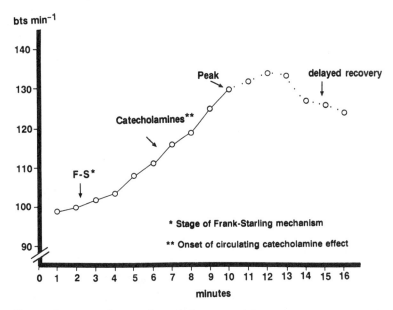

Figure 1   Typical transplanted denervated heart rate response to increasing effort. Note the high resting rate, the delayed rate of acceleration during effort, the delayed deceleration during recovery, and the tendency for the rate to continue to rise after the termination of effort (peak exercise).

common and disturbing finding (21). It is characteristically associated with an elevated peripheral vascular resistance; this may be a persistent response to the preoperative state of congestive heart failure and its resultant chronic elevation of plasma norepinephrine (22–24). The problem of increased vascular resistance is compounded by the presence of the healthy donor heart, with its normal cardiac output. In recent years, however, suspicion has centered increasingly on cyclosporine as the cause of hypertension in the transplant recipient (25,26). Prior to the introduction of that immunosuppressant in 1981, the incidence of hypertension in transplant patients was relatively low (27). High dosages may be a factor (27), and some have suggested that the hypertensive effect is increased by the concomitant use of steroids (28). The exact pathophysiology remains unclear, but is no doubt associated with the considerable adverse effects that cyclosporine has been noted to have on renal function (29,30).

The peak systolic blood pressure during maximal effort is reduced to approximately 80% of age-matched normal controls

Table 1 Initial Cardiovascular Status of Cardiac Transplant Patients Referred to the Toronto/Harefield Unit for Rehabilitation Compared With Age-Matched Normals (mean values ±SD)

	Age (yrs)	Heart rate (beats/min)		Systolic pressure (torr)		Diastolic pressure (torr)	
		rest	peak	rest	peak	rest	peak
Patients	47.3 ± 8.6	103.9 ±11.8	135.5 ±15.2	137.8 ±15.7	178.2 ±25.8	95.3 ±13.5	100.4 ±12.5
Age-matched Normal subjects	45.4 ± 7.2	76.8 ±13.7[a]	176.2 ±12.8[a]	128.6 ±16.5[a]	214.2 ±21.2[a]	83.8 ±10.0[a]	95.6 ±12.1

[a] $p < 0.001$.

Table 2 Physical Characteristics of Cardiac Transplant Patients Referred for Rehabilitation Compared with Age-Matched Normals (mean values ±SD) (TRC/Harefield)

	Age (yrs)	Height (cm)	Body mass (kg)	Lean mass	
				kg	kg/cm of stature
Patients	47.3 ±8.6	172.8 ±6.1	69.9 ±11.5	56.2 ±7.3	0.325 ±0.06
Age-matched Normal subjects	45.4 ±7.2	176.4 ±6.5[a]	80.7 ±10.9[b]	62.6 ±7.6[b]	0.355 ±0.07[b]

[a] $p < 0.01$.
[b] $p < 0.001$.

(18,19,31) (see Table 1). This is due to the loss of sympathetic stimulation with the resultant impairment of myocardial contractility (32). Presumably this impairment only manifests itself after the onset of moderately vigorous effort, since the heart transplant recipient's resting cardiac output is generally the same as age-matched controls. Furthermore, exercise radionuclide studies by Yusuf and coworkers (33) show patients to have normal systolic function and inotropic reserve during volume loading (leg elevation) and low-level supine exercise (a power output of 15 Ws on the cycle ergometer), but some impaired function at a power output of 45 Ws. A further explanation for the reduced peak systolic blood pressure is that chronically elevated levels of serum catecholamines may induce downregulation of the peripheral arterial α-receptors (34).

There is evidence of impairment of diastolic function after heart transplant (33–37) (see Table 1). Contributing factors could include impaired myocardial compliance, ischemia from accelerated coronary artery narrowing, the side effects of immunosuppressant drugs, or the ischemic time of the donor heart.

In our experience, the transplant recipient has a 10–15% reduction in lean body mass, likely the result of a prolonged preoperative period of physical inactivity, together with high steroid administration during the immediate postoperative period (18,38,32) (see Table 2). As a result, maximal work output is reduced. Whether the lower values for peak heart rate and systolic blood pressure previously referred to are contributing factors, or merely expressions of the muscle weakness, is still a matter of conjecture. In accord with the reduced exercise performance, we have also measured the maximal oxygen uptake (as defined by the attainment of an oxygen plateau) at approximately two-thirds that of the normal age-matched population. A direct consequence of the muscle wasting is early fatigue during physical effort, which in its turn discourages further physical activity and leads to a vicious circle of greater loss of muscle mass with even more fatigue.

In summary, then, orthotopic heart transplant patients have a typically high resting heart rate, with normal or near-normal resting cardiac output. However, at maximum effort they exhibit a significantly lower work output, heart rate, and systolic blood pressure (and thus double product) as well as oxygen uptake. Resting and maximal diastolic blood pressure are high compared with normals. At equivalent levels of submaximal effort oxygen uptake is the same, but minute ventilation, perceived exertion, and the ventilatory equivalent for oxygen are all higher than in normals; the absolute ventilatory threshold is lower, thus implying an earlier onset of anaerobic metabolism. Cardiac output increases linearly and in normal increments in response to increased in-work output on the cycle ergometer or treadmill, but absolute submaximal values are slightly lower than normal.

HETEROTOPIC CARDIAC TRANSPLANTATION

In heterotopic cardiac transplantation, the donor heart is implanted in the chest in parallel with the recipient heart. The arteries to both sinoatrial nodes are preserved as well as the nerves to the recipient heart, but not to the donor heart. Thus, the donor heart responds to acute exercise in the typically denervated manner, with the recipient heart still exhibiting the effects of autonomic innervation. Occasionally there is persistence of anginal pain and/or dysrhythmias in the recipient left ventricle. Apart from that, these patients share many of the features described for the orthotopic transplant recipient, including a loss of lean tissue, a low peak oxygen uptake, and peak work output.

Worldwide adoption of the heterotopic procedure has been very limited, with less than 1% of all cardiac transplants carried out being heterotopic in type (1). Nevertheless, such cases are encountered from time-to-time, and reference will be made later to their responses to an exercise rehabilitation training program.

HEART-LUNG TRANSPLANTATION

Combined heart-lung transplantation is now carried out for patients with end-stage cardiopulmonary disease. The majority (60%) of recipients are female, with an average age of 30 years. Experience with this procedure is less extensive than with cardiac transplantation; the 5-year survival rate is 55% (1). However, exercise capacity following surgery is similarly restricted, and therefore rehabilitation similarly indicated. In terms of responses to acute exercise, there are few differences from those of the orthotopic heart transplant recipient. Maximal work output, peak heart rate, peak systolic blood pressure, and peak oxygen uptake are all lower than normal, with the reductions being in the same order as for heart transplant patients. In response to submaximal effort, heart rate, systolic and diastolic blood pressures, and oxygen uptake behave similarly in both groups. However, there is a tendency for minute ventilation and respiratory rate to be higher in the heart-lung group, possibly owing to a loss of negative feedback from the pulmonary afferent nerves (19). This slight difference in cardiopulmonary response to acute exercise does not appear to affect exercise training results.

THE EXERCISE PROGRAM

Exercise Testing

The first step in establishing a safe and effective exercise rehabilitation program is an exercise test. Because this has been dealt with in detail elsewhere in this volume, only those aspects of testing which are particularly relevant to the heart transplant patient will be referred to here. The two most frequent modes of exercise in current use are, of course, the motor-driven treadmill and the cycle ergometer. The former is almost standard in North America and the United Kingdom, with the latter the method of choice in Europe. Hospital cardiology departments also tend to favor the treadmill, and respiratory laboratories the ergometer.

The advantages of the cycle are that the action is simple to perform and does not arouse anxiety, mechanical efficiency is largely independent of body mass, and the upper body remains stable, thus making it easier to obtain accurate metabolic and circulatory measurements. A possible disadvantage is early quadriceps fatigue, particularly in those unaccustomed to cycling. The treadmill, on the other hand, employs the more customary "natural" walking motion. However, in the absence of metabolic measurements, the use of the railings for support can reduce the energy cost of a given treadmill speed and slope, thus invalidating the tables which relate exercise duration time to oxygen uptake. Alternatively, preventing the use of the railings for support introduces an element of fear for the severely deconditioned patient.

The treadmill protocols generally used in testing heart transplant patients are continuous in type, and generally either modified forms of the Bruce or the Naughton protocol. Whatever protocol is used, the aim should be to achieve maximum effort in approximately 8–10 min, which implies work increments of 1–2 METs (metabolic equivalents of oxygen consumption) (3.5 ml kg min^{-1} to 7 ml kg min^{-1} oxygen uptake). Savin and coworkers have used 3-min stages, the first two at 2 mph and then 3 mph at 2.5% grade, with increases of 2.5% in grade for each stage thereafter (39).

The customary exercise test used at the Toronto Rehabilitation Centre and in the Rehabilitation Department of Harefield Hospital is carried out on the cycle ergometer and serves to measure peak heart rate, peak power output, and peak oxygen consumption, and to provide guidelines for the exercise prescription (18). Power outputs are increased stepwise by 100 kpm min^{-1} every minute (16.7 Ws) or, in severely deconditioned subjects, 50 kpm min^{-1} every minute (8.3 Ws) until the patient can no longer pedal at the required rate of 60 rpm. At each stage, the patient is asked to indicate perception of effort by pointing to a chart displaying the original Borg scale (40). The exercise electrocardiogram uses three leads (aVF, V_1, CM_5). For heterotopic transplant recipients we use leads V_6R, V_5, V_1, and aVF; the QRS complex from the donor heart produces the dominant positive vector in V_6R, whereas that from the recipient heart produces a dominant positive vector in V_5 and aVF (31) (Fig. 2). Blood pressure readings are taken at 2-min intervals, at peak effort, and during recovery. Expired air is collected and analyzed by means of a metabolic cart to determine peak oxygen uptake and ventilatory threshold.

The heart transplant recipient's atypical heart rate response to exercise precludes the use of age-related tables to predict aerobic power from the heart rate and work output; hence the advantage of direct measurement. Analysis of expired air also enables determination of the anaerobic threshold, which has generally been defined in relation to a number of ventilatory variables (41). These include, in respect to a progressive increase in oxygen uptake, a disproportionate increase in (a) the ventilatory equivalent for oxygen, (b) the minute ventilation, (c) the carbon dioxide output, and (d) the respiratory exchange ratio (42–44); the data are expressed in terms of the oxygen uptake at which the upward "breakpoint" of each plot occurs (Fig. 3). The attraction of the anaerobic threshold (or perhaps a better term, "ventilatory threshold") is that it occurs at approximately 60% of peak oxygen uptake (45–47), a level of effort which correlates well with the intensity required for endurance training, and is usually attainable even by those patients insufficiently motivated to exert maximal effort (48). Our practice is to use the disproportionate increase in the ventilatory equivalent for oxygen as our primary measure, with corroboration sought, where indicated, by the previously mentioned variables.

A maximal exercise test is one in which peak oxygen uptake has been demonstrated by the attainment of an oxygen consumption "plateau" of less than 2 ml/kg/min^{-1} when comparing the final and penultimate workstages (49). In the normal subject, this is a relatively stable measurement, which bears a clear relationship to maximal cardiac output (50), and has a high test-retest correlation (51). However, because of their severely deconditioned state, only about 50% of cardiac transplant patients are likely to meet the criterion of an oxygen plateau at the initial test (18). Corroborative evidence of maximal effort is therefore sought in a respiratory gas exchange ratio greater than 1.10 (52). The indications for stopping a test before the demonstration of a

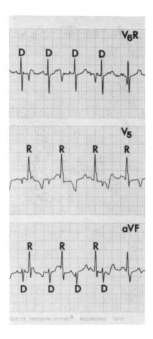

Figure 2 Electrocardiogram from a heterotopic cardiac transplantation patient showing separate identification of recipient (R) and donor (D) QRS complexes.

plateau are as recommended by the American College of Sports Medicine (53). However, it should be noted that the donor denervated heart cannot indicate an ischemic state by anginal pain. Particular attention has to be paid, therefore, to the symptoms of dyspnea, lightheadedness, and faintness as well as to the familiar electrocardiographic signs of increasing ectopy and ST segmental depression (54). Because the transplanted heart is invariably healthy, exercise electrocardiographic abnormalities are rare except during bouts of rejection. However, the late development of an accelerated form of coronary atherosclerosis in the donor heart is not uncommon, and therefore evidence of ischemia may eventually be seen in long-standing transplants (55–57). As mentioned previously, however, the heterotopic patient may experience occasional persistence of anginal pain and/or dysrhythmias in the recipient left ventricle.

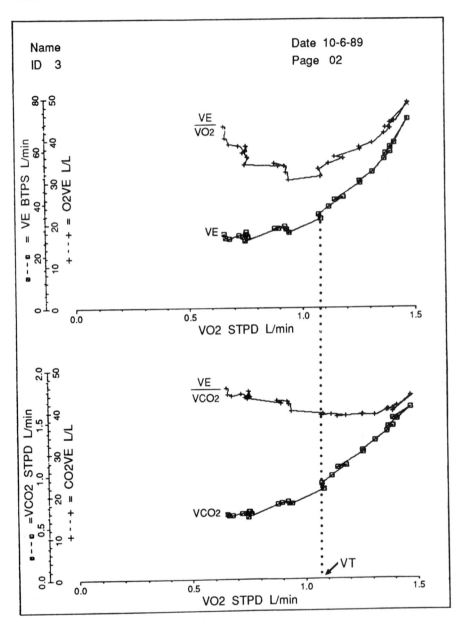

Figure 3 The ventilatory threshold (VT) is identified, relative to oxygen uptake, (VO_2) at the upward inflection of the curves for the ventilatory equivalent for oxygen (VE/VO_2); the minute ventilation (VE), and the carbon dioxide output (VCO_2); note that the ventilatory equivalent for carbon dioxide (VE/VCO_2) curve is still flat at the VT.

Inpatient Physical Therapy Program

Barring complications, cardiac transplant recipients are usually discharged from the hospital ward after approximately 3 weeks. During the first 24 hs they receive full reverse-barrier nursing in isolation rooms. Thereafter, rehabilitation takes the form of the customary physical therapy regimen. Passive range of motion, breathing, and postural exercises are followed by active upper and lower limb mobilization, initially in the supine position and then seated in a chair. Patients progress from sitting to standing exercises, and by the third to the fifth day are walking in the room. At this time they may also begin to use the cycle ergometer, pedaling at zero resistance for 3–5 min. During this early phase the blood pressure and electrocardiogram are monitored, and the perceived exertion held in the 11–13 range (fairly light to somewhat hard). As tolerance improves, the intervals of time and the power outputs of the ergometer are increased, corridor walking is permitted, and by the time of discharge a low-level incremental exercise test may be carried out either on the ergometer or on the treadmill, with power output increments of 1 MET. This would allow the prescription of a walking or stationary cycling program, which can be followed during the early outpatient phase of 4–8 weeks.

The major concerns during these early postoperative weeks include problems of rejection, infection, arrhythmias in the donor heart, neurological deficits, and renal dysfunction; in addition to intensive clinical monitoring for signs of rejection, there is also the need for frequent blood work, serial electrocardiograms, echocardiographic and Doppler assessments of heart size and function, and repeat endomyocardial biopsies. All of these must of necessity take precedence over an exercise rehabilitation program. Nevertheless, much can be done in these weeks by an enthusiastic therapist to attune the patient's mind to the restorative value of a long-term outpatient exercise rehabilitation regimen.

Outpatient Exercise Training Program

The activity prescribed for physical training will depend upon the experience and preference of the rehabilitation team, but should adhere to the accepted principle that cardiovascular fitness is achieved most consistently by dynamic activity which involves large muscle groups and which can be accurately quantified and monitored; e.g., walking/jogging, swimming, and circuit training. The customary training activity used by the author is walking, progressing to jogging, with stationary cycling or swimming either on a temporary or a permanent basis for those who have problems ambulating.

In the Toronto/Harefield program, the initial exercise prescription calls for 1.6 km, five times weekly. The intensity, or pace of the walk, is based on 60% of peak oxygen uptake, supported by the oxygen uptake level at which the ventilatory threshold is determined, and a perceived exertion of 14 on the Borg scale. This usually works out to an initial walking pace of between 11 and 14 min per km. The distance is then increased by 1.6 km every 2 weeks, maintaining the same pace until, by 6 weeks, the patient is walking 4.8 km, five times weekly. The pace is then quickened by 1 min/1.6 km until the 4.8 km is accomplished in 45 min (typically within 4 months of starting the program). Thereafter, 50-m bouts of slow jogging paced at 7.5 min/km are introduced at the start of every 800 ms, then every 400 ms, 200 ms, 100 ms, and so on until ultimately the entire 4.8 km is completed in 36 min. Finally, the more highly motivated and compliant individuals are progressed to 6.4 km, or 32 km weekly, maintaining the same pace of 7.5 min/km. After the first 6 weeks, and if the patient "sticks" at a given pace, then the exercise prescription is adjusted so as to obtain a training session which would last from between 30 and 60 min (58).

Because of the atypical heart rate response and the lack of angina as a symptom of myocardial ischemia, accurate pacing is emphasized as well as thorough familiarity with the concept of perceived exertion and correct interpretation of such symptoms of myocardial ischemia as excessive dyspnea, unusual fatigue, lightheadedness, and extrasystoles. Rejection episodes or intercurrent infections may interrupt the training program from time-to-time, and patients should be advised of this possibility at the outset.

Initially some patients may need regular supervision or even electrocardiographic monitoring during the exercise sessions, but these are a minority. Most will be able to train at home without risk, attending a supervised class only once a week, or even once monthly. During the first 6–12 months there are frequent return visits to the Transplant Unit or the local hospital for routine follow-up testing, and this gives ample opportunity for the appropriate rehabilitation team to carry out exercise testing and to assess the patient's progress and adherence to the training regimen.

Accelerated coronary atherosclerosis is a serious late complication after cardiac transplantation (59). By the third postoperative year, some 40% of patients will show angiographic evidence of this condition. Even this is probably an underestimate, since angiography is less sensitive in detecting the peculiar form of atherosclerosis which affects the transplanted heart; i.e., a diffuse concentric intimal thickening rather than the classic asymmetric and discrete atherosclerotic plaques.

As mentioned previously, anginal pain is absent in the orthotopic recipient with coronary artery disease, and so one has to be particularly vigilant for such signs of ischemia as undue exertional breathlessness, lightheadedness, or excessive fatigue. The exact cause of the condition is unknown, although it has been suggested that it is either due to prolonged use of cyclosporine and/or steroids, postoperative attacks of cytomegaloviral infection, or repeated bouts of rejection. Workers at Harefield report that the rate of coronary disease is lower in those patients who receive cyclosporine and azathioprine as opposed to those on prednisone and azathioprine (60). The Stanford group found a high association between elevated serum total and LDL cholesterol levels and graft atherosclerosis, and have advocated aggressive dietary, and if necessary, drug intervention (61,62). The rehabilitation program will, therefore, pay close attention to serum lipid and glucose levels, and will provide the necessary education to those who have problems in these areas.

From the viewpoint of exercise training, the transplant team's attitude toward the use of steroids as part of the postoperative immunosuppressant regimen is important. The long-term side effects of high-dosage oral steroids, which include osteoporosis, increased risk of infection, and adverse effects on glucose and lipid metabolism can constitute problems during a prolonged training program. To date, the majority of the transplant patients trained by the author have been receiving the customary Harefield immunosuppressant drug regimen, which utilizes cyclosporine in dosages to maintain a serum level of 100–200 ng/ml after the first month, and azathioprine in a dosage of 2 mg/kg/day. Oral steroids are not used routinely, but they are used temporarily if the patient has recurrent or persistent rejection or develops postoperative renal dysfunction. This approach has certainly been associated with the successful use of a vigorous and effective training program. On the other hand, patients taking the more conventional dosages of prednisone have also benefited from training, although we have found their progress has been slower.

Effects of Exercise Training

As might be expected, there are considerably fewer reports in the literature to date on the effects of training after heart transplantation than there are after acute myocardial infarction or coronary artery bypass graft surgery. The earliest was from Squires and coworkers (4), who trained two orthotopic transplantation recipients for 8 weeks, using a combination of treadmill walking and stationary cycling, three times weekly for 8 weeks at an intensity of 12–13 on the Borg scale. The exercise sessions were well tolerated. Comparison of treadmill test results at the beginning and end of the program showed a reduction in systolic blood pressures and ratings of perceived exertion at equivalent submaximal exercise levels, but no significant changes in resting, sub-maximal, or peak heart rates. One patient gained 0.9 kg and the other 3.5 kg in body mass over the 8-week period. The greater gain was felt to be due to fluid retention secondary to steroid therapy. Metabolic measurements were not carried out.

Shortly thereafter, Savin et al. (63) evaluated the effects of a 16-week stationary cycling program on five orthotopic patients. The duration of the exercise sessions was at least 30 min, they were repeated five times weekly, and the intensity was based on 75% of the peak heart rate. Cycle ergometry carried out at the end of the training period showed a 45% increase in peak work output, an 18% increase in peak oxygen uptake, and a 13% reduction in submaximal heart rates. Echocardiography failed to demonstrate any change in cardiac dimensions.

More recently, Niset followed 62 orthotopic transplants for 1 year (64). The exercise program consisted of stationary cycling and calisthenics, three to five times weekly, at an intensity of 60–70% of maximal working capacity. The physical benefits included a 30–40% increase in peak work output and oxygen uptake as well as an increase in peak heart rate and peak blood pressure. Submaximal heart rates and systolic blood pressures were unchanged, but there were significant reductions in the respiratory exchange ratio, minute ventilation, and blood lactates at equivalent levels of submaximal work. Keteyian and coworkers (65) have also reported the effects of a 12-week endurance training program on 21 orthotopic patients. Significant increases were observed in peak work output, peak oxygen uptake, and peak minute ventilation. There was a decrease in the rating of perceived exertion at submaximal levels of effort. There was no change in resting heart rate.

In a pilot study between the Toronto Rehabilitation Centre and the Cardiac Transplantation Unit of Harefield Hospital, England, Kavanagh et al. (18) trained 36 orthotopic transplant patients for an average duration of 16 months using a walk/jog program as described above. Compliance was very good, all patients progressing to an average distance of 24 km/week, at an average pace of 8.5 min/km. Eight of the patients were highly motivated, and achieved 32 km or more a week, at an average pace of 6.5 min/km. It was one of these eight who

entered and finished the 42-km Boston Marathon 12 months after join-
ing the program and 15 months after undergoing the transplantation
procedure (66). The group as a whole experienced only a few episodes
of rejection or infection, and these were of such a minor nature that
they had little effect on the training regimen.

After training there was a 5% increase in body mass, of which
3.2% was lean tissue (Table 3). The resting heart rate for all patients
was slightly reduced, but the greatest reduction occurred in those who
were highly compliant. The peak heart rate was significantly increased
in both highly compliant and moderately compliant patients.
Nevertheless, the final resting heart rates remained higher, and the
final peak heart rates lower than in a group of age-matched normal
subjects. Submaximal heart rates showed a small reduction in the
group as a whole. However, there was no change in the 28 moderately
compliant patients, whereas in the eight highly compliant patients the
effect was quite large (Fig. 4). Interestingly, the patient who completed
the Boston Marathon, averaging 65 km weekly in the final months of
training, showed the response closest to a true training bradycardia
(Fig. 5). Since the relationship of oxygen uptake to power output in all
patients, including the highly compliant eight, was unchanged during
submaximal effort, this reduction in submaximal heart rate could not

Table 3 Effects of an Exercise Training Program on 36 Orthotopic Cardiac
Transplant Patients (mean change ±SD)

	Physical characteristics	
	Body mass (kg)	Lean mass (kg)
All patients	$+4.0 \pm 6.7^a$	$+1.98 \pm 3.31^a$
	Heart rate (beats/min)	
	rest	peak
All patients	-3.6 $\pm 10.7^b$	$+12.7$ $\pm 16.7^a$
Highly compliant	-10.5 $\pm 4.9^a$	$+12.1$ $\pm 13.2^a$

[a] $p < 0.001$.
[b] $p < 0.05$.

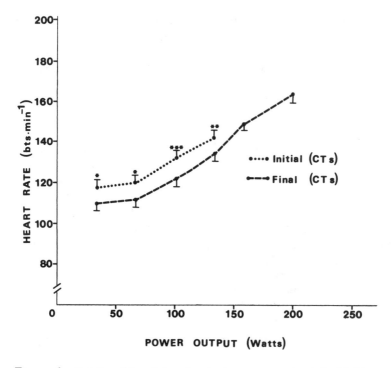

Figure 4 Relationship of heart rate to power output in highly compliant patients before and after conditioning. *p < 0.05; **p < 0.01; ***p < 0.001.

have been due to an improvement in mechanical efficiency on the ergometer (Fig. 6). There was also an overall and significant marked reduction in the rating of perceived exertion, minute ventilation, and diastolic blood pressure (Fig. 7) at equivalent work outputs.

The peak work output increased by 49% (65% in the 8 highly compliant), peak oxygen uptake by 27% (54% in the highly compliant), with all patients exercising to a larger respiratory minute ventilation and a higher maximal heart rate after training. Since changes in the respiratory gas exchange ratio and peak rating of perceived exertion were quite small, it is unlikely that greater voluntary effort was responsible for improved performance.

It was felt that the reduction in resting and submaximal heart rates seen in those who attained the greatest training distances was due to a drop in effort-induced levels of serum norepinephrine and/or downregulation in the sensitivity of cardiac β-adrenoreceptors. Both of

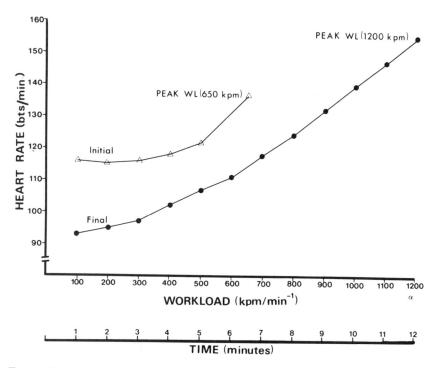

Figure 5 Development of training bradycardia in cardiac transplantation patient who completed the 1985 Boston Marathon.

these changes have been shown to occur in animals and humans exposed to vigorous training (67–70). The entire group's increase in the peak exercise heart rate was likely due to a strengthening of leg muscles. This peripheral adaptation would account for the improved power output, and because of a later onset of anaerobiosis, the reduced perception of effort and minute ventilation during submaximal exercise. Submaximal cardiac outputs, measured by the CO_2 rebreathing technique (71), did not change with training in relation to oxygen uptake (Fig. 8). This argues in favor of peripheral rather than central improvement, although it is tempting to infer that the reduction in submaximal diastolic blood pressures toward normal values is an indication of improved myocardial compliance.

The relative infrequency of the heterotopic transplantation procedure (less than 1% of the total) explains the paucity of reports on the rehabilitation of this group. Sieurat and his coworkers (72) trained

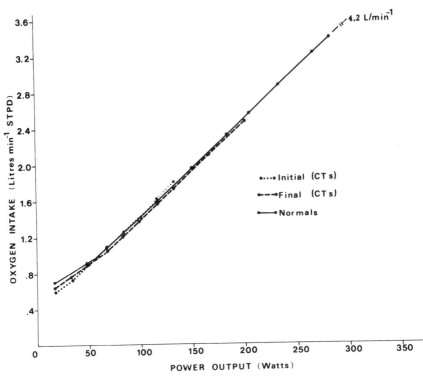

Figure 6 Relationship of oxygen intake to power output in a group of cardiac transplantation patients and age-matched controls.

eight heterotopic recipients and demonstrated an increase in peak work output and peak heart rate. This was associated with compliance to the program. Kavanagh et al. reported on 10 male heterotopes who followed a walk/jog training program for 18 months (32). Compliance was poorer than in orthotopic recipients, mainly because of a higher incidence of minor medical setbacks. Nevertheless, after training lean body mass increased by 4%, peak work output by 33%, peak oxygen uptake by 23%, and absolute ventilatory threshold by 16%. While the donor resting heart rate did not change significantly, the recipient resting heart rate fell significantly by 14 beats/min. The recipient submaximal heart rate showed a training bradycardia, and demonstrated less exercise-induced ventricular ectopy than at initial testing. Donor submaximal heart rates were unchanged.

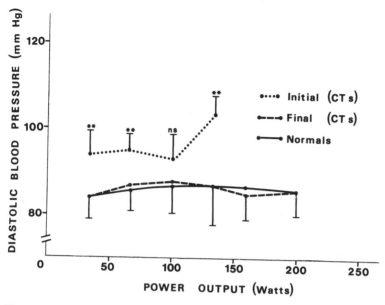

Figure 7 Relationship of diastolic blood pressure responses to power output before and after conditioning. *p < 0.05; **p < 0.01; ***p < 0.001.

PSYCHOSOCIAL ASPECTS

Psychological Changes

Information on the psychological effects of heart transplantation remains scant. Buxton et al. has used the Nottingham Health Profile to study the quality of life in 29 United Kingdom patients before, and then 3, 6, and 12 months after surgery (73). In all six dimensions (physical mobility, energy, pain, emotional reaction, sleep habits, and social isolation) there was very marked improvement by 3 months; the trend was continuing, although less pronounced, at the end of 1 year. Patients were uniformly enthusiastic about their progress, the following comments being typical: "It's a new lease on life"; "The best thing that has ever happened to me"; "A second chance"; "Every day a bonus."

Other workers have noted the high levels of anxiety and depression, the poor sense of well-being, and the negative body image frequently encountered in patients awaiting a new heart (74,75). This is hardly surprising when one considers that the patient is trying to cope

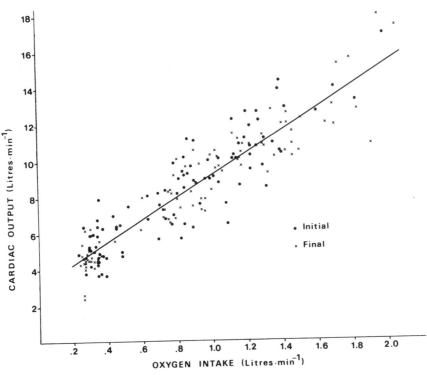

Figure 8   Relationship of individual cardiac output responses to VO₂ before and after conditioning.

with a life-threatening illness and all of its attendant social and financial consequences. Successful transplantation will inevitably bring about considerable improvement in mood state. Nevertheless, the posttransplantation months can also be highly stressful. In a group of Australian heart recipients, a greater proportion (43%) were more anxious at 1 year than at discharge (19%) (76). Causes for their concern included financial problems and being a burden on the family (50%), fear that overexertion would harm the new heart (43%), excessive weight gain (36%), and an inability to exercise (29). These findings would suggest that a comprehensive rehabilitation program should have a major role to play in terms of psychosocial benefit. Again, no prospective randomized controlled trial to investigate this possibility has been carried out to date, and therefore conclusions must be drawn from observational reports.

Degre has carried out psychological assessment on 100 transplant patients who participated in a structured exercise rehabilitation program for 1 year (77). He found that acceptance of the new heart and improved quality of life was apparent in the early phases of the program, but that psychosocial items (anxiety, coping ability, social interaction, and mental alertness) took longer to recover. Ultimately, however, there was complete return to normality in all areas and in almost all patients. Kavanagh et al. have investigated the influence of a 2-year exercise training program upon the psychological status of 30 male patients (23 orthotopic and seven heterotopic recipients). Although the average time elapsing between surgery and entry to the program was 6 months, initial testing showed significant depression together with high scores for the neurotic triad (hypochondriasis, hysteria, and psychasthenia) as well as significant anxiety, feelings of fatigue, and loss of vigor. These findings were more apparent in the heterotopes than in the orthotopes, perhaps because the former experienced more frequent, although mild, bouts of infection and rejection. Training was accompanied by a lessening of depression and the neurotic triad, a decrease in anxiety and fatigue, and an increase in vigor. It could be argued that some of the improvement might have arisen as part of the natural recovery process. Against this is the fact that the initial observations were made at a time when most of the spontaneous recovery could be expected to have occurred, and second by the failure to find any correlation between initial scores and the postoperative interval (78).

Return to Work

Given the high cost of the transplantation procedure and the average age of the recipients, return to work is a highly desirable goal. In those who have not been entered into a formal rehabilitation program, the proportion obtaining work after surgery has been variously reported as being anywhere between 32 and 64% (79–82). The reasons for failure to find employment are rarely medical, and include age, preillness employment pattern, type of work, and availability of disability payments. Degre's experience with a group attending the rehabilitation program was that 71% of those who were working 6 months before surgery had returned to work (76). Age seemed to be a factor in that the return rate was 82% for those under 45, 76% for those between 46 and 55 years, and 10% for those over 55 years. While a high proportion of those who were working before their illness returned (73%), only 10% of those who were unemployed prior to their illness managed to do so. Psychological profile was important, with 85% of nondepressed returning to work, but only 27% of those who were depressed went back to work. Similarly, 72% of those with a "Type A" personality were successful in finding work, whereas only 44% of those with "Type B" did so. Nevertheless, the high proportion of patients returning to work, i.e., 71%, suggests that a comprehensive rehabilitation program is of value. Similarly, 69% of patients attending the Toronto/Harefield program returned to work, 8% took early retirement, and only 3% were finally unemployed for medical reasons (83).

CONCLUSIONS

The routine use of a comprehensive exercise rehabilitation program following cardiac transplantation is fully justified on physiological, psychological, and vocational grounds. It is a safe and effective way to maximize the benefits of surgery, and can be applied not only after orthotopic cardiac transplantation, but also after the heterotopic procedure and heart-lung transplantation. There is, of course, still a considerable scope for further research. Questions remaining to be answered include the precise nature of the training adaptations and the contribution made by central and peripheral factors. It is also tempting to speculate on the favorable effects of a rehabilitation program, which includes exercise training, dietary advice, and weight control on: (a) the incidence and severity of posttransplant coronary atherosclerosis, (b) the extent and degree of posttransplantation hypertension, and (c) the incidence of bouts of intercurrent infection and rejection in the immunosuppressed patient.

REFERENCES

1. Heck, C.F., Shumway, S.J., and Kaye, M.P., *J. Heart Transplant*, 8: 271–276 (1989).
2. Stinson, E.B., Griepp, R.B., Schroeder, J.S., Dong, E., and Shumway, N.E., *Circulation*, 45: 1183 (1972).
3. Pope, S.E., Stinson, E.B., Daughters, G.T., Schroeder, J.S., Ingels, N.B., and Alderman, E.L., *Am. J. Cardiol.*, 46: 231 (1980).
4. Squires, R.W., Arthur, P.R., Gau, G.T., Muri, A., and Lambert, W.B., *J. Cardiac Rehabil.*, 3: 570 (1983).
5. Jose, A., and Collision, D., *Cardiovasc. Res.*, 4: 160 (1970).
6. de Marneffe, M., Jacobs, P., Haardt, R., and Englert, M., *Eur. Heart J.*, 7: 662 (1986).
7. Alexopoulos, D., Yusuf, S., Johnston, J.A., et al., *Am. J. Cardiol.*, 61: 880 (1988).

8. Donald, D.E., and Shepherd, J.T., *Am. J. Physiol.*, *25*: 393 (1963).
9. McLaughlin, P.R., Daughters, G.T., Ingels, N.B., et al., *Circulation, 58*: 476 (1979).
10. Yusuf, S., Mitchell, A., and Yacoub, M., *Br. Heart J.*, *54*: 173–178 (1985).
11. Degre, S.G., Niset, G.L., De Smet, J.M., et al., *Am. J. Cardiol.*, *60*: 926–928 (1987).
12. Sarnoff, S.J., Gilmore, J.P., and Wallace, A.G., *Neural Control of the Heart* (W.C. Randall, ed). Williams & Wilkins, Baltimore (1965).
13. Donald, D.E., Ferguson, D.A., and Milburn, S.E., *Circ. Res.*, *22*: 127 (1968).
14. Cannom, D.S., Rider, A.K., Stinson, E.B., et al., *Am. J. Cardiol.*, *36*: 859 (1975).
15. Bexton, R., Milne, J.R., Cory-Pearce, R., English, T.A.H., and Camm, J.A., *Br. Heart J.*, *49*: 584–588 (1983).
16. Yusuf, S., Theodoropoulos, S., Dhalla, N., Mathias, C.J., Teo, K.K., Wittes, J., and Yacoub, M., *Am. J. Cardiol.*, *64*: 636–641 (1989).
17. Pflugfelder, P.W., Purves, P.D., McKenzie, F.N., and Kostuk, W.J., *J. Am. Coll. Cardiol.*, *10*: 336–341 (1987).
18. Kavanagh, T., Yacoub, M., Mertens, D.J., Kennedy, J., Campbell, R.B., and Sawyer, P., *Circulation, 77*(1): 162–171 (1988).
19. Banner, N.R., Lloyd, M.H., Hamilton, R.D., Innes, J.A., Guz, A., and Yacoub, M., *Br. Heart J.*, *61*: 215–223 (1989).
20. Quigg, R.J., Rocco, M.B., Gauthier, D.F., Creager, M.A., Hartley, L.H., and Colucci, W.S., *J. Am. Coll. Cardiol.*, *14*: 338–344 (1989).
21. Banner, N.R., Fitzgerald, M., Khaghani, A., et al., *Clinical Transplants 1987* (P. Teraski, ed.). UCLA Tissue Typing Laboratory, Los Angeles, pp. 17–26 (1987).
22. Zelis, R., and Flaim, S.F., *Mod. Concepts Cardiovasc. Dis.*, *51*: 79 (1982).
23. Borow, K.M., Neumann, A., Arensman, F.W., and Yacoub, M.E., *Circulation, 71*: 866 (1985).
24. Greenberg, M., Uretsky, B.F., Reddy, P.S., et al., *Circulation, 71*: 487–494 (1985).
25. Thompson, M.E., Shapiro, A.P., Johnsen, A.M., et al., *Transplant Proc.*, *15*(Suppl. 1): 2573 (1983).
26. Barrett, A.J., Kendra, J.R., Lucas, C.F., et al., *Br. Med. J.*, *285*: 162 (1982).
27. Jarowenko, M., Flechner, S., Van Buren, C., et al., *Am. J. Kidney Dis.*, *10*: 98 (1987).
28. Loughran, T.P., Jr., Deeg, H.J., Dahlberg, M.S., et al., *Br. J. Hematol.*, *59*: 547 (1985).
29. Murray, B.M., Paller, M.S., and Ferris, T.F., *Kidney Int.*, *28*: 767–774 (1985).
30. Kaham, B.D., *Am. J. Kidney Dis.*, *3*: 332–337 (1986).
31. Kavanagh, T., Yacoub, M., Mertens, D.J., Campbell, R.B., and Sawyer, P., *J. Cardiopulmon. Rehabil.*, *9*: 303–310 (1989).
32. Shaver, J.A., and Gray, S., *Clin. Res.*, *17*: 518 (1969).

33. Yusuf, S., Aikenhead, J., Theodoropoulos, S., Shalla, N., Wittes, J., and Yacoub, M., *J. Am. Coll. Cardiol.*, *7*: 225A (1986) (Abstr.).
34. Borow, K.M., Neumann, A., Arensman, F., and Yacoub, M., *Circulation*, 72(Suppl. III): 111–129 (1985).
35. Dawkins, K.D., Jamieson, S.W., Hunt, S.A., et al., *Circulation*, *71*: 919–926 (1985).
36. Leachman, R.D., Cokkinos, D.V.P., Rochelle, D.G., et al., *J. Thorac. Cardiovasc. Surg.*, *61*: 561–569 (1979).
37. Hausdorf, G., Banner, N.R., Mitchell, A., Khaghani, A., Martin, M., and Yacoub, M., *Br. Heart J.*, *62*: 123–132 (1989).
38. Ehrman, J., Keteyian, S., Fedel, F., and Relyea, B., *Responses of Heart Transplant Patients to Exercise*. American College of Sports Medicine 35th Annual Meeting, Dallas, May 25–28, 1988. Abstract no. 156, p. S26 (1988).
39. Savin, W.M., Haskell, W.L., Schroeder, J.S., and Stinson, E.B., *Circulation*, *62*: 55 (1980).
40. Borg, G., *Physical Performance and Perceived Exertion*. Gleerup, Lund, Sweden, p. 1 (1962).
41. Jones, N.L., and Ehrsam, R.E., *Exerc. Sports Sci. Revs.*, *10*: 49–83 (1982).
42. Caiozzo, V.J., Davis, J.A., Ellis, J.F., et al., *J. Appl. Physiol.*, *53*: 1184–1189 (1982).
43. Wasserman, K., *Am. Rev. Respir. Dis.*, *129*(Suppl.): S35–S40 (1984).
44. Wasserman, K., *Circulation*, *76*(Suppl. VI): 29–39 (1987).
45. Wasserman, K., Whipp, B.J., Koyal, S.N., and Beaver, W.L., *J. Appl. Physiol.*, *35*: 236–243 (1973).
46. Wasserman, K., and McIlroy, M.B., *Am. J. Cardiol.*, *14*: 844–852 (1964).
47. Koyal, S.N., Whipp, B.J., Huntsman, D., Bray, G.A., and Wasserman, K., *J. Appl. Physiol.*, *40*: 864–867 (1976).
48. Lipkin, D.P., *Br. Heart J.*, *58*: 559–566 (1987).
49. Taylor, H.L., Buskirk, E., and Henschel, A., *J. Appl. Physiol.*, *8*: 73–80 (1955).
50. Wade, O.L., and Bishop, J.M., *Cardiac Output and Regional Blood Flow*. Davis, Philadelphia (1962).
51. Wright, G.R., Sidney, K.H., and Shephard, R.J., *J. Sports Med. Phys. Fitness*, *18*: 33–42 (1978).
52. Cummings, G.R., and Borysyk, L.M., *Med. Sci. Sports*, *4*: 18–22, (1972).
53. Hanson, P., *Resource Manual for Guidelines for Exercise Testing and Prescription* (S.N. Blair, P. Painter, R.R. Pate, L.K. Smith, and C.B. Taylor, eds.). Lea & Febiger, Philadephia (1988).
54. Gao, S.Z., Schroeder, J.S., Hunt, S.A., Billingham, M.E., Valantine, H.A., and Stinson, E.B., *Am. J. Cardiol.*, *64*: 1093–1097 (1989).
55. Hunt, S.A., *Heart Transplant*, *3*: 70–74 (1981).
56. Cooper, D.K.C., Novitsky, O., Hassoulas, J., Chi, B., and Barnaard, C., *Heart Transplant*, *2*: 78–83 (1982).
57. Uretsky, B.F., Murali, S., Reddy, P.S., et al., *Circulation*, *76*: 827–834 (1987).

58. Kavanagh, T., *The Healthy Heart Program*. 3rd ed. Key Porter Books, Toronto (1985).
59. Billingham, M.E., *Transplant Proc.*, *19*(Suppl. 5): 19 (1987).
60. Banner, N.R., Khaghani, A., Fitzgerald, M., Mitchell, A.G., Radley-Smith, R., and Yacoub, M., in *Assisted Circulation 3* (F. Unger, ed.). Springer-Verlag, Berlin, Heidelberg, pp. 448–467 (1989).
61. Gao, S.Z., Schroeder, J.S., Hunt, S., and Stinson, E.B., *Am. J. Cardiol.*, *62*: 876–881 (1988).
62. Kuo, P.C., Kirshenbaum, J.M., Gordon, J., et al., *Am. J. Cardiol.*, *64*: 631–635 (1989).
63. Savin, W.M., Gordon, E., Green, S., et al., *J. Am. Coll. Cardiol.*, *1*(2): 722 (1983) (Abst.).
64. Niset, G., Coustry-Degre, C., and Degre, S., *Cardiology*, *75*: 311–317 (1988).
65. Keteyian, S.J., Ehrman, J.K., Fedel, F.J., and Rhoads, K.L., *Med. Sci. Sports Exerc.*, *21*: S55 (1989).
66. Kavanagh, T., Yacoub, M.H., Campbell, R., and Mertens, D., *Cardiopulm. Rehabil.*, *6*: 16 (1986).
67. Hartley, L.H., Mason, J.W., Hogan, R.P., et al., *J. Appl. Physiol.*, *33*: 602 (1972).
68. Sylvestre-Gervais, L., Nadeau, A., Nguyen, M.H., Tancrede, G., Rousseau-Migneron, S., *Cardiovasc. Res.*, *16*: 530 (1982).
69. Butler, J., O'Brien, M., O'Malley, K., and Kelly, J.G., *Nature*, *298*: 60 (1982).
70. Butler, J., Kelly, J.G., O'Malley, K., and Pidgeon, F., *J. Physiol.*, *344*: 113 (1983).
71. Jones, N.L., and Campbell, E.J., *Clinical Exercise Testing*. 2nd Ed. Saunders, Philadelphia, p. 130 (1982).
72. Sieurat, P.P., Roquebrune, J.P., Grinneiser, D., et al., *Arch. Mal Coeur*, *79*: 210–216 (1986).
73. Buxton, M., Acheson, R., Caine, N., Gibson, S., and O'Brien, B., *Costs and Benefits of the Heart Transplant Programmes at Harefield and Papworth Hospitals*. Her Majesty's Stationery Office, London, 91–106 (1985).
74. Mai, F.M., McKenzie, F.N., and Kostuk, W.J., *Br. Med. J.*, *292*: 311–313 (1986).
75. Christopherson, L.K., *Circulation*, *75*(1): 57–62 (1987).
76. Jones, B.M., Chang, V.P., Esmore, D., et al., *Med. J., Aust.*, *149*: 118–122 (1988).
77. Degre, S., *Rehabilitation and Psychosocial Factors After Heart Transplantation*. Presented at the XIth Congress of the European Society of Cardiology, Nice, France, September 10–14 (1989).
78. Kavanagh, T., Tuck, J.A., Yacoub, M., Shephard, R.J., Kennedy, J., and Mertens, D.J., The influence of a rehabilitation exercise program on mood and personality following cardiac transplantation. In preparation.
79. Wallwork, J., et al., *Quality Life Cardiovasc Care 4*: 137–142 (1985).

80. Evans, R.W., Mannimer, D.L., Overant, T.D., et al., The National Heart Transplantation Study. Seattle Battelle Human Affairs Research Centres, Seattle, Washington (1984).
81. Meister, M.D., McAlster, R.W., Meister, J.S., et al., *J. Heart Transplant*, 5: 154–161 (1986).
82. Harvison, A., Jones, B.M., McBride, M., et al., *J. Heart Transplant*, 7: 337–341 (1988).
83. Kavanagh, T., Yacoub, M., and Tuck, J.A., *Circulation*, 74(Suppl. II): 10 (1986) (Abst.).

9

Exercise Prescription in the Rehabilitation of Patients Following Coronary Artery Bypass Graft Surgery and Coronary Angioplasty

Carl Foster and Hoshedar P. Tamboli

University of Wisconsin Medical School
Sinai Samaritan Medical Center
Milwaukee, Wisconsin

INTRODUCTION

Exercise and risk factor education programs designed for the rehabilitation of patients with myocardial infarction have a generation-long history. Their beneficial effect on the general clinical outcome of these patients is well accepted. The benefit of these programs relative to hard clinical outcomes, including mortality and reinfarction, has been demonstrated by combining results of independent randomized clinical trials (1,2). Beginning about 15 years ago, patients have been referred to rehabilitation programs following coronary artery bypass graft surgery (CABGS). The general clinical experience in this population has been favorable and has been reviewed by Foster (3). More recently, patients have been referred to risk factor and rehabilitation programs following percutaneous transluminal coronary angioplasty (PTCA). As yet, there is no summary experience in this population, although preliminary results appear favorable (4).

The purpose of this chapter is to (a) review briefly the overall clinical expectations following CABGS and PTCA, and how they might be influenced by participation in risk factor– and exercise-based rehabilitation programs, (b) briefly review the physiological sequelae of successful CABGS and PTCA, and how they may be used to evaluate the success of these procedures, (c) briefly discuss our experience concerning the general problems of rehabilitation in patients following

CABGS and PTCA, and (d) present in some detail an approach to exercise prescription that we have developed, and discuss how it might be useful with post-CABGS and post-PTCA patients.

Clinical Expectations Following CABGS and PTCA

Symptomatic relief following CABGS is usually favorable, with most patients reporting elimination or reduction of anginal symptoms. The CABGS procedure is of established benefit relative to survival in patients with three-vessel or left main coronary artery disease (5) and in patients with exercise-induced left ventricular dysfunction while on medical therapy (6).

Return to work following CABGS has been shown to be less frequent than might be expected on the basis of improvements in functional capacity and symptoms (7). Previous work status and the nature of the occupation seem to have a significant impact on the likelihood of returning to work. Although PTCA is significantly less traumatic to the patient, there are also surprisingly unfavorable statistics relative to return to work following PTCA (8). Job classification, concurrent myocardial infarction, and low-self efficacy all relate to the likelihood of returning to work following PTCA. Although documentation is lacking, available evidence suggests that improved self-efficacy following rehabilitation may favor return to work following either CABGS or PTCA.

Solymoss et al. (9) have demonstrated that 15–25% of saphenous vein grafts close during the first postoperative year. Much of this early graft closure is attributable to thrombus secondary to endothelial damage at the time of surgery (10). After the first year, bypass grafts close at the rate of 0.5–3.0% of grafts per year through year 7. After year 7, the rate of closure is increased to 1.5–9.0% per year. Internal mammary artery grafts apparently have a greater patency rate than saphenous vein grafts.

The risk of closure of grafts is related to a number of variables, including mechanical problems with the graft itself, and with conventional risk factors for atherosclerosis. Both postoperative dyslipidemia and smoking (10) have been shown to be associated with an increased risk of graft closure. There are no published data from randomized clinical trials documenting the effect of participation in exercise therapy on the fate of bypass grafts or on hard clinical endpoints following CABGS. Common sense argues for a favorable effect of exercise and risk factor reduction. This finding awaits documentation.

The risk of restenosis following PTCA varies between 15 and 50% at 1 year in the general population (11). This risk is increased in patients with narrow vessels or in the presence of total occlusion prior to PTCA. There are no convincing data regarding the influence of either exercise or risk factor management on the long-term fate of dilated vessels. Smoking has been associated with an increased-risk of restenosis from approximately 38% in nonsmokers to 55% in continuing smokers (12). Data from Emory University (S. King, unpublished) suggests that restenosis rate is increased in patients with hypercholesterolemia.

In spite of the generally favorable experience with rehabilitation programs following myocardial infarction, and the generally favorable subjective response to these programs in post-CABGS and post-PTCA patients, there is little documentation of the benefit that might be derived relative to patency or to hard clinical outcomes in these patients.

Consequences of Myocardial Revascularization

Responses during exercise testing conducted both before and after CABGS and PTCA have been reviewed by Dubach et al. (13). They observed that although CABGS patients had a much greater incidence of multivessel disease than PTCA patients (80 versus 28%), the relief of anginal symptoms was similar (70 to 18% versus 68 to 14%) and the reversal of exercise-induced ST-segment depression was similar (70 to 35% versus 60 to 16%). They pointed out that direct comparison of the interventions using exercise testing is complicated by the usual time course of exercise testing following the procedures. Although patients can safely perform symptom-limited exercise testing by the time of hospital discharge following CABGS ($\sim$ 11 days postsurgery) (14), they most often are not tested until 2–3 months following surgery, when grafts destined to close early have already closed. Alternatively, PTCA patients may be exercise tested within days of the procedure.

Functional capacity usually improves following both CABGS and PTCA, although the time course following surgery is often delayed secondary to recovery from the surgical procedure. In Figure 1 are presented maximal oxygen uptake ($VO_{2\,max}$) data obtained during treadmill exercise during 24 weeks following surgery in patients participating in a randomized clinical trial of exercise based rehabilitation following CABGS (15). The improved functional capacity in the control group in this population indicates the magnitude and time course of

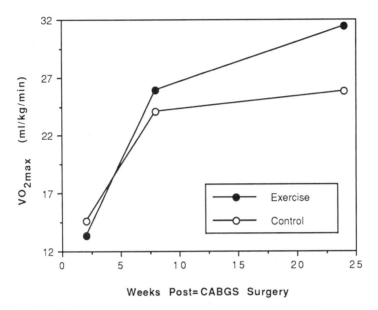

Figure 1   Time course of changes in $VO_{2\,max}$ in post-CABGS patients randomly assigned to an exercise-based rehabilitation program or to a control group using deep muscle relaxation exercises (15). Participation in a rehabilitation program accelerates the rate of recovery, and increases the total magnitude of the improved $VO_{2\,max}$ postoperatively.

the improved functional capacity secondary to CABGS alone. As can be seen from the figure, participation in an exercise-based rehabilitation program increases the eventual change in $VO_{2\,max}$ by about (60%) and accelerates the time course of changes in $VO_{2\,max}$. The 6-month postoperative level of functional capacity in the control group was reached by 7 weeks postoperatively in the exercise group. This directly measured $VO_{2\,max}$ data is consistent with other published reports using estimated $VO_{2\,max}$ in CABGS patients (16). Although functional capacity improves significantly following PTCA (17), we have seen comparatively small changes when exercise testing is conducted relatively soon following PTCA, and have noted similar improvement in functional capacity in patients with unsuccessful PTCA (not requiring emergency surgery) versus those with angiographically successful procedures (17). In view of the presumed importance of coronary blood flow as a limiting factor for exercise cardiac output, the failure to note bigger differences between the successful and unsuccessful PTCA groups is surprising.

Isolated exercise testing following CABGS, without a preoperative control study, has proven to be disappointing in that there are a substantial number of normal tests despite the continued presence of anatomically significant disease (18,19). An isolated observation of abnormal ventricular function during exercise testing using either radionuclide (18) or echocardiographic (20) methods following surgery is, however, better correlated with angiographic evidence of incomplete revascularization. Our attitude to the use of exercise testing is that the absence of functional abnormalities during exercise testing indicates that anatomically significant coronary artery disease may be insignificant relative to limiting myocardial blood flow.

The peak exercise left ventricular ejection fraction usually improves significantly following successful CABGS (16). If exercise radionuclide angiographic studies are conducted at the time of hospital discharge, the magnitude of improvement in exercise ejection fraction is overestimated (16). Participation in an exercise-based rehabilitation program does not significantly influence the exercise ejection fraction (16), although from the magnitude of increase in functional capacity, the calculated cardiac output is significantly greater following exercise training. Exercise left ventricular function is improved following successful PTCA based on the results of both radionuclide (21) and echocardiographic (22) studies. There appears to be a tendency for participants in post-PTCA exercise programs to have higher values for resting ejection fraction versus patients assigned to usual care (4). The effect of therapeutic exercise has not been studied in a randomized trial which included measures of left ventricular function.

As demonstrated in the Coronary Artery Bypass Surgery Study, CABGS improves survival only in patients with three-vessel disease, exercise-induced ischemia, and limited functional capacity (5). Other studies have demonstrated that survival in medically treated patients is good, so long as exercise left ventricular function remains normal (6). In patients who become symptomatic after CABGS, the prognostic information available from exercise testing is low, although patients with better functional capacity and an adequate heart rate reserve have a low mortality (23). To the degree that the functional capacity and heart rate reserve measure the same thing as the exercise left ventricular ejection fraction, the results of this study indicate that good pump performance is a favorable prognostic index.

Experience with Postsurgical/Angioplasty Patients

In general, post-CABGS patients may be treated more aggressively than postmyocardial infarction patients, and post-PTCA patients may be treated more aggressively than post-CABGS patients. The risk of exercise-induced catastrophic events is related mostly to the presence of myocardial ischemia during exercise training (24). In the revascularized patient, this risk factor is largely absent. Thus, the primary limitation of the postoperative patient is related to sequelae of the sternotomy, which may limit upper extremity exercise for some weeks and may hamper ventilatory efforts until 6 months postoperatively (25). There are generally fewer medical problems observed during rehabilitation with postsurgical patients despite the more aggressive approach taken with this population (26). There have been several studies demonstrating a high frequency of dysrhythmias in the postsurgical population (27–29), although these dysrhythmias are often not severe and may not require intervention (30). Despite the lack of serious medical problems, one important and continuing role of rehabilitation programs is to provide for physician surveillance, and to identify early postoperative problems before they evolve into situations requiring intervention.

There is limited experience in the rehabilitation of post-PTCA patients. The general attitude seems to be that these patients are like postsurgical patients without the residual effects of surgery. As such, the basic need to recover strength and endurance from the acute clinical event is minimal. These patients can be approached largely from the standpoint of secondary prevention. Given the fairly high rate of restenosis following PTCA (11), early surveillance for the reemergence of exercise-induced ischemia would seem to be justified. The value and yield of this approach is yet to be documented.

Exercise Prescription

The basic concept of exercise prescription for post-CABGS and post-PTCA patients is the same as for any other patient (or for a healthy individual). In general, exercise effects and side effects follow a dose-response curve as do medicines. The prescriptive markers for exercise can be remembered by the acronym FIT, meaning frequency, intensity, and time. The combination of frequency, intensity, and time necessary to provoke physiological adaptations in healthy individuals are well documented (31). As a general rule, more acutely debilitated patients, such as recent postoperative patients, cannot tolerate either intensity or time of exercise, but may do very well with frequent (three to four times daily) exercise bouts. As the patient recovers, the exercise prescription is increased first relative to total time and later relative to intensity and eventually evolves toward maintenance guidelines. For the post-PTCA patient, an exercise prescription not unlike that for healthy sedentary controls may be appropriate, with the understanding that surveillance for ischemia secondary to restenosis is desirable. The overall time course of the total exercise dose, presented against that recommended for healthy controls and for postmyocardial infarction patients is shown in Figure 2.

In our inpatient program, we employ a modification of the step approach of Wenger (31). During the last 5 years, with the progressive reduction in the duration of hospitalization, we have given our inpatient staff great latitude to adjust the step schedule and to respond to the patient's present clinical condition and needs. This has included the administration of a routine lifting task for all suitable patients in order to familiarize them with the practical implications of the 10-lb lifting limitation that we recommend at the time of hospital discharge (32). In our experience, patients seem surprised at how light 10 lb feels; they have a low self-efficacy for lifting at the time of hospital discharge. Thus, in addition to providing behaviorally meaningful guidelines, lifting during the inpatient phase may help improve self-efficacy and remove one of the primary impediments to return to work in post-CABGS and post-PTCA patients (7,8).

Several years ago we became concerned that patients were fairly unskillful at taking pulse rates despite considerable effort training in this skill. They also frequently asked more behaviorally meaningful questions such as how fast to walk, how hard to ride the ergometer, or whether they could participate in recreational activities such as tennis or skiing. For patients in our outpatient program, it was relatively easy to define workloads on common ergometric modes. For patients whom we only saw for predischarge instructions, for clinic visits, or for patients interested in recreational activities, the process was more difficult. Accordingly, we have spent some time and effort to develop a method for "translating" exercise test information into specific guidelines for exercise prescription (33–35).

Our efforts with the functional translation of exercise responses began with a simple assumption (Fig. 3). We assumed that twin brothers, one fit and one not so fit, would have different heart rate responses during a standard graded exercise test. We also assumed that their heart rate responses to different rates of level ground ambulation would also be different. We further assumed that there would be some proportionality between the time during a graded exercise test that they passed through their target heart rate and the speed of level ground ambulation necessary to elicit the same heart rate under

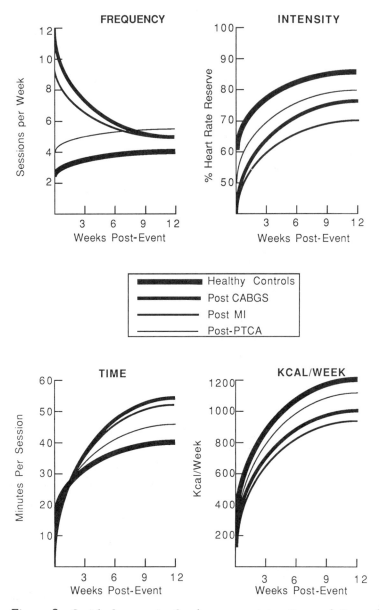

Figure 2 Serial changes in the frequency, intensity, and time of exercise recommended for healthy individuals, postmyocardial infarction patients, post-CABGS, and post-PTCA patients. Also presented is a global index of the total exercise load presented as kilocalories expended per week.

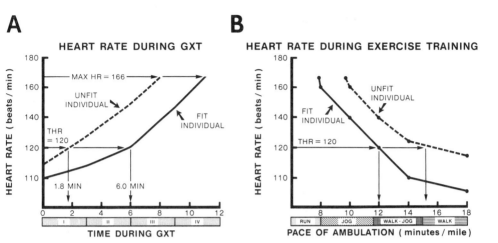

Figure 3 Expected heart rate responses during: (A) a standard exercise test protocol in fit and unfit individuals, and (B) level ground ambulation in the same two individuals. The more fit person passes through a given submaximal target heart rate later during the exercise test and at a greater speed of ambulation. The quantitative linkage between these phenomena form the conceptual foundation of the functional translation approach (33).

steady-state conditions during exercise training. We have shown that these assumptions can be defended for level ground ambulation, for cycle ergometry, and for exercise on an arm-leg ergometer (Fig. 4). The use of this approach allows us to generate behaviorally meaningful information that we can use to show a patient the proper level of exertion. This further reduces (but does not eliminate) the burden on the patient's accuracy in taking his or her pulse rate, since they have additional perceptual information regarding the proper exercise intensity. Originally, we had also made the assumption that appropriate recreational activities could be identified on the basis of published metabolic equivalent data for walking-cycling and various recreational activities (Fig. 5). A recent test of this assumption, however, has demonstrated that recreational activities are generally less demanding than would be predicted on the basis of published data. Activities that would be expected to elicit target heart rate, or even to be too hard (require >90% of heart rate reserve), are in fact quite moderate (35). While disappointing as a test of our functional translation method, these results suggest that most recreational activities can be attempted without undue fear of violating the target heart rate in patients who

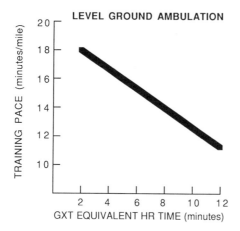

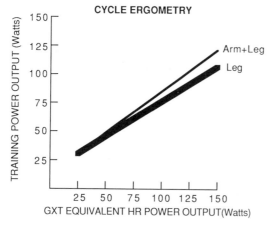

Figure 4 Functional transition relationships for level ground ambulation and leg cycle ergometry (33) and combined arm-leg ergometry (34). A given submaximal heart rate will be observed at the workloads defined by connecting perpendicular lines to the diagonal regression line drawn in the figure.

can use conventional ergometry. Certainly, patients who have ischemic responses during exercise testing should not participate in these recreational activities, since exceeding the target heart rate even briefly can be associated with untoward events (24). Our belief is that if exercise testing fails to reveal ischemic responses under truly maximal provocation, then participation in recreational activities should not

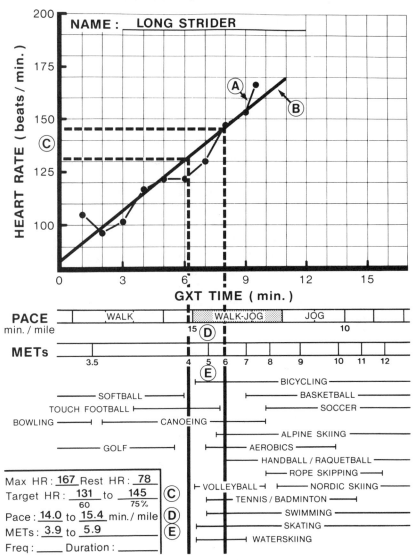

Figure 5 Hypothesized functional translation relationship between time during exercise testing, the pace of level ground ambulation, and the appropriateness of various recreational activities. (From Ref. 49; used with permission.)

be discouraged, since the recreational activities seem to be self-limiting in terms of intensity, and the better compliance with these activities may contribute to the other health benefits of exercise.

We have also used perceived exertion as an important adjunct to the target heart rate in our rehabilitation program (31). For the majority of patients (>90%), perceived exertion is well correlated with physiological responses (36). We particularly use perceived exertion to adjust the percentage of heart rate reserve used for defining the target heart rate and try to keep perceived exertion in the range of 3–4 (moderate to somewhat hard). We have also made some minor modifications of Borg's category ratio perceived exertion scale (37) that seem to improve the ease with which patients use the scale (Fig. 6). Recent evidence from our laboratory (unpublished), however, suggests that merely recommending that patients exercise at 3–4 on the perceived exertion scale does not guarantee achieving the target heart rate. Many patients may need to approach 5 (hard) by the end of a 20–30 min training session to ensure achieving the target heart rate. The need for this kind of intensity in the early postoperative patient is marginal, since aerobic conditioning is not essential to regaining the ability to conduct activities of daily living successfully. However, after 4–6 weeks post-CABGS or 2–3 weeks post-PTCA, aerobic conditioning becomes an important goal in the secondary prevention efforts.

During the past decade, there has been an increased interest in the use of resistance training in patients with cardiovascular disease. This topic has been well reviewed recently (38–43). Except for the need to allow for healing of the sternotomy, there is no reason why CABGS patients should not respond favorably to resistance training. Despite the substantial pressor response during resistance exercise (39,44), guidelines for selection of patients for resistance training are, basically, the same as for vigorous aerobic training; that is, in clinically stable patients without active exercise-induced ischemia (24) and with comparatively normal left ventricular function (43,44). Although there is some suggestion that patients with poor left ventricular function may respond acutely less well to resistance exercise, the overall favorable effect on psychological status and improved self-efficacy resulting from resistance training (41) may make it a reasonable risk to assume in the monitored setting. Certainly, programs employing significant amounts of upper extremity and resistive exercise have not reported an increased incidence of unfavorable side effects (45). Our recent clinical experience with higher-intensity training, including resistance training in all nonischemic patient populations, is also demonstrative of the safety of this mode of exercise.

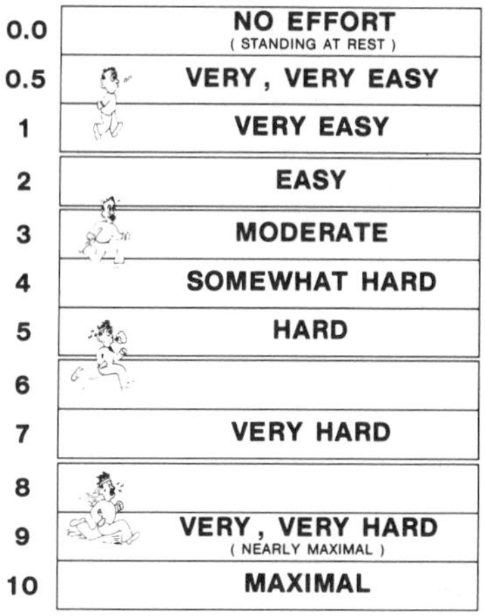

0.0		**NO EFFORT** (STANDING AT REST)
0.5		**VERY , VERY EASY**
1		**VERY EASY**
2		**EASY**
3		**MODERATE**
4		**SOMEWHAT HARD**
5		**HARD**
6		
7		**VERY HARD**
8		
9		**VERY , VERY HARD** (NEARLY MAXIMAL)
10		**MAXIMAL**

Figure 6 Modification of Borg's perceived exertion scale designed to facilitate use by patients. As an additional aid, colors can be added to the figure, green for the lower numbers evolving through yellow and orange to red for the upper numbers.

With post-CABGS and, particularly, post-PTCA patients there is an inevitable problem of thinking that their heart disease has been "cured" or can be "fixed" relatively easily. Accordingly, understanding factors which can influence compliance with the rehabilitation regimen, and particularly factors which can enhance compliance, are of particular importance. Oldridge (46) has reviewed factors associated with compliance and dropout from rehabilitation programs. Generally, about 60–70% of participants may be expected to be involved 1 year following enrollment. Dropouts are particularly likely in certain classes of patients: blue collar workers, continuing smokers, the overweight, the habitually sedentary, patients with continuing symptoms, and patients with low self-motivation. In effect, those patients who need rehabilitation most are the most likely to drop out. None of these factors are controllable by the rehabilitation staff. However, factors such as a pleasant staff and facilities may enhance compliance. Scheduling of classes and the location of classes may also be important, particularly for patients who have already returned to work. Strategies such as contracting with patients, a self-monitored mini-exercise test, and daily activity logs may improve compliance. The method of payment for the program, particularly some form of contingency contract allowing the patient to recover all or part of the cost of the program by virtue of their behavior, may also be important (47). These factors are, of course, important for all classes of patients but may be more important in situations where the patient may feel "cured" (48).

CONCLUSIONS

Post-CABGS and post-PTCA patients may respond favorably to participation in an exercise- and risk factor reduction-based rehabilitation program. Although there is not hard evidence regarding the effect on subsequent morbidity/mortality, there is enough supportive evidence to hypothesize an effect as great as that documented in postmyocardial infarction patients. The basic principles of exercise prescription are similar to those accepted for myocardial infarction patients. Generally, post-CABGS and post-PTCA patients may be progressed more aggressively than postmyocardial infarction patients. Some care is required to adjust upper extremity exercise in post-CABGS patients until the sternotomy has healed. Surveillance for the reemergence of ischemia secondary to graft closure or restenosis of dilated arteries remains an important feature of the rehabilitation program in this population. Given the negative impact on compliance from patients thinking that they are "cured," aggressive use of compliance enhancing strategies is particularly important following CABGS and PTCA.

REFERENCES

1. Oldridge, N.B., Guyatt, G.H., Fischer, M.E., and Rimm, A.A., *J.A.M.A.*, 260: 945–950 (1988).
2. O'Connor, G.T., Buring, J.E., Yusef, S., Goldhaber, S.Z., Olmstead, E.M., Paffenburger, R.S., and Hennekens, C.H., *Circulation, 80*: 234–244 (1989).
3. Foster, C., *Exerc. Sports Sci. Rev., 14*: 303–323 (1986).
4. Ben-Ari, E., Rothbaum, D.A., Linnemeir, T.J., Landin, R.J., Steinmetz, E.F., Hillis, S.J., Noble, J.R., Hallam, C.C., See, M.R., and Shiner, R., *J. Cardiopulmon. Rehab., 7*: 281–285 (1989).
5. Weiner, D.A., Ryan, T.J., McCabe, C.H., Chaitman, B.R., Sheffield, L.T., Fisher, L.D., and Tristani, F., *J.A.C.C., 8*: 741–748 (1986).
6. Jones, R.H., Floyd, R.D., Austin, E.H., and Sabiston, D.C., *Ann. Surg., 197*: 743–754 (1983).
7. Gutmann, M.C., Knapp, D.N., Pollock, M.L., Schmidt, D.H., Simon, K., and Walcott, G., *Circulation, 66*(Suppl. III): *111*: 33–42 (1982).
8. Fitzgerald, S.T., Becker, D.M., Celentano, D.D., Swank, R., and Brinker, J., *Am. J. Cardiol., 64*: 1108–1112 (1989).
9. Solymoss, B.C., Nedeau, P., Millette, D., and Campeau, L., *Circulation, 78*: 140–143 (1988).

10. Angelini, G.D., and Newby, A.C., *Eur. Heart J., 10*: 273–280 (1989).
11. McBride, W., Lange, R.A., and Hillis, L.D., *N. Eng. J. Med., 318*: 1734–1737 (1988).
12. Galan, K.M., Deligonnul, V., Kern, M.J., Chaitman, B.R., and Vandormael, M.B., *Am. J. Cardiol., 61*: 260–263 (1988).
13. Dubach, P., Lehmann, K.G., and Froelicher, V.F., *Am. J. Cardiol., 64*: 1039–1040 (1989).
14. Rod, J.L., Squires, R.W., Pollock, M.L., Foster, C., and Schmidt, D.H., *J. Cardiac Rehabil., 2*: 100–205 (1982).
15. Pollock, M.L., Foster, C., Anholm, J.D., Squires, R.W., Ward, A., Rod, J., Johnson, W.D., Saichek, R., and Schmidt, D.H., *Med. Sci. Sports Exerc., 13*: 133 (1981) (Abst.).
16. Foster, C., Pollock, M.L., Anholm, J.D., Squires, R., Ward, A., Dymond, D.S., Rod, J.L., Saichek, R.P., and Schmidt, D.H., *Circulation, 69*: 748–755 (1984).
17. Rod, J.L., Foster, C., and Schmidt, D.H., *J. Cardiac Rehabil., 4*: 70–73 (1984).
18. Pollock, M.L., Foster, C., Anholm, J.D., Rod, J.L., Wolf, F.G., Akhtar, M., Al-Nouri, M.B., and Schmidt, D.H., *Cardiology, 69*: 358–365 (1982).
19. McConahay, D.R., Valdes, M., McCallister, B.D., Crockett, J.E., Conn, R.D., Reed, W.A., and Killen, D.A., *Circulation, 56*: 548–552 (1977).
20. Sawada, S.G., Judson, W.E., Ryan, T., Armstrong, W.F., and Feigenbaum, H., *Am. J. Cardiol., 64*: 1123–1129 (1989).
21. O'Keefe, J.G., Layre, A.C., Holmes, D.R., and Gibbons, R.J., *Am. J. Cardiol., 61*: 51–59 (1988).
22. Labovitz, A.J., Lewen, M., Kern, M.J., Vandormael, M., Mrosek, D.G., Byers, S.L., Pearson, A.C., and Chaitman, B.R., *Am. Heart J., 117*: 1003–1008 (1989).
23. Dubach, P., Froelicher, V.K., Klein, J., and Detrano, R., *Am. J. Cardiol., 63*: 530–533 (1989).
24. Hossack, K.F., and Hartwig, R., *J. Cardiac Rehabil., 2*: 402–408 (1982).
25. Foster, C., Pollock, M.L., Anholm, J.D., Squires, R.W., Ward, A., Rod, J.L., Lemberger, K., Rasansky, M., Oldridge, N.B., and Schmidt, D.H., *Circulation, 85*: 1004 (1985) (Abst.).
26. Sennett, S.M., Pollock, M.L., Pels, A.E., Foster, C., Dolatowski, R., Laughlin, J., Patel, S., and Schmidt, D.H., *J. Cardiopulm. Rehabil., 7*: 458–465 (1987).
27. Dion, W.F., Grevenow, P., Pollock, M.L., Squires, R.W., Foster, C., Johnson, W.D., and Schmidt, D.H., *Heart Lung, 11*: 248–255 (1982).
28. Silvidi, G.E., Squires, R.W., Pollock, M.L., and Foster, C., *J. Cardiac Rehabil., 2*: 355–362 (1982).
29. Dolatowski, R.P., Squires, R.W., Pollock, M.L., Foster, C., and Schmidt, D.H., *Med. Sci. Sports Exerc., 15*: 281–286 (1983).
30. Muth, J.W., Adams, G.E., Kaufman, J.A., Quinn, E.J., Pima, V., and Arcotta, K.F., *Med. Sci. Sports Exerc., 18*: 409 (1986) (Abst.).

31. Pollock, M.L., Pels, A.E., Foster, C., and Ward, A., in *Heart Disease and Rehabilitation*. 2nd Ed. (M.L. Pollock and D.H. Schmidt, eds.). Wiley, New York, pp. 477–515 (1986).

32. Grevenow, P., Foster, C., Dion, W., Adashek, M., and Schmidt, D.H., *J. Cardiopulm. Rehabil.*, *9*: 409 (1989) (Abst.).

33. Foster, C., Lemberger, K., Thompson, N.N., Sennett, S.M., Hare, J., Pollock, M.L., Pels, A.E., and Schmidt, D.H., *Am. Heart J.*, *112*: 1309–1316 (1986).

34. Foster C., Thompson, N.N., and Bales, S., *J. Cardiopulm. Rehabil.*, in press.

35. Thompson, N.N., and Foster, C., *Med. Sci. Sports Exerc.*, *21*: S113 (1989).

36. Pollock, M.L., Foster, C., Rod, J.L., and Wible, G., *Adv. Cardiol.*, *31*: 129–133 (1982).

37. Borg, G., Ljunggren, G., and Ceci, R., *Eur. J. Appl. Physiol.*, *54*: 343–349 (1985).

38. Goldberg, A.P., *Med. Sci. Sports Exerc.*, *21*: 669–674 (1989).

39. Keleman, M.H., *Med. Sci. Sports Exerc.*, *21*: 675–677 (1989).

40. Stewart, K.L., *Med. Sci. Sports Exerc.*, *21*: 678–682 (1989).

41. Ewart, C.K., *Med. Sci. Sports Exerc.*, *21*: 683–688 (1989).

42. Hurley, B.F., *Med. Sci. Sports Exerc.*, *21*: 689–693 (1989).

43. Effon, M.B., *Med. Sci. Sports Exerc.*, *21*: 694–697.

44. Hanson, P., and Nagle, F., *Cardiol. Clin.*, *5*: 157–170 (1987).

45. Franklin, B.A., Hellerstein, H.K., Gordon, S., and Timms, G.C., in *Exercise in Modern Medicine* (B.A. Franklin, S. Gordon, and G. Timms, eds.). Williams & Wilkins, Baltimore, pp. 44–80 (1989).

46. Oldridge, N.B., *J. Cardiac Rehabil.*, *4*: 166–177 (1984).

47. Pollock, M.L., Foster, C., Salisbury, R., and Smith, R., *Physician Sportsmed.*, *10*(1): 898–100 (1982).

48. Donahue, P.R., and Liu, C.Y., *Circulation, 80*: 418 (1989) (Abst.).

49. Foster, C., in *Cardiac Rehabilitation and Clinical Exercise Programs: Theory and Practice* (N.B. Oldridge, C. Foster, and D.H. Schmidt, eds.). Mouvement Publications, Ithaca, New York, pp. 169–177 (1988).

10

The Role of Exercise in the Prevention and Management of Diabetes Mellitus and Blood Lipid Disorders

Arthur S. Leon

University of Minnesota
Minneapolis, Minnesota

INTRODUCTION

Diabetes mellitus (DM) affects 3–5% of the population (or 11–15 million people) in the United States, and it is an important contributor to morbidity and mortality. It directly causes about 40,000 deaths/year, or 10 deaths per 100,000 population; however, this represents only the tip of the iceberg, since about 90,000 more deaths/year in diabetic individuals are attributed to complications, particularly cardiovascular disease (CVD). Diabetes mellitus also is the principal cause of nontraumatic lower limb amputations accompanying peripheral vascular disease. It is also a major contributor to visual impairment and new blindness, renal failure requiring renal dialysis and transplant, and neuropathies. The disease accounts for at least 10% of all acute hospital days. The gross overall economic impact of DM in this country is estimated to be over $10 billion per year.

This chapter discusses the pathophysiology of DM, its complications, and preventive and management strategies with an emphasis on the contributions of exercise. Included is information on the management of dyslipidemias that frequently accompanies DM and are a prime contributor to atherosclerotic complications.

PATHOPHYSIOLOGY AND CLASSIFICATION

Diabetes mellitus is not a single disease. It is a metabolic disorder of heterogeneous origin in which hyperglycemia, its principal landmark, and associated metabolic dearrangements stem from either an absolute deficiency of circulating insulin or a relative insufficiency of insulin in terms of the ability to normalize blood glucose levels (4,5). Insulin is a large peptide consisting of 2 attached amino acid chains secreted by the beta islet cells of the pancreas (4). Circulating insulin binds to specialized cell plasma membrane receptors to stimulate uptake and oxidation of circulating glucose as a fuel substrate by the liver, muscle, and other tissues. In addition, insulin affects specific rate-limiting cell enzymes promoting anabolic biosynthetic processes, whereas inhibiting catabolic ones. The synthesis and storage of glycogen, protein, and triglycerides are promoted, while glycogen breakdown and release of its glucose-building blocks from the liver are inhibited. Furthermore, triglyceride lipolysis and release of free fatty acids from adipocytes also are inhibited by insulin.

A deficiency of insulin results in hyperglycemia because of both tissue failure to clear glucose from the blood and excess glucose release from the liver. In addition, insulin deficiency initiates a series of catabolic processes. These include accelerated lipolysis of triglycerides in adipocytes with an increased release of free fatty acids (FFA) and their utilization by tissues for fuel. Formation of ketone bodies results from an inability by the liver to utilize excess acetyl coenzyme A generated from the metabolism of FFA, which leads to ketacidosis. There also is a reduced uptake of amino acids by cells and increased proteolysis with conversion of released amino acids to glucose by the liver. Dehydration and electrolyte disturbances may result from an excess loss of fluid and electrolytes owing to an accompanying diuresis. Diabetes mellitus also is accompanied by an excess secretion of hormones that antagonize the action of insulin, i.e., the so-called counterregulatory hormones, which contribute significantly to the metabolic dearrangements. These include cortisol, growth hormone, and particularly glucagon, from the alpha islet cells of the pancreas accompanying a deficiency of insulin.

Diabetes mellitus is commonly classified into at least four clinically and pathologically distinct clinical types (4,6): (a) idiopathic insulin-dependent, or type I DM (IDDM), formerly referred to as juvenile-onset DM; (b) non–insulin-dependent, or type II DM (NIDDM), formerly referred to as adult- or maturity-onset DM; (c) malnutrition-related DM; and (d) secondary DM. The latter results from specific conditions and syndromes that reduce the availability of insulin or that increase the levels of counterregulatory hormones, such as destructive disease of the pancreas or syndromes of excess secretion of hormones antagonistic to insulin (e.g., Cushing's syndrome or acromegaly). In addition, gestational DM refers to DM first recognized during pregnancy, which if it persists after pregnancy is subsequently reclassified. Further, impaired glucose tolerance is used to describe the condition in which there are above normal levels of plasma glucose in the fasting or postprandial rate or following an oral or intravenous glucose challenge, but glucose levels are not high enough to be diagnostic of DM. However, glucose intolerance is associated with an increased future risk of NIDDM as well as of cardiovascular complications (5,7).

The underlying pathophysiology of the two major types of diabetes, IDDM and NIDDM, are quite different (4,8,9). IDDM accounts for 10% or less of all cases of DM in the United States. This form of DM usually results from an idiopathic physical destruction of pancreatic beta cells. It is commonly associated with an autoimmune process in which antibodies to islet cells cause or contribute to their destruction. It is hypothesized that anything that damages beta cells (e.g., viruses and chemicals) results in antigen release, which can initiate this autoimmune destructive process in genetically susceptible people (10). Supporting evidence for this hypothesis is the demonstration of antibodies to islet cells in the blood of newly diagnosed patients with IDDM; the fact that IDDM is much more likely to occur in people with certain inherited major classes of human histocompatibility leukocyte antigen complexes (HLA types); and the reported effectiveness of experimental immunosuppression with cyclosporine in enhancing and preserving beta cell function (11).

EPIDEMIOLOGY

Commonly, IDDM first becomes clinically evident before age 30 and particularly during childhood or adolescence (4,5,8). The incidence of IDDM is about 15 per 100,000 in people under 20 years old with no gender predominance; however, IDDM may occur at any age. Victims are usually of normal weight or underweight, and often have a family history of DM, suggesting a genetic predisposition. Because of the absolute deficiency of circulating insulin, individuals with IDDM usually are symptomatic at the onset of the disease and require exogenous insulin replacement to control associated metabolic dearrangements and improve survival.

Much more prevelant than IDDM, NIDDM accounts for about 80% of all cases of DM in the United States (5,9,94). It generally presents after age 40 and is much more common in women than men. It is usually associated with obesity, as well as with a strong family history of DM. In contrast to IDDM, antibodies to islet cells are not present in the plasma of patients with NIDDM, and there is no association with any particular HLA type. Thus, hyperglycemia with NIDDM is not secondary to autoimmune destruction of insulin-secretory cells and there is an absence or absolute insulin deficiency at least early in the course of the disease. However, beta cell failure may develop later, particularly in obese individuals (12). Not only is circulating insulin always detectable initially in patients with type II DM, but plasma insulin levels are often higher than in nondiabetic individuals; i.e., hyperinsulinemia may be present. The implication of these findings is that a defect exists in patients with NIDDM in the ability of insulin to maintain glucose hemostatis; i.e., they are insulin resistant. A great deal of experimental evidence supports this conclusion. Cellular mechanisms appear to be responsible for the insulin resistance. A reduction in the number of cell membrane insulin receptors, reduced insulin-receptor binding, or postreceptor activity may be present in liver, muscle, adipocytes, and other insulin-sensitive tissues. In addition, a defect in insulin-mediated glycogen synthesis by skeletal muscle may contribute to the development of NIDDM (13), and a delayed or relatively insufficient responsiveness of beta cells may coexist with peripheral insulin resistance, particularly in older patients with NIDDM (12). Although oral hypoglycemic agents or insulin administration may be required in patients with NIDDM to control severe hyperglycemia and associated symptoms, including hypermolar coma, it is extremely unusual for patients with this form of DM to develop ketoacidosis in the absence of medication. Insulin also may be required for glycemic control under special circumstances, such as acute injuries, infections, surgery, pregnancy, or when there is an allergic response to sulfonylurea oral hypoglycemic agents (8).

Although a genetic predisposition appears to play an important role in NEDDM (14), there is strong evidence that lifestyle is more important in the etiology of this condition. This is hopeful in terms of the potential for primary prevention. Both epidemiological and experimental data indicate that obesity usually plays a critical role in the pathogenesis of this form of diabetes (1,4,5,9,15). About 80% of individuals with NIDDM are obese and the incidence of this disease is extremely low in lean populations. Recent research has shifted attention from obesity per se to the differential distribution of body fat. A centralized or abdominal-type of fat predominance as indicated by waist-to-hip ratios of >1.0 in men or >0.8 or 0.9 in women is associated with an increased incidence of hyperinsulinemia and disorders of glucose metabolism (as well as disorders of lipid metabolism and risk of hypertension, cardiovascular complications, and premature death) (16,17). Experimentally, overeating and weight gain both in animals and humans have been demonstrated to cause insulin resistance associated with a loss of insulin receptors in distended adipocytes (1,18). This process can be reversed by weight loss.

A sedentary lifestyle also appears to be another important risk factor for NIDDM, independent of its relationship to weight gain and obesity. In fact, peripheral insulin resistance, hyperinsulinemia, and glucose intolerance can be induced experimentally in healthy volunteers by just a few days of bed rest (19,20).

In our society, the incidence of NIDDM is much greater in women than men, and the risk increases with parity and aging (1,4,5,15), with the majority of victims being women over 40 years of age. The usual decline in physical activity and associated weight gain that occurs after attainment of physical maturity, particularly in women, undoubtedly contributes to this disease pattern. A decline in lean body mass during aging may be another contributing factor which can be attenuated by regular exercise. Thus, a strong, consistent body of evidence suggests that weight maintenance or management and regular physical activity are the keys to prevention or reducing risk of NIDDM. Such preventive measures are particularly important for overweight middle-aged women with a family history of diabetes and a tendency for central accumulation of fat.

CLINICAL COURSE AND LONG-TERM COMPLICATIONS

The natural course of DM is extremely variable. Many individuals (probably about 20–30%) with even severe IDDM remain free of major complications; however, as a rule, late complications are common in people who have had DM for many decades. There usually is a lag period of several years before chronic complications occur, and the risk of complications increases with duration of the disease. The late complications elaborated on below are the principal contributors to morbidity and mortality in the diabetic population. There is suggestive evidence that "tight" glycemic control will reduce the incidence and severity of these complications. A controlled multicenter clinical trial is currently under way to test this hypothesis (21). Major sites for late complications of DM include the eyes, kidneys, nervous system, cardiovascular system, and feet (1,4).

Ocular Complications

Diabetes mellitus is the leading cause of significant visual impairment in the United States. Visual loss may result from diabetic retinopathy, premature cataracts, glaucoma, or optic neuropathy (4). Of these, retinopathy is the major contributor to new blindness. Despite major recent advances in the management of diabetic retinopathy about 5000 new cases of blindness occur annually in the United States and 30,000–40,000 cases worldwide (22). Diabetic retinopathy is a microvascular disorder specific for DM, involving the capillaries and veins of the retina. The associated lesions include microaneurysm, small hemorrhages, intraretinal lipid infiltrates, and a proliferation of newly formed exudates. Accelerated proliferative retinopathy, consisting of a proliferation of microvascular abnormalities arising from the retinal veins, develops in about 5% of all diabetic individuals. Vitreous hemorrhages from the fragile new vessels, resulting in scarring and retinal detachment, may lead to blindness. Treatment of proliferative retinopathy consists of photocoagulation of the new vessels by a xenon photocoagulator or argon laser light beam and vitrectomy to remove vitreous hemorrhages (4,22). Although some degree of visual impairment is common with long-term DM, less than 2% of diabetic individuals become completely blind; nevertheless, the presence of ocular complications in patients with DM are significant predictors of a reduced survival rate (23).

Renal Complications

Renal failure is a significant cause of both morbidity and mortality among patients with DM (4,91). About 30–40% of people with IDDM and 10% of those with NIDDM develop renal failure within 25 years after the onset of DM (24,25). Further, about 20–30% of all newly diagnosed cases of end-stage renal disease in the United States is related to DM. The underlying cause of renal failure is usually diabetic nephropathy, which often accompanies diabetic retinopathy. The risk of diabetic end-stage renal disease is much higher among blacks, as compared to white diabetic individuals, particularly among those with NIDDM (26). The death rate from renal disease in the diabetic population is 18 times greater than in the nondiabetic population. At the onset of hyperglycemia, before any pathological lesions are evident, there is an increase in the glomerular filtration rate accompanied by microalbuminuria, which is detectable only by radioimmunoassay for protein. The earliest morphological renal lesions visible under the microscope are microvascular changes involving the afferent and efferent arterioles of the glomeruli. This is followed by diffuse intracapillary glomerulosclerosis, and glomerular obliteration with secondary interstitial and tubular atrophy and fibrosis. As with retinopathy, these renal microvascular changes are believed to be related to hyperglycemia and associated metabolic disorders which accompany poor diabetic control, particularly the glycosylation of tissue proteins (27). The initial evidence of clinically significant renal lesions is progressive gross albuminuria detectable by "dipstick" methods. Urinary tract infections and pyellonephritis may contribute to the development of renal insufficiency. Hypertension is a concomitant finding in most diabetic patients with renal insufficiency, and its presence accelerates the progression of the nephropathy (245,250).

At present, there is no known treatment to prevent the progression of proteinuria and renal failure, however, the investigational use of angiotensive-converting enzyme (ACE) inhibitors appears promising (28,29). End-stage renal disease eventually requires hemodialysis, peritoneal dialysis, or renal transplantation.

Neurological Changes

Diabetic neuropathy is another chronic condition related to hyperglycemia and its associated intracellular biochemical abnormalities. Multiple metabolic abnormalities are believed to promote nerve dysfunctions, which may be similar to those contributing to the development of diabetic retinopathy, cataracts, and nephropathy (4,27,30). Diabetic neuropathy usually occurs in patients with more than a 15-year history of DM, and may affect the peripheral sensory and motor nerves, cranial nerves, or the autonomic nervous system. Although moneuropathy may occur, symmetrical polyneuropathy is more common. The initial symptoms of peripheral neuropathy typically involve the distal extremities, particularly the legs and feet. These include a gradual loss of deep tendon reflexes, proprioception, and especially sensory functions. Accompanying symptoms may include paresthesias, numbness, and burning or lancinating pain, usually greater at night (4,30). With time, some patients also develop symmetrical muscular atrophy and weakness. Complications may include painless arthropathy (Charcot's joints) and plantar foot ulcerations which may develop secondary infections. Cranial neuropathies with motor deficits of nerves III, IV, and VI are less common than peripheral neuropathies. Older individuals with mild DM sometimes develop a progressive atrophy and weakness (amyotrophy) involving the muscles of the pelvic girdle and proximal thigh; however, this neuromuscular complication is uncommon.

Autonomic neuropathy usually occurs only in association with significant peripheral polyneuropathy and other major complications in patients with long-standing DM. Diabetic autonomic neuropathy presents with a wide variety of clinical manifestations. Symptoms include postural hypotension, gastrointestinal dysfunctions (especially of the stomach, esophagus, and small intestine) that cause a variety of gastrointestinal symptoms, a neurotropic or atoic urinary bladder, and impotence. Autonomic neuropathy is associated with a high morbidity rate and poor prognosis. Complications resulting from the neuropathic bladder dysfunction include urinary tract infections, ureteral reflux, hydronephrosis, and pyelonephritis which can contribute to loss of renal function. Abnormal sweating patterns, ranging from anhidrosis (absence of sweating) to hydrohidrosis (excess sweating), are other possible manifestations of autonomic dysfunction. Autonomic dysfunction also may reduce warning symptoms or awareness of hypoglycemia in patients on insulin therapy as well as of myocardial ischemia (30). This is one of multiple reasons to carefully evaluate a diabetic patient with neuropathy prior to prescribing an exercise regimen.

The Diabetic Foot

The foot is another common site of diabetic complications (4,31). Generally, foot complications are due to a combination of diabetic neuropathy, vascular impairment, and infection. Neuropathy makes the foot more vulnerable to damage and ulceration in response to injury or even normal pressure during walking conditions. Absence of sweating and loss of sensation may be other contributing factors. Atherosclerotic peripheral vascular disease (to be discussed in more detail later) and probably hyperglycemia itself make the injured foot more susceptible to infection. Because of the absence of pain sensation, the infection may remain untreated and spread throughout the foot. The associated increase in metabolic demands and blood flow requirements of the involved tissues may not be met because of the vascular insufficiency, and the end result may be gangrene requiring amputation. From 50 to 70% of all nontraumatic amputations in this country are attributed to DM (31). It is estimated that about 80 per 10,000 diabetic individuals per year require amputations, with the rate increasing to over 1000 per 10,000 patients in those over age 65 years. The potential for prevention of serious foot problems in diabetic individuals is illustrated by a preventive program reported by a large diabetic clinic (31). The amputation rate was halved simply by having all diabetic patients remove their shoes for foot inspection at each clinic visit and referring those with early evidence of potential foot problems for education and advise about proper foot care and shoe fitting.

Cardiovascular Complications

The advent of insulin replacement therapy 70 years ago was followed by a shift in the pattern of mortality accompanying type I DM. A marked decline in deaths from diabetic coma unfortunately has been accompanied by a progressive rise in the proportion of deaths from CVD. In part, this may reflect an improved survival rate related to insulin therapy. However, a more important contributing factor is the increased prevalence of maturity-onset NIDDM with the aging of the population. About 70% of patients with NIDDM die of CVD. There also is a high rate of cardiac mortality with juvenile-onset, IDDM with the risk increasing with the duration of the disease.

Observational epidemiological and necropsy studies have demonstrated that coronary atherosclerosis and its clinical manifestations are more frequent, more severe, occur at an earlier age, affect men and women similarly, and are the principal contributor to CVD mortality in people with either major type of DM, as compared to matched nondiabetic subjects (32–35). In addition, diabetic individuals over age 35 also are more likely than matched nondiabetic individuals to have detectable silent ischemia during an exercise tolerance test and silent myocardial infarctions (35). Perhaps this is related to the absence or attenuation of myocardial ischemic pain, as a manifestation of damage to the cardiac nerves, associated with autonomic neuropathy. In addition, diabetic individuals who sustain a myocardial infarction have a poorer prognosis than matched nondiabetic individuals due to a higher incidence of congestive heart failure, cardiogenic shock, serious arrhythmias, and myocardial rupture. A lower survival rate and an increased recurrence of heart attacks also are more common in patients with DM sustaining a myocardial infarction as compared to nondiabetic patients.

Even in the absence of significant coronary artery atherosclerosis, the individual with DM is at increased risk for the development of cardiac problems. This is because diabetics are susceptible to a specific type of cardiomyopathy presenting with enlargement of the heart, impaired left ventricular function, and congestive heart failure (5,36). This condition is apparently due to myocardial microangiopathy, involving small branches of the coronary vessels, analogous to that found in the retinae and kidneys. Coexisting hypertension also may be a contributing factor (35,36).

Atherosclerosis involving the cerebral and peripheral arteries of the lower extremities are other common cardiovascular manifestations in individuals with DM. Atherothrombotic cerebrovascular accidents or strokes account for 6 and 15% of deaths in IDDM and NIDDM patients, respectively (33). Occlusive peripheral vascular disease resulting in intermittent claudication, gangrene, and amputations involving the lower extremities also is much more common in patients with DM as compared to the general population (4,32,37,38). Occlusive peripheral artery disease has its highest prevalence in the sixth and seventh decades of life.

Mechanisms

Multiple mechanisms appear to contribute to accelerated atherosclerosis and coronary heart disease (CHD) events in diabetic individuals (Table 1). These may be classified as (a) factors increasing injury and dysfunction of the artery lining endothelium cells, (b) blood lipid-lipoprotein disturbances, and (c) hemostatic (platelet and clotting factor) abnormalities (Table 1). Injury or dysfunction of the vessel wall endothelium may be related to premature cell aging, increased permeability to plasma proteins, and osmotic damage due to the accumulation of abnormal metabolites (as with microvascular disease) (39). In addition, endothelial damage is accelerated by elevated blood pressure levels commonly found in people with DM (35,40). Diabetic individuals not only have a higher prevalence of hypertension, but also appear to generally have as a group higher than average blood pressure levels than matched nondiabetic individuals. Coexisting renal or renovascular disease may further contribute to the blood pressure elevations associated with DM. In addition, hyperinsulinemia, by increasing sodium reabsorption by the kidney tubules and obesity, both commonly associated with NIDDM, also are believed to contribute to blood pressure elevations (40).

Blood lipid abnormalities. Abnormal blood lipid and lipoprotein concentrations as well as alterations of the structure of certain lipoproteins and altered metabolism of apolipoproteins appear to play important roles in accelerated atherosclerosis with DM (34,35,39,41–44). However, lipid and lipoprotein abnormalities are not inevitable conse-

Table 1 Possible Contributing Factors to Accelerated Atherosclerosis and Coronary Artery Occlusions in Diabetic Individuals

---

I. Injury and dysfunction of the artery endothelial lining
   A. Premature endothelial cell aging
   B. Increased permeability to plasma proteins
   C. Osmotic damage
   D. Accumulation of abnormal metabolites
   E. Elevated blood pressure
   F. Excess smooth muscle proliferation at injury sites

II. Blood lipid-lipoprotein disturbances
   A. Uncontrolled IDDM
      1. hypertriglyceridemia
      2. elevated VLDL levels
      3. reduced lipoprotein lipase activity
      4. impaired removal of chylomicrons
      5. reduced HDL (esp. HDL_2) levels
      6. increased total and LDL cholesterol levels (less common)
      7. glycosylation of LDL
      8. blood lipid abnormalities potentiated by nephropathy
   B. Controlled IDDM: Normalization of blood lipid-lipoprotein profile
   C. NIDDM
      1. Variable changes:
         a. possible hypertriglyceridemia
         b. possible elevated VLDL levels
         c. possible reduced HDL levels
         d. possible elevated total cholesterol and LDL levels
      2. blood lipid-lipoprotein abnormalities more likely in the presence of obesity, high waist-to-hip ratio, a high fat diet, and physical inactivity
      3. abnormal blood lipid-lipoprotein profile improved by glycemic control

III. Hemostatic abnormalities
   A. Increased platelet adhesiveness and aggregation in response to injury or physiological stimuli
   B. Increased platelet thromboxane (TXA_2) to endothelial prostacyclin (PGI_2) ratio promotes thrombosis and coronary artery smooth muscle reactivity
   C. Increased plasma protein coagulation factors (VI, VIII, von Willebrand factor)
   D. Deficiency of certain coagulation inhibitors
   E. Diminished tissue plasminogen activator (TPA) levels, reducing fibrinolytic activity

---

quences of this disease. Variability in blood lipid-lipoprotein levels is understandable considering the heterogeneity of DM, and the large number of biological and host factors which may affect lipid metabolism. These include the type of DM, the gender of the patient, body fatness and fat distribution, diet, physical activity, alcohol consumption, cigarette smoking, the concomitant use of various types of medication, and extent of diabetic control. The prevalence and pattern of blood lipid and lipoprotein disturbances differ between IDDM and NIDDM (41,44). Patients with an untreated insulin deficiency, particularly if it is associated with ketoacidosis, commonly present with moderate to severe hypertriglyceridemia. This is primarily due to the elevation of levels of very low–density lipoprotein (VLDL). An elevation in chylomicron levels, sometimes also present in the fasting state, gives the plasma a lactescent appearance. An elevation in triglyceride-rich lipoprotein levels is generally due to overproduction of triglycerides by the liver. This results from the excess release of free fatty acids (FFA), by adipocytes and uptake by the liver, associated with a deficiency in insulin and an excess of counterregulatory hormones. In addition, there often is an accompanying impairment in removal of VLDL and chylomicrons from the blood due to deficient activity of lipoprotein lipase (LPL) in tissue capillaries, another manifestation of insulin deficiency. The excess production of VLDL and deficient activity in LPL are believed to contribute to a reciprocal reduction in levels of high density lipoprotein (HDL), especially the HDL_2 fraction. Apparently, HDL is a lipid scavenger (particularly its HDL_2 fraction) that helps prevent or reverse atherosclerosis by transporting cholesterol away from peripheral tissues to the liver for excretion into the gut as bile salts. Numerous epidemiological studies, including a recent 10-year follow-up of the Lipid Research Clinic Prevalence Study (45), have confirmed the inverse relationship between plasma HDL cholesterol levels and the risk of CHD.

A less consistent finding in patients with poorly controlled IDDM is an increase in the levels of serum total cholesterol and its principal carrier, low-density lipoprotein (LDL). An increase in serum total and LDL cholesterol when it occurs may be secondary to an elevation in VLDL, since LDL is derived primarily from the catabolic breakdown of VLDL by LPL. In turn, LDL delivers cholesterol to tissue cells. It is well known that high levels of LDL are strongly related to the severity of atherosclerosis and the risk of CHD.

It also has been postulated that elevated levels of plasma VLDL and chylomicrons promote atherogenesis (44,46). It is postulated that cholesterol-rich catabolic remnants of these lipoproteins become incorporated into the artery wall and stimulate atherosclerotic lesion formation.

Another factor which may contribute to accelerated atherogenesis is impaired removal of LDL from the plasma in the presence of poor glycemic control of DM. The major pathway for LDL removal from the plasma is by binding to LDL receptors present on cell membranes of the liver and various other tissues initiating cellular uptake. The LDL receptor recognizes apoprotein B-100 on LDL and after binding LDL is taken up by either the liver or extrahepatic tissues for degradiation by an endocytotic process (44). A deficiency of receptors or chemical alterations of apoprotein B-100 or of the LDL particle itself results in a decreased rate of LDL clearance and catabolism. Elevated levels of blood sugar causes glycosylation of LDL by glucose-binding to amino acids on apoprotein B-100 molecules. This reduces "recognition" of LDL by cell receptors and decreases cellular uptake and degradation. Glycosylation of LDL–apoprotein B also is believed to promote LDL uptake by arterial wall macrophages, which are precursors of foam cells involved in the formation of atherogenic lesions (43).

Diabetic nephropathy may further contribute to disturbances in lipid-lipoprotein metabolism with elevated plasma levels of triglycerides; total, VLDL, and LDL cholesterol; and reduced levels of HDL cholesterol, thus increasing severity of atherosclerosis (44). Dietary and insulin therapy in patients with uncomplicated IDDM can normalize these blood lipid abnormalities through maintenance of good or at least moderate glycemic control (41–44).

Although patients with NIDDM are more likely to have lipid-lipoprotein disturbances than those with IDDM, blood concentrations are highly variable for similar reasons as outlined for type I diabetic individuals. The most common lipoprotein abnormalities with type II DM is elevation of plasma VLDL and associated triglyceride levels as a result of increased hepatic VLDL secretion. In this case, it may be a consequence of excess levels of circulating endogenous insulin due to peripheral insulin resistance. The levels of HDL cholesterol vary inversely with those of VLDL levels. Slightly or moderately increased levels of plasma total and LDL cholesterol also has been reported in some studies in patients with NIDDM. However, in other studies the prevalence of hypercholesterolemia in type II diabetic patients was similar to matched nondiabetic controls. Improved diabetic control by loss of excess weight, diet, exercise, insulin, or oral antidiabetic agents all may favorably affect the blood lipid-lipoprotein profile in patients with NIDDM. For many patients however, antilipidemic drug therapy will be required (43). It is hoped that the management of these lipid disorders will reduce the risk of CVD in patients with DM as it has in nondiabetic populations; however, this remains to be proven by controlled clinical trials.

Hemostatic Abnormalities. A "hypercoagulable state" appears to contribute to the high incidence of occlusive arterial disease accompanying DM (47,48). An array of hemostatic abnormalities appear to be involved, an understanding of which requires a general review of hemostatic mechanisms.

The initial coagulation response to injury is rapid adhesion of platelets to areas of endothelial damage. A platelet-fibrin plug occurs at the injury site as a result of a sequence of complex physiochemical changes in which platelets, endothelial cells, clotting factors, and inhibitors all make important contributions. Normal hemostatis depends upon the proper interaction of these systems, and an alteration in any one of them can increase the tendency for either vascular thrombosis or hemorrhage. In addition, there appears to be a relationship between altered platelet activity at an injury site and the development of atherosclerotic platelet adherence to areas of denuded endothelium. Injured endothelial cells also release substances which promote platelet aggregation, reduce blood flow by vasoconstriction, and promote thrombus formation. The most potent of such substances is thromboxane A_2 (TXA_2). Other substances released by platelets stimulate smooth muscle cell proliferation and promote migrations of smooth muscle cells and macrophages to injury sites. Both smooth muscle cells and macrophages have a great avidity for the uptake of LDL and in the presence of elevated plasma of LDL they are converted to foam cells, the focal elements in atheromata formation. Smooth muscle cells also serve as precursors of fibroblasts, thereby, also contributing to the "sclerosis" component of atherosclerotic lesions.

In vitro studies have found increased platelet adhesiveness and aggregability in response to usual chemical agonists in some, but not all, diabetic individuals, as well as in experimental animal models of DM. Diabetic individuals often have elevated plasma levels of β-thromboglobulin (BTG), a specific protein released from platelets during aggregation, believed to be a marker for increased in vivo platelet activation. Particularly, high levels of BTG are found in diabetic patients with either atherosclerosis or microangiopathy; however, nondiabetic individuals with atherosclerosis also have elevated levels of this platelet-specific protein, suggesting that accelerated in vivo platelet aggregation may be a result rather than a causative factor in vascular complications. Nevertheless, diabetic children with no overt evidence of vascular disease also have been found to have elevated levels of BTG (48). Furthermore, glycemic control in newly diagnosed diabetic patients reduces blood levels of this platelet protein.

Prostaglandin synthesis by platelets and endothelial cells also plays a role in hemostasis. As previously mentioned, platelet synthesize and secrete TXA_2, which is a prostanoid derivative of the polyunsaturated fatty acid arachidonic acid. Thromboxane is an extremely potent, but short-lived, promoter of platelet aggregation and vasoconstriction. Its generation is one of the principal mechanisms for the platelet aggregation response to endothelial injury. The activity of TXA_2 is counteracted by another prostanoid metabolite of arachidonic acid, prostacyclin (PGI_2), which is generated by endothelial cells. Prostacyclin is the most potent naturally occurring inhibitor of platelet adhesion and aggregation, as well as being a potent vasodilator. In patients with DM, there is evidence of the increased production of TXA_2 by platelets and reduced synthesis of PGI_2 by endothelial cells (47,48). However, controversy exists as to whether the excess production of TXA_2 in patients with DM is the result rather than the cause of vascular complications. A recent study of patients with type I diabetes who lacked evidence of microvascular or atherosclerotic complications failed to find any abnormality in TXA_2 biosynthesis or increased platelet aggregability (48).

In addition to platelet abnormalities, a number of other coagulation factor dysfunctions as well as disturbances in fibrinolytic or thrombolytic activity have been demonstrated to contribute to the hypercoagulable state in DM (47). These include increased plasma concentrations of coagulation factors VII and VIII, fibrinogen, and the von Willebrand factor, necessary for binding of platelets to subendothelium in the process of platelet adhesions; a deficiency of antithrombin II and of other physiological inhibitors of coagulation; and diminished levels of plasminogen activators in blood vessels, required to activate plasmin in order to initiate fibrinolytic activity.

Much additional work is required to study the relationship of disturbances of blood platelet function, coagulation factors, and fibrinolytic activity to vascular complications of DM. This should include assessment of the effects of improved metabolic control of DM by diet, exercise, and drugs affecting platelet reactivity on TXA_2-PGI_2 balance, bleeding time, fibrinolysis, and subsequent rate of complications.

MANAGEMENT OF DIABETES MELLITUS

Initial Evaluation

General steps involved in the management of DM are summarized in Table 2. The initial diagnosis of DM is made in a nonpregnant adult by the presence of classic symptoms and unequivocally elevated plasma glucose levels of >140 mg/dl or 2-h postprandial plasma glucose level of ≥200 mg/dl (4,6,8,9). If the fasting glucose concentration is icreased, but less than diagnostic (i.e., a fasting plasma glucose level between 115 and 140 mg/dl), an oral glucose tolerance test should be performed to confirm the diagnosis. The finding of two elevated plasma glucose levels (i.e., ≥200 mg/dl) during the glucose tolerance test, including the 2-h specimen, is diagnostic of DM. The diagnosis of gestational diabetes requires a fasting plasma glucose level of ≥105 mg/dl or a plasma glucose level of 190 mg/dl at 30, 60, or 90 min of an oral glucose tolerance test plus a 2-h concentration of 165 mg/dl.

The determination of glycosylated hemoglobin, particularly Hgb A_{1C} at baseline, is useful for monitoring metabolic control. This test is based on the glycosylation reaction between the terminal amino acid of red blood cell hemoglobin and the number 2 carbon of glucose. This reaction increases with the blood glucose concentration. Since the reaction is irreversible and persists for the duration of the life of the red blood *cell*, (about 120 days), the glycosylated hemoglobin concentration reflects the average blood glucose control for the previous 120 days, and serial changes are useful for monitoring the adequacy of long-term glycemic control during subsequent treatment. Normal glycosylated hemoglobin values range between 3.5 and 8.5% (49). Poor control is generally associated with values greater than 12%.

Table 2 Steps in Management of Diabetes Mellitus

I. Initial evaluation
    A. Rule out secondary causes and contributing factors
    B. Classification
    C. Evaluate for diabetic complications
    D. Screen for other atherogenic risk factors

II. Glycemic control/normalization of metabolic state
III. Prevention or attenuation of microvascular and atherosclerotic complications

Radioimmunoassay for levels of plasma insulin and determinations of serum or urinary C peptide levels at the time of diagnosis of DM may help distinguish an absolute deficiency of pancreatic insulin secretory activity (type I DM) from a relative insulin deficiency state (type II DM) (50). In addition, pancreatic islet cell antibodies are present in the blood of a majority of patients with IDDM at the time of initial diagnosis, although this may only be a transitory phenomenon.

Medical evaluation of the diabetic patient should include ruling out secondary causes or contributing factors for the metabolic abnormalities. These may include obesity, other endocrine disturbances, pancreatic disease, or diabetogenic drugs such as glucocorticoids or thiazide diuretics. Evaluation should also include screening for evidence of diabetic complications, accelerated atherosclerosis, and risk factors for CHD. As a minimum, in addition to a general physical examination, the evaluations should include ophthalmological and neurological examinations; careful inspection of the feet and skin; assessment of peripheral pulses; auscultation for carotid, abdominal, and femoral bruits; complete urinalysis; blood for determination of urea nitrogen, creatinine, total cholesterol, triglycerides, and HDL cholesterol; a resting ECG; and a chest X-ray. Relative weight for height and desirable weight should be determined as well as the waist-to-hip circumference ratio. Patients should also be questioned about smoking habits, alcohol consumption, and dietary and physical activity habits. A progressive exercise stress test also is advised to screen patients age 35 and over and younger patients with a history of DM for 10 years or longer for asymptomatic coronary heart disease, as well as to determine their functional capacity and exercise tolerance. This is particularly important for those who are physically active on-the-job or during leisure time or plan to initiate a strenuous exercise program.

Glycemic Control and Prevention of Complications

The two major therapeutic goals in the management of DM are (a) to achieve glycemic and metabolic control of the disease, and (b) to prevent, slow the progression, or attenuate microvascular and atherosclerotic complications. Three treatment approaches act in concert toward accomplishment of these two goals. These are dietary modification (including weight management), increased physical activity, and pharmacological intervention with insulin or an oral hypoglycemic agent. As previously indicated, it is hoped that good metabolic control by these approaches will reduce the rate of diabetic complications. However, this remains to be proven by a conclusive clinical trial. A multicenter clinical trial of this nature, the Diabetes Control and Complications Trial (DCCT), is currently in progress (21).

Multiple risk factor intervention in conjunction with metabolic control of DM is crucial to reduce the risk of atherosclerotic cardiovascular complications. This includes smoking cessation, weight loss, and dietary changes. In addition, an increase in physical activity may not only improve glycemic control, but also may reduce blood pressure levels and improve the blood lipid profile. Finally, drug therapy is indicated if these nonpharmacological measures fail to achieve glycemic control, sufficiently reduce blood pressure levels, and correct blood lipid abnormalities. An intensive patient education program is the cornerstone for successfully carrying out these life-long diabetic management requirements.

The Diabetic Diet

General nutritional objectives for management of DM are listed in Table 3, and are discussed below. With the exception of the symptomatic patient with IDDM and ketosis, nutritional management is generally the initial treatment and cornerstone for management of hyperglycemia as well as associated blood lipid disorders. Generally, dietary therapy is attempted for at least a month alone or in combination with exercise for glycemic control prior to the initiation of insulin or an oral hypoglycemic agent. It is estimated that nutritional therapy alone will control hyperglycemia in about one-third of ketosis-resistant patients with DM. In ketosis-prone type I patients for whom insulin is required, a diabetic diet is generally begun simultaneously with insulin therapy, and insulin dosage is adjusted to balance the glycemic affects

Table 3   General Objectives of Nutritional Care of the Diabetic Patient

1. Provide an adequate intake of essential nutrients throughout the life cycle.
2. Adjust energy intake (and physical activity) to achieve or maintain proper body weight.
3. Restore blood glucose, blood lipids, and blood pressure levels to normal.
4. Maintain a consistent timing of meals and snacks in patients receiving insulin therapy to prevent large fluctuations in blood glucose levels.
5. Individualize a person's eating (and physical activity). Plan to fit his/her lifestyle.

of meals. Timing of the IDDM patient's meals and snacks are influenced by the type(s) and dosage of insulin prescribed.

Basic Requirements

Food exchange system. The basic meal structure, usually required for the diabetic patient after attaining glycemic control with insulin, is three main meals a day plus snacks at mid morning, mid afternoon, and bedtime. A food-exchange system is an excellent educational tool commonly employed for making dietary recommendations (4,49,51). This involves selection of food choices for daily menus from six lists of different food types: (a) milk, (b) vegetables, (c) fruit, (d) bread, (e) meat, and (f) fat exchanges. In addition, lists are provided of food items that should generally be avoided and of items permitted in unlimited quantities. Selection of a properly prescribed number of food items from each of the food-exchange lists should provide a proper blend of essential vitamins, minerals, and protein to meet recommended dietary allowances as well as to meet daily energy requirements.

Desirable body weight and energy requirements. Two other basic considerations necessary for designing a nutritional program are to determine the individual's "desirable" body weight and daily energy requirements for achieving or maintaining desirable weight. A number of standards for desirable weight for height have been proposed. The National Institute of Health's Consensus Conference on obesity and health (52) recommended the 1959 Metropolitan Life Insurance Tables (53), which are based on the mortality survival rate in an insured population. The National Research Council's Food and Nutrition Board alternate recommendations, on the other hand, are based on actual weights for height of adults in the United States observed by the Second National Health and Nutrition Examination Study (NHANES II) (54). A commonly used rule of thumb for estimating desirable body weight, which approximates values from the Metropolitan tables, is to allow for adult men 106 lb for the first 60 in. of height and 6 lb for each additional inch (49,51). For women, 100 lb is allowed for the first 60 in and 5 lb for each additional inch. Adjustments can be made for body frame size by subtracting or adding 10% to the estimated weight for small and large frames, respectively.

Energy needs are affected by body weight and height, age, gender, and most importantly physical activity habits. Approximate energy expenditure values for adults and children are available in the National Research Council's book *Recommended Dietary Allowances* (54).

These are based on estimates of the resting metabolic rate for age and physical activity status for average sized men and women. Another rule of thumb that can be used to estimate daily energy requirements for adults is as follows (49): resting energy requirement (kcal/day) = desirable body weight (DBW) in pounds × 10. Then add the following in kilocalories for usual physical activity status:

Sedentary: DBW × 3
Moderately active: DBW × 5
Very active: DBW × 10

For women *over* age 50 years, it is necessary to subtract 200 kcal from the total and for men *under* age 50 years to add 200 kcal. For patients who are underweight, an additional 500 kcal per day will provide for a pound a week weight gain or will meet the requirement for pregnancy or lactation.

On the other hand, if the patient is overweight, a 500-kcal deficit per day should provide for approximately a pound a week weight loss. An alternative system for estimating adult energy needs, which takes DBW and physical activity status into consideration, is as follows (49).

Weight status	Daily energy needs by physical activity classification (kcal/kg of actual body weight)		
	sedentary	moderate	very active
Above DBW	20–25	25–30	30–35
At DBW	25–30	30–35	35–40
Below DBW	30–35	35–40	40–45

Table 4 lists the usual range of energy requirements for age and gender for adolescents and adults based on the National Research Council recommendations (NCR) (54). For children, energy recommendations can be estimated as follows:

Age 4–6 years: 90 kcal/kg
7–10 years: 80 kcal/kg

The following is a brief review of current recommendations for micronutrient intake by diabetic individuals.

Protein Requirements. The American Diabetic Association (ADA) (55) recommends that the diabetic plan contain a daily protein intake in

Table 4   Usual Range of Daily Energy
Requirements by Age and Gender

Gender and age group	kcal/day
Males	
adolescents	2000–3000
19–50 years	2500–3300
51–75 years	2000–2800
Females	
adolescents	1500–3000
19–50 years	1700–2500
51–75 years	1400–2200

Source: From Ref. 54; used with permission.

adults of 0.8 g/kg of body weight, the same as recommended for non-diabetic individuals. For most diabetic adults, this allowance means that protein will contribute 15–20% of the total daily energy requirements. In patients with diabetic nephropathy, the protein intake may be reduced in an attempt to slow the progression of the disease. In general, protein sources should be provided by foods which are relatively low in total fat, saturated fat, and cholesterol. This is because of the well-documented relationship of dietary cholesterol, total fat, and saturated fat intake to levels of plasma total and LDL cholesterol, severity of atherosclerosis, and risk of CHD (56–59). Thus, animal sources of protein should be limited to 6 oz or less daily and should consist of leaner types of red meat, fish, and poultry (without skin). Complementary plant sources of protein sources should also be used as often as possible in place of animal sources; e.g., a combination of beans and grains.

Carbohydrate Intake.   The place of carbohydrates in the diet of diabetic individuals has long been a subject of controversy. Substantial data supports recent recommendations by the American Diabetic Association (55) for a diet high in complex carbohydrates (i.e., 55–70% of calories) and dietary fiber (about 40 g/day). This should primarily be obtained by an increased consumption of whole-grain cereals and bread, starchy roots, legumes and other vegetables, and fruits rather than the use of dietary supplements. The basis of these recommendations are findings of both epidemiological and short-term metabolic experiments. These studies have shown the *adverse effects* of a diet low in complex carbohydrates and dietary fiber and high in fat on both glucose tolerance (51) and blood lipid levels (58–61). Conversely, glucose tolerance and insulin sensitivity is generally improved and blood cholesterol levels are significantly reduced with no adverse effects on triglyceride levels by a diet high in complex carbohydrate and fiber and low in fat. Although, most of the blood cholesterol change is due to the reduced saturated fat intake, soluble components of dietary fiber may make a modest independent contribution (61).

Further support for such a dietary plan comes from population studies, which show that diabetic individuals who habitually consume low-fat diets with carbohydrates contributing up to 70% of calories, such as those in Japan and China, have an extremely low incidence rate of CHD even in the presence of DM (1,58). However, when they adopt a Western style diet (e.g., Japanese diabetic men living in Hawaii) their CHD rates increase markedly. Furthermore, there is recent evidence in patients with CHD who have had coronary artery bypass surgery that a high-carbohydrate, low-fat diet can reduce the progression of atherosclerotic lesions on serial coronary arteriograms (62). Additional studies are required to determine if similar beneficial dietary effects on atherogenesis occur in diabetic individuals.

Another recommendation by the American Diabetic Association (55) is to liberalize the consumption of sucrose and fruit containing simple carbohydrates by diabetic individuals. The basis for this is that the postprandial glycemic effects of sucrose and starch are similar when consumed as part of a meal by individuals with type I or II DM (51). However, a high intake of sucrose (17–35% of total calories) may have at least short-term adverse metabolic effects in some diabetic and nondiabetic individuals (63). These include the possibility of impaired insulin binding and sensitivity and increases in the plasma levels of fasting triglyceride and VLDL cholesterol levels and a significant reduction in the levels of HDL cholesterol. However, since there are no controlled metabolic studies in the literature lasting longer than 6 weeks (1), it is unknown whether these metabolic changes are permanent (63). Another reason to restrict the intake of sucrose and other simple sugars is the strong association between sugar consumption and dental caries. Thus, the current consensus is that sucrose and other glucose-containing disaccharides should not account for more than 10% of the total dietary energy (51). Since the current average American is believed to obtain 16% of their calories in their diets from sucrose, this recommendation may require an actual reduction in sucrose intake for most diabetic individuals.

Fat Intake. The American Diabetic Association (ADA) (55) also recommends that the total fat content of the diabetic diet should provide no more than 30% of the daily energy intake. This is in contrast to the usual American's intake of 38–40% of calories from fat. The ADA further recommends that the proportion of saturated, polyunsaturated, and monounsaturated fats be approximately equal and that dietary cholesterol consumption be limited to less than 300 mg/day. These recommendations are identical to those of the American Heart Association's Step 1 diet advocated by the National Cholesterol Education Program (NCEP) for individuals with elevated blood cholesterol levels (64).

For NIDDM patients with hyperlipidemia, the ADA advocates further restrictions of dietary fats to 20% of total energy intake and of dietary cholesterol to 100–150 mg/day. This reduction in saturated fats and cholesterol intake requires a restriction on sources and quantities of animal protein, limiting egg yolks to only a few per week, using only low-fat dairy products, and avoiding commercially prepared baked goods and other products which contain animal fat, hydrogenated oils, or tropical oils (palm and coconut), all rich in saturated fatty acids. Good sources of polyunsaturated oils, which lower blood cholesterol levels, are safflower, sunflower, corn, and soybeans. In addition, olive and canola oils are good sources of monounsaturated fatty acids, which have a neutral effect on blood cholesterol levels, while being low in saturated fatty acids. Soft margarines containing these oils as the principal ingredients are excellent substitutes for butter and hard, hydrogenated fat-containing margarines.

In individuals who do not tolerate a high carbohydrate intake or have at least a temporary worsening of hypertriglyceridemia, it is possible to substitute more monounsaturated fat; an intake up to 18% of total calories does not adversely affect the blood cholesterol–lowering power of the AHA Step 1 Diet (60,65). In addition, the consumption of a monounsaturated fat–enriched diet can either prevent the decrease in plasma concentration of HDL cholesterol, which frequently occurs with a marked reduction in total fat intake, or it may actually raise HDL cholesterol levels (43,65).

Another dietary issue related to lipid ingestion for the diabetic patient pertains to the appropriate dietary content of omega-3 polyunsaturated (n-3 PUFA) fatty acids and their possible role in the prevention of diabetic complications. Fish oils are a rich source of two of these highly unsaturated fatty acids; i.e., eicosapentaenoic acid (EPA) (22:6) and docosahexaenoic acid (DCA) (22:6). In addition, another n-3 PUFA, alpha-linoleic acid (C16:3), is present in certain vegetable oils, particularly canola and soybean oils, and can be converted in the body to EPA and DCA.

Epidemiological studies have reported that a high intake of seafood rich in n-3 PUFA is associated with a reduced risk of cardiovascular disease (66). Most of the earlier studies which were performed in the 1970s involved eskimos who consumed a diet composed predominantly of seafood. However, a more recent retrospective study from the Netherlands by Kromhut et al. (67) reported that subjects who consumed on the average of 30 g of fish per day also had a reduced death rate from CHD. To put this quantity of fish in perspective, the mean daily per capita consumption of fish in the United States is about half that amount. These epidemiological observations have stimulated animal and human feeding trials using either fatty fish, fish oils, or purified n-3 PUFA to examine the metabolic and biochemical effects related to the development of atherosclerotic cardiovascular disease. A number of these findings discussed below may have relevance to the diabetic patient, although the amounts or n-3 PUFA required for these effects would require the administration of fish oil or n-3 PUFA supplements, since the quantity of fatty fish that would have to be consumed regularly to achieve these desirable physiological effects is not commonly practiced in Western societies (68).

There is consistent evidence that 5–10 g/day of n-3 PUFA can reduced elevated plasma triglyceride and VLDL levels with no change, or at least a transient increase in HDL cholesterol levels (66,68). These studies include preliminary observations in patients with NIDDM. However, these changes may be associated in hyperlipidemic patients with an undesireable actual *increase* in the levels of plasma LDL cholesterol and in LDL-apoprotein B. The possibility also exists that n-3 PUFA may have adverse effects on glycemic control in NIDDM patients (68).

In addition to its effects on blood lipid levels, n-3 PUFA have a profound effect on platelet aggregation and blood coagulability (66). Decreased platelet aggregation in response to usual stimuli has been demonstrated in both animal and human feeding studies with n-3 PUFA apparently due to their ability to reduce platelet TXA_2 formation. This results in prolongation of bleeding time. These blood platelet changes theoretically should counteract increased platelet aggregability and increased TXA_2 release by patients with DM and the reduced risk of thrombosis in narrowed atherosclerotic arteries; however, these possibilities remain to be proven.

In addition, a recent large dietary-supplementation trial has demonstrated the effectiveness of 6 g/day of 85% EPA and DCA in reducing elevated blood pressure levels in nondiabetic individuals with hypertension (69). Furthermore, a fish oil supplement (cod liver oil) has been shown in IDDM patients to reduce the renal transcapillary escape rate of albumin, independent of its effect on blood pressure (70). These intriguing observations of the potential beneficial effects of n-3 PUFA in reducing diabetic renal complications require confirmation. In the meantime, the routine use of n-3 PUFA supplements for diabetic patients is not currently recommended beyond encouraging fish consumption several times a week.

Concerns about the nutritional adequacy of a fat-restricted high-carbohydrate diet in patients with DM have been addressed in the literature. Hollenbeck et al. (71) and others have demonstrated that such diets even when self-selected can provide adequate amounts of essential micronutrients. A modest restriction of sodium intake to less than 3 g/day also is generally recommended for diabetic patients. This is to reduce the propensity for high blood pressure and perhaps of diabetic nephropathy. Sodium intake can be minimized by the avoidance of table salt and grossly salty foods and reducing the intake of processed foods. Alcohol should be avoided in individuals whose blood glucose is out of control, in those attempting weight loss, in those who are pregnant, and in those who have hypertriglyceridemia or hypertension. In other diabetic individuals, alcohol may be used prudently; i.e., up to 2 oz once or twice a week. However, because of the possibility of alcohol-induced hypoglycemia in people with IDDM on insulin alcohol should be consumed only along with food.

In summary, nutritional management is a major pillar in the control of DM and in the prevention and management of associated blood lipid disorders and associated elevated blood pressure levels. Its potential role in the prevention of atherosclerosis and thrombotic complications appears promising, but remains to be confirmed by clinical trials. In patients receiving insulin therapy, the timing of meals and snacks is crucial for the prevention of hypoglycemia, particularly in physically active type I diabetic individuals, as will be discussed in greater detail later in this chapter.

Insulin Therapy

Candidates

About one-third of all diabetics in the United States require insulin for treatment. Patients with IDDM characterized by a near-absolute deficiency in endogenous insulin require daily insulin replacement to treat or avoid ketoacidosis. Insulin therapy also is useful in both types I and II diabetic patients to control symptoms accompanying marked hyperglycemia (i.e., >250 or 300 mg/dl) in the absence of ketoacidosis and for glycemic control in asymptomatic type I or II patients. Insulin also is being more widely used routinely in an attempt to reduce future chronic complications, or for initial pharmacological intervention in type II patients as an alternate to oral hypoglycemic agents, if diet and exercise fail to normalize blood glucose levels or when oral hypoglycemic agents are ineffective or contraindicated because of allergic problems or the presence of significant renal or hepatic disease. It may also be used as a short-term measure to control the exacerbation of diabetic metabolic dearrangements accompanying trauma, surgery, infections, pregnancy, myocardial infarctions, or when diabetogenic drugs or other "glycemic stressors" are required (4,8,9). It should be noted that large doses of insulin (i.e., >100 U/day) are likely to be required for the glycemic control in obesity-related type II diabetic patients owing to marked peripheral insulin resistance.

Goals

The immediate goals of insulin therapy are to alleviate diabetic symptoms and correct metabolic disorders while returning blood glucose (and glycosylated hemoglobin) levels as close to normal as possible, while avoiding hypoglycemia due to overdosage. Improved metabolic control in type I diabetic individuals with insulin therapy generally is accompanied by the correction of associated blood lipid abnormalities, including raising plasma HDL levels (44,72).

Details on Administration

Insulin therapy usually is initiated in a hospital setting with insulin doses correlated with the patient's blood glucose responses, and are related to body weight and physical activity status. The usual starting dose for a normal-weight sedentary adult is 0.2–0.5 U/kg of body weight of an insulin with an intermediate duration of actions (e.g., NPH insulin) administered subcutaneously in an arm (49). Adolescents usually require a larger initial dose. In the presence of ketoacidosis, the initial dose may be as high as 2–4 U/kg. Following hospital discharge, subsequent management of insulin dosage is based on home self-monitoring of capillary blood glucose levels in drops of blood obtained by fingerstick using an automated lance. Details for self-monitoring of DM have been extensively reported (4,8,73). As previously mentioned, periodic glycosylated hemoglobin determinations are useful in gauging the adequacy of long-term glycemic control during therapy. Suggested algorithms for insulin dosage adjustments based on blood glucose levels are available (49,73).

Most commercial insulin preparations consist of a mixture of beef and pork insulins obtained by pancreatic extraction; however, pure pork insulin, which is less antigenic than beef insulin because its amino acid sequence is closer to human insulin, also is available. In addition, human insulin is now manufactured by recombinant deoxyribonucleic acid (DNA) techniques or by chemical modification of the pork insulin molecule. Although, less antigenic than pure pork insulin, the subcutaneous administration of human insulin still elicits some antibody response. The purified pork and human preparations are much more costly than the mixture of beef and pork insulin and generally are only prescribed to patients who develop significant immunological or local skin complications.

A complete list of insulins sold in the United States has been published by the American Diabetic Association (9). In general, insulins may be classified by their duration of action as short-, intermediate-, and long-acting (49,73). The longer-acting preparations have had certain materials added in order to prolong their pharmacological activity in order to reduce the required number of daily injections for glycemic control.

Table 5 lists the expected duration of action of representative animal insulins from each class (49,73); however, since the actual rates of absorption may vary up to 25% from day-to-day owing to variations in local subcutaneous tissue conditions and other factors influencing insulin pharmacokinetics, the clinician should not rely too heavily on textbook descriptions of insulin activity. Adjustments of insulin dosage

Table 5 A Comparison of Time Course of Action of Different Classes of Insulins of Animal Origin

Insulin type	Preparation	Onset (h)	Peak (h)	Duration (h)
Short-acting	Regular	0.25–0.5	2–4	5–7
(rapid onset)	Semi-lente	0.5	3–6	12–16
Intermediate	NPH[a]	1–2	6–12	18–24
	Lente	1–2	6–12	18–24
	Globin	1–2	4–8	12–18
Long-Acting	Ultralente	4–6	14–16	24–36

[a] NPH, neutral protamine Hagedorn.
Source: Adapted from Ref. 73; used with permission.

should be based on actual blood glucose values obtained by self-monitoring by the patient of blood glucose levels before and after meals and exercise and during the night. Frequent self-monitoring of glucose levels is particularly important when initiating or intensifying insulin therapy or adjusting dosage because of hypoglycemic reactions. As previously mentioned, insulin therapy usually is initiated in a nonemergency situation with a dose of an intermediate-acting insulin well below the amount likely to be required for glycemic control and the dose is gradually increased in order to minimize the risk of hypoglycemia. For example, a usual safe starting dose of insulin is 15–20 U of NPH or lente (U-100 containing 100 U/ml) given subcutaneously 30 min before breakfast. The maximal blood glucose–lowering effect with intermediate-acting insulins is 4–12 h after administration, with the ability to lower blood glucose concentration waning overnight, and reaching a nadir in the early morning hours. A 2- to 5-day observation period is recommended prior to adjustments in the dose of intermediate-acting insulin because of the variability in the rate of insulin absorption and the day-to-day variation in food intake and physical activity. Optimal glycemic control is unlikely with a single daily insulin dose. Usually two or more doses of intermediate-acting insulin or the addition of regular insulin to the intermediate-acting insulin generally is required. An advantage of using regular insulin in combination with an intermediate-acting insulin is that the peak effect of regular insulin (2–4 h after administration) may abort midmorning hyperglycemia, which is common when an intermediate-acting insulin is used alone. However, regular insulin should only be added after the appropriate dose of intermediate-acting insulin has been established. Usually 5–10 U of regular insulin is administered in the same syringe with the intermediate-acting insulin. If postprandial hyperglycemia persists, additional doses of regular insulin alone may be administered 30 min before meals. In general, 1 U of regular insulin will lower the blood glucose level 40–50 mg/dl, if the blood glucose concentration is in the range of 150–200 mg/dl. For example, 2 U of regular insulin would be expected to reduce a plasma glucose level of 200 mg/dl to 100–120 mg/dl.

A typical multidose regimen might consist of an injection of a mixture of NPH or lente insulin with regular insulin in the morning at a half hour prior to breakfast, and another injection of the same mixture in the evening, a half hour before the evening meal. The recommended ratio of intermediate-acting to regular insulin in the morning is 2:1 and in the evening 1:1. Adjustments of the dosage and amounts of each type of insulin can be made to further reduce blood glucose levels at appropriate times of the day; however, the clinician should be aware that mixing different types of insulin may alter the time of the peak effect and duration of action of insulin, especially when regular insulin is mixed with lente insulin (8,9).

Goals for plasma or capillary glucose concentrations considered to reflect excellent or "tight" glycemic control are 70–120 mg/dl in the fasting state or before meals and 100–140 mg/dl 1 h after meals. Control is considered poor if the fasting and preprandial glucose levels are >150 mg/dl and if the postprandial level(s) is greater than 200 mg/dl.

Usual sites for the subcutaneous administration of insulin include over the quadriceps muscle, the deltoid and the abdominal muscles, or the gluteal regions. Injection of insulin into a region of the body (upper or lower extremities) soon to be involved in physical activity should be avoided because of the resulting accelerated absorption of insulin (74). This can cause a rapid onset of insulin action, resulting in a greater reduction than expected of blood glucose levels during exercise, which increases the risk of hypoglycemia as well as reduces the duration of insulin activity. Avoiding exercise for an hour immediately after insulin injection or using the abdominal region for insulin administration usually alleviates these problems. Using a single anatomical site for all insulin injections rather than rotation of anatomical sites was recently reported to reduce the variability in blood glucose levels in type I diabetic subjects (75).

Side Effects

The side effects of insulin therapy include a loss of subcutaneous fat at injection sites, local skin reactions, systemic allergic reactions, insulin resistance (>100 U of insulin required daily), and hypoglycemia (insulin reaction) (4,8,9,73). In actuality, hypoglycemia (blood glucose level <60 mg/dl) is actually an exaggerated therapeutic response and occasional mild episodes are unavoidable during intense insulin therapy, especially in someone who exercises regularly. The symptoms and signs of hypoglycemia include one or all of the following: anxiety, tremulousness, tachycardia, sweating, tingling of the digits, dizziness, headache, and hunger (4). Sympathoadrenal system stimulation is primarily responsible for these initial warning symptoms, and their suppression by the concomitant use of β-adrenergic drugs used for the management of hypertension or CHD may mask the onset of hypoglycemia. Hypoglycemia also may occur in some diabetic individuals in the presence of normal or even elevated glucose levels as a result of a rapid insulin-induced reduction in blood glucose levels. However, the presence of true hypoglycemia constitutes a medical emergency, since cerebral dysfunction may result if glucose is not promptly administered. Symptoms at the stage of advanced hypoglycemia may include faintness, visual disturbances, mental disturbances, slurred speech, coordination problems, personality changes or bizarre behavior, drowsiness, and unconsciousness or coma. Because of the resemblance of these cerebral symptoms to alcohol or drug intoxication, it is imperative for a diabetic individual receiving insulin to wear a medical alert identification. Delayed or skipped meals, decreased food intake, or an unexpected increase in physical activity uncompensated for by extra food intake or reduced insulin dosage may contribute to the development of hypoglycemia.

Every diabetic individual receiving insulin therapy must be cognizant of their individualized early warning symptoms of hypoglycemia, respond by promptly checking their capillary blood glucose level, and have an existing plan for combating low blood glucose levels. Food containing 10–15 g of simple carbohydrates, such as 1 cup (8 oz) of orange juice, or seven to eight hard candies (such as Life Savers) may be sufficient to abort a mild insulin reaction. This should be repeated within 20 min if symptoms persist. Since avoiding hypoglycemia is a major concern of the diabetic individual participating in sports or on an exercise program, additional discussion is included in the section on exercise for the diabetic individual.

Recent developments which can significantly improve the metabolic control of the diabetic individual receiving insulin and make life easier and nearer normal are external or implantable battery-powered insulin infusion devices (4). Insulin pumps are refillable reservoirs which deliver short-acting crystalline zinc insulin subcutaneously, usually in the abdominal wall or directly into a vein. The external pumps are worn on a belt and require refilling and a needle change every 2 days. The more sophisticated implantable infusion pumps have glucose-sensing devices which monitor the blood glucose concentration and provide insulin "on demand." These are often referred to as an artificial endocrine pancreas. At present, they are regarded as experimental, are cumbersome in size, and require two patient intravenous lines. Potential serious risks with either type of infusion devise may be associated with pump damage or malfunction, catheter-related problems, infections, and severe hypoglycemia. However, in the future as technology advances, these devices have great potential for improving diabetic control and the quality of life.

Another important development which holds great promise for the future control of IDDM is the progressive improvement in the success of transplanting in diabetic individuals of a whole or partial pancreas or islet beta cells.

Oral Hypoglycemic Drug Therapy

Types of Agents

Oral hypoglycemic drugs are commonly prescribed in the United States; they account for 1% of all prescriptions filled. About 40% of patients with NIDDM are currently receiving one of these drugs. Detailed guidelines for their use have been published (8,9,76). In the United States, there are currently six orally administered hypoglycemic drugs available, all of which are members of the sulfonylurea class (Table 6). Three of these agents, chloropromide, glyburide, and glipizide, account for about 75% of those prescribed (76). In addition, a biguaride-type of oral hypoglycemic agent, metaformin, is undergoing clinical trial in the United States. This drug is already marketed and widely prescribed in Canada and Europe. As is true with the different types of insulin preparations, sulfonylurea drugs may be classified by their duration of action. Table 6 lists the six available sulfonylurea agents by progressive duration of action and their usual required dosage range.

Table 6   Available Sulfonylurea Oral Hypoglycemic Agents by Duration of Action and Usual Dosage

Drug	Daily dose range (mg)	No. of doses (per day)	Duration of action (h)
Tolbutamide (Orinase)	500–3000	2–3	6–10
Acetohexamide (Dymelor)	250–1500	2	12–18
Tolazamide (Tolinase)	100–1000	1–2	16–24
Glipizide (Glucotrol)	2.5–40	1–2	16–24
Glyburide (Mironase, Diabeta)	1.25–20	1–2	18–24
Chlorpropamide (Diabonese)	100–500	1–2	27–72

Source: From Ref. 76; used with permission.

Pharmacological Actions

The principal pharmacological action of the sulfonylurea drugs is stimulation of pancreatic islet cells to release more insulin, apparently by increasing their sensitivity to glucose (76). They do not increase the rate of insulin synthesis, however. High-affinity sulfonylurea receptors have been demonstrated on pancreatic beta cells. The order of potency of binding of these drugs to pancreatic beta cells approximates their potency in stimulating the release of insulin. Sulfonylurea drugs may also inhibit the secretion of the counterregulatory hormone, glucagon, from the pancreatic alpha islet cells. Possible extrapancreatic effects of these drugs include improved peripheral tissue sensitivity to insulin and reduced clearance of insulin from the blood by the liver (76). The net result of these actions is increased effectiveness of available endogenous insulin.

Candidates

Sulfonylurea drugs are primarily used to treat patients with type II DM who fail to adhere or respond to nonpharmacological measures, including diet, weight reduction, and exercise therapy. Although these drugs are contraindicated in patients with type I DM who are prone to ketoacidosis, persons with mild IDDM capable of insulin production and requiring less than 20 U of insulin per day for control also may be suitable candidates for sulfonylurea therapy. Further, some patients who fail to achieve adequate glycemic control with a sulfonylurea drug may achieve better control on the addition of insulin. The rationale for this combination approach is that failure of response to sulfonylurea therapy may be due primarily to impaired beta islet cell functioning; however, the effect of the sulfonylurea on improving insulin sensitivity may still occur, and this may potentiate the effectiveness of concomitant insulin administration. Factors involved in the selection of a specific sulfonylurea have previously been described (9) and are beyond the scope of this chapter.

Therapy should begin with the lowest doses possible and increase as necessary at weekly intervals until satisfactory glycemic control is attained or the highest recommended dose is reached. Patients who respond satisfactorily to sulfonylurea therapy should undergo periodic assessment to determine whether the drug dose can be reduced. A ''bonus'' associated with improved glycemic control with sulfonylurea treatment is generally a decrease in plasma levels of total and LDL cholesterol, triglycerides, VLDL triglycerides and cholesterol, and either no change or an increase in HDL cholesterol levels (77).

Side Effects

Sulfonylurea drugs are generally well tolerated, with less than 2% of patients having to discontinue therapy because of side effects (76). The most common serious side effect of sulfonylurea therapy is an insulin-like hypoglycemic reaction. Its frequency appears to be related to the potency and duration of drug action. The highest incidence occurs with glyburide and chloropromide and the lowest with tolbutamide (77). The hypoglycemia produced may be prolonged and require intravenous glucose infusions for several days to correct. Severe sulfonylurea-induced hypoglycemia is associated with about a 10% mortality rate. Other less common side effects, occurring with a similar frequency with all of the available agents, include gastrointestinal disturbances, skin rashes, bone marrow suppression, hyponatremia, mild intolerance to alcohol (disulfran-like reaction), and interactions with other drugs which may include potentiation of the action of sulfonylurea drugs (76). Weight gain is common in patients who improve glycemic control, but this also occurs with insulin therapy and is presumably the result of reduced energy loss with clearing of glycosuria. This weight gain in turn may cause secondary therapeutic failure in patients with good initial glycemic control with sulfonylurea drugs. Sulfonylurea drugs also cross the placental barrier in pregnant women and can cause severe hypoglycemia in the fetus or newborn.

The relationship of the use of these agents to the risk of CHD has been the subject of a great deal of controversy. The results of a large multicenter research study in the 1970s, the University Group Diabetic Program (UGDP), appeared to indicate that tolbutamide was no more effective in prolonging life than diet alone and was associated with an increased risk of cardiovascular mortality (77). Subsequently, the UGDP study design was criticized and the results questioned. Furthermore, the results of other large-scale studies have not supported the conclusions of the UGDP (76). Nevertheless, the FDA still requires that packages of tolbutamide include an insert warning of the possibility of associated increased risks of cardiovascular mortality.

Exercise Therapy

Acute Exercise Effects

Exercise conditioning has been promoted since ancient times as a treatment for DM, and this topic has previously been reviewed (78–82). Familiarization with the metabolic effects of acute exercise on substrate utilization is required to better understand its potential benefits for glycemic control as well as associated hazards for patients with DM. During physical exertion, energy demands of muscular work necessitate an accelerated delivery of fuels and oxygen to the contracting skeletal muscles. These demands are met by major metabolic, hormonal, and cardiovascular adjustments. The principal fuels or substrates utilized by the contracting muscles are carbohydrates (in the forms of muscle glycogen and blood-borne glucose) and circulating free fatty acids (FFAs), derived primarily from the lipolysis of triglycerides in adipose tissue. The relative contribution of carbohydrates and FFAs to oxidative energy production depends both on the intensity and duration of muscular exertion. The more strenuous the exercise, i.e., the greater the percentage of maximal oxygen uptake ($\dot{V}O_{2\,max}$) achieved, the greater the dependence of the participating muscles on carbohydrates for fuel. Strenous high-intensity exercise also results in an increase in the blood glucose level, since glucose production by the liver exceeds peripheral utilization. Light- to moderate-intensity dynamic or endurance exercise which can be sustained for long intervals of time, such as walking, running, cycling, and swimming, results in an orderly sequence of fuel utilization. During the first few minutes of exercise, muscle glycogen provides the chief source of energy for muscle contraction. After about 5–10 min, blood glucose and FFAs become increasing more important as substrates. Glucose utilization may increase 20-fold over the basal rate and contribute 25–40% of the total oxidative fuel requirements. An increase in blood flow to the exercising muscle contributes to the increased glucose uptake, but exercise also has a proinsulin effect on facilitating uptake of glucose by muscle. Despite increased utilization, the blood glucose level generally remains unchanged or only shows a slight decrease even after hours of dynamic exercise in the nondiabetic individual. What makes this possible is a continuous replacement of the blood glucose pool through an increase in the rate of glucose production and release by the liver. For at least the first 40 min of dynamic exercise, increased liver glucose production is derived primarily from the breakdown of hepatic glycogen (i.e., glycogenolysis); however, liver glycogen stores are limited, particularly in diabetic individuals. During more prolonged exercise, the formation of new hepatic glycogen and glucose becomes an increasingly more important contributor to glucose released by the liver by a process called gluconeogenesis.

Diabetic individuals are more effective than undiabetics in using gluconeogenesis for maintaining glucose homeostasis. Substrates for gluconeogenesis include blood-borne lactate, pyruvate, glycerol, ketone bodies, and certain amino acids. Eventually after many hours of endurance activity even this process begins to fail, and blood glucose levels fall. However, this is accompanied by a progressive shift from dependence on carbohydrate to FFA for oxidative metabolism as a compensatory mechanism. Again diabetic individuals show superior efficiency for utilization of FFA as fuels compared with nondiabetic individuals. Exercise conditioning further improves the ability to use FFAs as a fuel, thereby having a muscle glycogen and glucose-sparing effect. Despite this shift during prolonged exercise to the increased use of FFA for fuel, the utilization of muscle glycogen for fuel remains essential to maintain muscle contraction. Initial stores of glycogen are thereby an important limiting factor for performing prolonged dynamic exercise. This may prove to be a problem for diabetic individuals who generally have reduced muscle glycogen stores. A reduction of muscle and liver glycogen stores stimulates activity of glycogen synthetase an enzyme essential for glycogen synthesis. Increased activity of this enzyme appears to be related to the accelerated, noninsulin-dependent uptake of glucose by muscle and liver which persists up to 48 h following prolonged exercise, whereas glycogen stores continue to be replenished (82). During this prolonged recovery period, there is a temporary improvement of glucose tolerance and insulin sensitivity in both diabetic and nondiabetic individuals. It now is generally believed that improved glycemic control of DM in people who regularly exercise is primarily due to an overlap of acute exercise. However, exercise conditioning also improves the ability to store glycogen.

A number of hormones contribute to the regulation of fuel availability, rate of utilization, and glucose hemostasis during exercise (79). Of these, insulin plays the critical role. It promotes glucose uptake and utilization by muscle. An important adaptation to prolonged exercise in both nondiabetic and type II diabetic individuals is a decline in endogenous circulating insulin levels. Increases in tissue insulin receptor activity, cell membrane glucose transport proteins, and in blood flow to exercising muscle contribute to increased uptake of substrate despite the reduction in plasma insulin concentration (83). As previously indicated, improved insulin sensitivity and increased muscle glucose uptake may persist for several days following a single acute prolonged exercise session. With endurance exercise conditioning the effects on the glucose-insulin dynamics appear similar, but they may persist longer, perhaps up to 7 days after the last exercise session (80).

A consequence of reduced levels of circulating endogenous insulin during prolonged exercise is stimulation of hepatic glycogenolysis and gluconeogenesis with an increased glucose release by the liver. However, the type I diabetic individual receiving insulin replacement therapy does not experience the physiological decline in blood insulin levels during prolonged exercise. Persistence of blood insulin concentration limits the liver's ability to release glucose in response to a fall in blood glucose levels during prolonged exercise and poses a risk of hypoglycemia in diabetic individuals on insulin therapy. This translates into the necessity of having diabetic individuals on insulin who do prolonged exercise either reduce their dosage of insulin or increase their intake of carbohydrates before, during, and after prolonged physical exertion in order to avoid hypoglycemia. Prevention of hypoglycemia during exercise in IDDM will be discussed further later in this chapter.

The usual decline in circulating insulin levels during prolonged exercise in both the nondiabetic and type II diabetic individuals promotes lipolysis of adipose tissue fat and increased release of FFA. A concomitant increase in the release of epinephrine and glucagon and other counterregulatory hormones during exercise also profoundly affects carbohydrate and lipid availability, and their contributions are the opposite of those associated with insulin (80). Increased secretion of these hormones along with reduced circulating insulin levels promotes the release of glucose by the liver and of FFA from adipose tissues.

The metabolic response to acute exercise is profoundly influenced by the adequacy of diabetic control, particularly in those with type I DM. With poorly controlled DM (fasting plasma glucose levels >250 or 300 mg/dl with or without ketoacidosis), there is an excess secretion of counterregulatory hormones which is potentiated by exercise. The end result may be a worsening of metabolic dysfunctions and aggravation of ketoacidosis (78–82). When the DM is under adequate control or if only mild hyperglycemia is present, an acute prolonged exercise session usually improves glycemic control and reduces requirements for exogenous insulin or oral hypoglycemic drugs for up to 48 h similarly to the improved insulin sensitivity in nondiabetic individuals. However, if exercise is performed when exogenous insulin level or the activity of an oral hypoglycemic drug is at its peak, a hypoglycemic reaction may result either during or more commonly several hours following exercise. Again, this appears to be primarily due to insulin suppression of the release of glucose from the liver. Accelerated insulin-enhanced glucose uptake by active skeletal muscle may also be a contributing factor.

Exercise Training Effects

The basis of the common recommendation of regular dynamic exercise as adjunctive therapy for patients with DM (particularly those with

NIDDM) are summarized in Table 7. Supporting data for each of these proposed areas of benefits are discussed below.

Improved Glucose-Insulin Dynamics. Historically, the demonstration that exercise can improve glycemic control of DM preceded the discovery of insulin. As previously mentioned, acute exercise potentiates the effect of insulin on glycemic control in IDDM as a result of enhanced glucose uptake by working skeletal muscle both during exercise and for a prolonged period following exercise recovery (84). In addition, an exercise-induced increased rate of absorption of a recently injected insulin dose into an exercising limb may contribute to glucose reduction (74). Further, it is well documented experimentally that exercise conditioning can improve insulin sensitivity and glucose intolerance, particularly in obese individuals with insulin insensitivity and hyperinsulinemia or glucose intolerance (80,81,85,86).

In addition, an increase in skeletal muscle mass, capillary density and blood flow, enhanced mitochondrial oxidative capacity, and glycogen synthesis with exercise conditioning theoretically should further contribute to "disposal" of excess blood glucose levels (80,81). Both observational and experimental data support the potential role of regular exercise in the prevention of NIDDM. These include population-based data relating a sedentary lifestyle to increased risk of NIDDM, $\dot{V}O_{2\,max}$ levels to insulin-stimulated glucose disposal (87), and the development within a few days of forced inactivity of insulin insensitivity and impaired glucose tolerance in healthy individuals (19,20).

There is a paucity of controlled clinical studies involving either type I or type II diabetic individuals to determine whether there are chronic effects of exercise on glucose-insulin dynamics and glycemic control beyond those resulting from repeated bouts of acute exercise or an accompanying weight loss. The few chronic exercise studies involving subjects with IDDM have yielded contradictory results (80,81,88–

Table 7 Possible Beneficial Effects of Dynamic Exercise Training in Patients with Diabetes Mellitus

1. Improved glucose-insulin dynamics and glycemic control
2. Prevention or reduction of obesity
3. Improved physical fitness
4. Improved blood lipid profile
5. Reduced risk of coronary heart disease
6. Psychosocial benefits

93). However, most studies involving children and adolescents with type I DM have demonstrated substantially improved metabolic control of IDDM with regular vigorous dynamic exercise (88–90). In these studies exercise was performed at least for 30 min, three times a week for up to 12 weeks, and was associated with a significant increase in $\dot{V}O_{2\,max}$ levels. Exercise conditioning in type I diabetic youngsters in these studies was reported to either substantially reduce daily insulin requirements (88), to lower fasting blood glucose and glycosylated hemoglobin concentrations (89), or to improve insulin sensitivity as measured by the euglycemic clamp technique (90). Variability in the type of metabolic responses in these studies is believed to be related to the extent of control of DM prior to the exercise program, changes in energy intake during the exercise program, extent of improvement in $\dot{V}O_{2\,max}$, and whether there was an accompanying increase in lean body mass.

On the other hand, at least four controlled exercise studies involving adults with a type I DM yielded mixed results (78,91–93). In these studies, training generally consisted of moderate-intensity exercise sessions done three to four times a week on a cycle ergometer for 12 or more weeks. None of these studies were able to demonstrate improved glycemic control beyond that of the acute effects of exercise. However, two of these studies did report improved peripheral insulin sensitivity (92,93), which was associated in one of these studies (92) with a modest 6% reduction in daily insulin requirements (i.e., 2 U/day). Increased energy intake primarily as carbohydrates on exercise days was postulated to be a likely cause of the failure to improve glycemic control with exercise training in these studies despite the acute glucose-lowering effect with each exercise session (78).

There also have been few controlled studies evaluating the effects of exercise training on metabolic control of NIDDM. These studies also yielded contradictory results in terms of effect on glycemic control and glucose-insulin dynamics. In a large-scale study in our laboratory (94), the metabolic effects of moderate-intensity treadmill walking for 30 or 60 min per session, two to four times a week, for 12 weeks were studied in 48 overweight, previously sedentary, middle-aged men with poorly controlled mild or moderately severe type II DM or significant glucose intolerance, not on glucose-lowering medications. Body weight was kept constant in an attempt to distinguish the effects of exercise from weight reduction. The exercise regimen resulted in a mean 5.5% increase in $\dot{V}O_{2\,max}$, and a significant reduction in skin-fold thickness, despite the maintenance of baseline body weight. However, there was no associated improvement in either fasting glucose or glycosylated hemoglobin levels, glucose tolerance, basal plasma insulin levels, or in the insulin response to oral glucose, all measured repeatedly within 48 h after an exercise session. These negative findings are in agreement with those of a smaller study by Ruderman et al. (95) involving six middle-aged, obese type II diabetic patients who performed cycle ergometer exercise, 5 days per week for 6 weeks. This exercise program resulted in a modest improvement in the mean $\dot{V}O_{2\,max}$ level, but no change in body weight, glucose levels, glucose tolerance, or insulin sensitivity. Bogardus et al. (96) also failed to find any metabolic improvement in carbohydrate metabolism with exercise training in a small group of patients with either NIDDM or glucose intolerance. While Kovisto and DeFranzo (97) noted a reduction in the insulin response to an oral glucose challenge; i.e., improved insulin sensitivity, there was no significant improvement in either fasting plasma glucose levels or glucose tolerance after a 6-week training program in subjects with NIDDM.

On the other hand, several studies reported an improvement in glucose tolerance and/or insulin sensitivity in patients with NIDDM or glucose intolerance in the absence of improvement in fasting glycemic control (98–104). Saltin et al. (98) subjected 11 sedentary nonobese, middle-aged men with glucose intolerance to twice weekly 60-min sessions of vigorous exercise for 12 weeks and demonstrated a substantial (20%) increase in $\dot{V}O_{2\,max}$ with body weight remaining constant. Exercise conditioning resulted in improvement in oral glucose tolerance, but surprisingly not in insulin sensitivity. An additional 25 men, also with impaired glucose tolerance, received a similar exercise conditioning program along with a weight-reduction diet, and experienced a 4.5-kg weight loss. This latter group demonstrated both an improvement in glucose tolerance and a reduction in plasma insulin levels during the oral glucose challenge, which were reversed after 2 weeks of discontinuing exercise. An additive metabolic effect of weight loss and exercise on enhanced glucose tolerance and insulin sensitivity also has been demonstrated in nondiabetic obese people in our laboratory as well as by others (85). Krotkiewski et al. (99) subjected a group of 46 type II diabetic men and women to a 3-month, three times a week combined walking, jogging, calisthenics, and cycle ergometer exercise program. A 14% increase in $\dot{V}O_{2\,max}$ was observed with no associated change in body weight. This was accompanied by an improvement in both glucose tolerance and insulin sensitivity. In a more recent study, normalization of glucose tolerance and reduced insulin resistance were observed 18 h after the last exercise bout in 13 men with mild NIDDM or abnormal glucose tolerance, who were subjected to vigorous training for 50–60 min, 5 days a week, for 1 year at an intensity of 70–85% of $\dot{V}O_2$ (160). In another recent study from the same laboratory, Rodgers (101) reported that moderate-intensity walking and running programs (68% $\dot{V}O_{2max}$), performed 50–60 min for 7 consecutive days also substantially improved glucose tolerance and insulin sensitivity in 10 middle-aged men with either mild NIDDM or glucose intolerance. There was no reported change in $\dot{V}O_{2max}$ levels or body composition during this short period of training.

Improved diabetic control also has been reported in some studies involving subjects with type II DM after endurance exercise training (102–104). Trovati et al. (102) evaluated the effects on glucose-insulin dynamics of moderate-intensity (50–60% $\dot{V}O_{2max}$), cycle ergometer exercise, 1 h a day, 7 days a week, for 6 weeks in five patients with type II DM. Training resulted in a mean 15% improvement in $\dot{V}O_{2max}$, but no change in body weight. This was associated with a significant reduction in fasting plasma glucose and glycosylated hemoglobin levels measured 48 h after the last exercise session. Glucose tolerance and insulin sensitivity also were improved.

Schneider et al. (103) also demonstrated a significant decline in fasting plasma glucose and glycosylated hemoglobin levels in 14 type II diabetic patients who exercised for 6–10 weeks; however, surprisingly this was not accompanied by an improvement in either glucose tolerance or insulin sensitivity. Reitman et al. (104) likewise demonstrated improved glycemic control with exercise training. In this well-controlled study, six obese native American men and women with recently diagnosed NIDDM were hospitalized on a clinical research ward and subjected to a vigorous exercise program. This consisted of intermittent exercise on a cycle ergometer at 60–90% $\dot{V}O_{2max}$ for 20–40 min, 5 to 6 days per week, for 6–10 weeks, with body weight maintained constant. There was an average increase in $\dot{V}O_{2max}$ of 17%. All patients experienced a significant decline in fasting plasma glucose levels measured 36 h after the last exercise session, and five of the six subjects also showed an improvement in oral glucose tolerance; however, the effect of training on insulin sensitivity during euglycemic clamp studies was extremely variable.

Inconsistency in changes in glucose-insulin dynamics with endurance exercise conditioning in subjects with type I or II DM or glucose intolerance may be related to a number of factors. These include (a) the heterogeneity of study populations, (b) baseline differences in disease severity, (c) differences in relative weight, body fatness, and initial physical fitness of study subjects, (d) the variability in control of diet composition, (e) the presence or absence of weight changes, (f) the type, intensity, frequency, and duration of exercise, (g) the magnitude of the resulting improvement in $\dot{V}O_{2\,max}$, and (h) how long after the last exercise session the metabolic measurements were made. None of the studies reporting metabolic benefit with exercise could exclude the possibility that the observed changes may have at least partially been due to the last bout of exercise, since most measurements were made 36–48 h after the last exercise session. Additional research is needed to clarify the discrepancies among exercise studies in diabetic individuals, taking the above variables into consideration.

Although the bulk of the evidence indicates that regular moderate-intensity exercise can improve glucose-insulin dynamics in people with type I DM, type II DM, glucose intolerance, or obesity-related insulin resistance, a recent National Institute of Health (NIH) consensus development conference (105) concluded that the effects of exercise alone on the metabolic control of glucose metabolism are of *minor importance* in the overall management of DM. This ignores the contributions of regular exercise to loss of excess weight and its associated potentiations of the effects of diet and medications on diabetic control as well as its substantial effects on the physical and mental well-being and quality of life of the individual, as will be elaborated on below.

Prevention or Reduction of Obesity.   The contribution of obesity to insulin resistance, the etiology of type II DM and its associated effects on blood lipids and blood pressure levels, and the risk of CHD have been discussed previously. Physical inactivity is often a major contributor to obesity in modern societies. Increased physical activity, including regular exercise, can reduce the susceptibility to DM by weight maintenance in addition to the independent contribution of exercise to improve glucose-insulin dynamics. Regular walking is the most popular form of physical activity for people of all ages in the United States. Its value for helping normalize body weight and reduce adiposity in obese women and men has been demonstrated even in the absence of dieting (85,86,106–110). The loss of lean body mass commonly associated with dieting does not occur during weight reduction by exercise alone or exercise combined with mild to moderate caloric restriction in obese individuals. In addition, body fat may be lost more rapidly from the central or abdominal region of the body than elsewhere with exercise (83). It will be recalled that fat distribution in this region is associated with an excess risk of DM, hyperlipidemia, hypertension, CVD, and premature mortality (16,17). Moreover, weight loss through exercise may slightly exceed levels anticipated through direct energy expenditure during exercise (109). Mechanisms for this include temporary suppression in appetite, a distraction from snacking, and an increase in the resting metabolic rate for 1 or more hours after exercise. However, despite these potential contributions of an exercise program to weight reduction and maintenance, there are no studies to demonstrate the long-term effectiveness of exercise alone in managing obesity in people with NIDDM. A more feasible weight reduction plan for most obese type II diabetic patients would be to combine a moderate increase in physical activity with a moderate reduction in energy intake as recommended by American College of Sports Medicine guidelines (110).

Improved Physical Fitness. Physical fitness has been defined as the ability to carry out daily tasks with vigor and alertness without fatigue and with ample reserve energy to enjoy leisure time pursuits and to meet unforeseen emergencies, as well as to respond to physical and emotional stress without an excessive increase in heart rate and blood pressure (111). The measurable components of physical fitness may be derived into two major groups; one related to *health* and the other related to *skills* primarily pertaining to athletic performance.

Cardiorespiratory endurance or aerobic power, the most important health-related component of physical fitness, is defined as the maximal ability of the circulatory and respiratory systems to supply oxygen and fuel to the skeletal muscles and other organs and to eliminate metabolic waste products. It is determined by measuring $\dot{V}O_{2\,max}$ during all-out exercise on the treadmill or cycle ergometer. An increase in $\dot{V}O_{2\,max}$ not only enhances the maximal capacity for endurance types of physical exertion, but it also reduces fatigue and the level of perceived exertion during performance of sustained moderate-intensity activities. This can greatly enhance the quality of life, particularly in people with chronic diseases such as DM.

In order to increase $\dot{V}O_{2\,max}$, it is necessary to perform dynamic endurance-type physical activities regularly, which increase the heart and respiratory rates, such as walking, running, bicycling, or swimming. It has been repeatedly demonstrated that to obtain a significant improvement in $\dot{V}O_{2\,max}$ (typically 5–30%), 20–60 min of training activities are required, at least three times a week, at an intensity of 50–85% of a person's baseline $\dot{V}O_{2\,max}$. This level of exercise corresponds to about 60–90% of maximal heart rate. The same intensity and volume of dynamic exercise appears to be required to improve carbohydrate and lipid metabolism in both diabetic and nondiabetic people. An inverse relationship also exists between the intensity and the duration of exercise necessary to improve $\dot{V}O_{2\,max}$. In other words, to perform moderate-intensity exercise at 60% $\dot{V}O_{2\,max}$ requires a longer duration and frequency of exercise sessions than is necessary with higher-intensity exercise. A trade-off is that moderate exercise is less likely to result in musculoskeletal injury as compared with high-intensity exercise, and adherence is generally better. Attention should also be called to the fact that the relative improvement in aerobic power after a training program is inversely related to baseline $\dot{V}O_{2\,max}$ levels. Improvement in $\dot{V}O_{2\,max}$ with exercise training results from increases in the maximal arteriovenous oxygen difference, the maximal stroke volume of the heart, or both. To maintain one's existing level of $\dot{V}O_{2\,max}$, only twice-a-week endurance exercise is generally required; however, this may not be of sufficient quantity to obtain the other physiological and metabolic benefits of regular exercise described below.

Improved Blood Lipid Profile. The effects of exercise on blood lipid and lipoprotein levels have been extensively reviewed (112–114), and only the highlights will be summarized here. Attempts to correlate endurance fitness or $\dot{V}O_{2\,max}$ levels with HDL cholesterol have met with mixed results (112). Cross-sectional observational studies report a dose-response association between habitual physical activity and plasma HDL cholesterol levels, ranging from extreme inactivity associated with quadraplegia to the high volume of training required for marathon running (115). The increase in HDL cholesterol levels with activity status parallels the usual mean levels of $\dot{V}O_{2\,max}$ expected for the various activity groups. For example, endurance exercise trained men and women athletes, such as long-distance runners and Nordic skiers, generally are found to have plasma HDL cholesterol levels 20–35% higher than values for matched healthy sedentary individuals (116). Higher levels of HDL_2 cholesterol generally accounts for most of the differences in HDL cholesterol levels between endurance athletes and sedentary people, although in some studies higher levels of both HDL_2 and HDL_3 cholesterol were observed in the athletes. In contrast, strength-trained athletes, such as weight lifters, as a group have been reported to have HDL cholesterol levels similar to those of nonathletes (116). However, it is possible that this may be confounded by the adverse effects of anabolic steroids on blood lipid levels. Further, American men and women selected from the general population for the Lipid Research Clinics Prevalence Study who reported vigorous occupational or recreational physical activity were found to have slightly higher (+5 mg/dl) HDL cholesterol levels than those who reported no such heavy activities (117).

In respect to other blood lipid components, cross-sectional comparison studies show that plasma triglyceride and VLDL cholesterol levels are significantly lower in more active people, especially endurance athletes, as compared to matched inactive individuals (113). Typically, endurance athletes in these studies had plasma triglyceride levels below 100 mg/dl, but had either similar or only slightly lower LDL cholesterol levels, as compared to sedentary subjects. In general, major problem in interpreting cross-sectional comparisons of athletes versus nonathletes is the failure of most of these studies to adjust for potential confounding variables, which can contribute to differences in blood lipid levels between athletes and nonathletes; i.e., differences in body weight and composition, dietary habits, cigarette usage, alcohol consumption, and the use of oral contraceptives and other drugs as well as other variables.

Experimentally, *acute* prolonged endurance exercise generally results in significant changes in blood lipid levels probably related to increased energy needs by working muscles (118). These changes include reductions from baseline levels in plasma triglycerides and VLDL and LDL cholesterol and a substantial (10.0–17.5%) increase in HDL cholesterol levels. These changes persist for several days following prolonged exercise. In actuality, it appears that at least some of the reported effects on blood lipid levels of chronic exercise training may actually reflect acute adaptations remaining from the last exercise session, reminiscent of the postexercise effects on glucose metabolism. In addition, studies to determine the effects of endurance exercise conditioning on blood lipid levels have yielded mixed results in both nondiabetic and diabetic subjects. Differences in responses probably reflect baseline differences or changes in some of the same variables mentioned in the discussion of the cross-sectional studies, such as physical fitness and body fatness, as well as differences in the exercise programs, baseline fitness and fatness levels, accuracy of the laboratory measurements, seasonal fluctuations in blood lipid levels, and how long after the last exercise session blood was drawn for lipid assays.

In nondiabetic individuals, there is relatively consistent evidence that endurance exercise conditioning can significantly reduce *elevated* levels of fasting and postprandial plasma triglycerides, but not generally triglyceride levels in the normal range (112–114,119). Reductions in fasting and postprandial triglyceride levels reflect the increase during exercise in lipoprotein lipase activity in skeletal muscle and adipose tissue with a resulting increase in the rate of catabolism of the triglyceride-rich lipoproteins, VLDL, and chylomicrons both in the fasting and postprandial state. The relevance of these changes to the risk of CHD is the possible atherogenicity of catabolic products of remnants of these triglyceride-rich lipoproteins (47,119).

In addition, about half of all published endurance exercise training studies involving nondiabetic men have demonstrated a significant exercise-induced increase in plasma HDL cholesterol concentration (112). In most of the positive studies, the increase in HDL cholesterol levels generally ranged from 3 to 8 mg/dl, or 5 to 16%. Theoretically, an increase in plasma HDL cholesterol levels of this magnitude should reduce the risk of CHD 15–40%. One of the largest reported studies was a 1-year randomized trial involving 48 previously sedentary middle-aged men. In this study, Wood et al. (120) observed a significant increase in plasma HDL and HDL_2 cholesterol levels in only 25 (52%) of the participants, who averaged at least 4.8 km (8 miles) a week of running for at least 9 months. Their reported average increase in HDL cholesterol levels was 4.4 mg/dl, or about 9%. Statistically, significant correlations also were observed between weekly running mileage and both an increase in plasma HDL cholesterol levels and a reduction in body fatness. However, surprisingly, the men who self-selected higher volumes of running generally had higher baseline levels of plasma HDL cholesterol as well as significantly lower baseline levels of triglycerides as compared to less active runners. This raises the intriguing possibility that unmeasured factors, such as higher tissue lipoprotein lipase activity, generally associated with elevated HDL cholesterol levels, improve the ease of participation in endurance activities, perhaps by reducing perceived exertion levels, thereby enhancing compliance (121). Based primarily on data from this 1-year exercise study, Haskell (113) postulated that the lowest threshold of energy expenditure to produce an increase in HDL cholesterol values for healthy but previously sedentary men over a 9- to 12-month period of time is 1000 kcal/week of exercise.

In our laboratory, we have consistently demonstrated increases in plasma HDL cholesterol concentrations of 15% or more in previously sedentary and overweight men within 12–16 weeks of brisk treadmill walking with or without accompanying weight loss. In these studies, exercise was distributed over 4–5 days per week and the weekly energy expenditure was 2000–5000 kcal. In the best controlled of these studies (122), diet composition was kept constant and all meals and exercise were provided in the laboratory. One group of men walked 5 days a week on a treadmill (about 14 km/week) at an approximately energy cost of 3500 kcal/week with body weight kept constant by increasing food energy intake. This group experienced a 12% mean increase in the HDL cholesterol concentration over a 15-week training period. A similar increase in the mean HDL cholesterol level was

achieved by a physically inactive second group which lost 6.1 lb of
body weight over a 12-week period by dietary restrictions followed by
3 weeks of weight stabilization by increasing food intake. A third
group performed a similar amount of exercise per week as group 1,
but were not provided additional food and lost a similar amount of
weight as the groups which lost weight by dieting. This third group
experienced a more rapid rate of increase in HDL cholesterol levels
than the other two groups, and the total increase in plasma HDL
cholesterol levels was 22% above baseline levels, almost twice the
increase found in the other two treatment groups. These findings suggest an additive effect of exercise and weight reduction on HDL
cholesterol levels. Schwartz (123), in an uncontrolled study, essentially
confirmed our findings. Wood et al. (124) also compared weight loss
through dieting and exercise in a less well-controlled experiment than
in our laboratory, and found that a 7.8-kg weight loss associated with
either dieting or exercise was accompanied by similar increases (11–
12%) in the HDL cholesterol level. The reason for the discrepancies
between studies is uncertain. The increase in the HDL cholesterol level
with exercise training regresses to baseline levels within 4 weeks after
cessation of training or with regaining of lost weight.

Endurance exercise training appears less likely to increase plasma
HDL cholesterol levels in nondiabetic women than men (112–
114,125,126). In our laboratory, we were unsuccessful in increasing
plasma HDL cholesterol levels in previously sedentary women age
20–40 years with four different modes of moderate-intensity endurance
exercise training (i.e., treadmill walking or jogging, minitrampoline
rebounding, and simulated cross-country skiing) for periods of 16–40
weeks. In one of these studies (125), women either walked or jogged
on a treadmill 7.2 km a week, divided into 4 weekly sessions, for 20
weeks at exercise intensities of 52 or 70% $\dot{V}O_{2\,max}$ and a weekly energy
cost of about 1400 kcal. No mean change in plasma lipid or lipoprotein
levels were found with either mode of exercise, as compared to the
sedentary control group, despite marked improvements in $\dot{V}O_{2\,max}$ levels with both walking and jogging. Body weight and composition also
were unaltered during training in this study, which probably contrib-
uted to the stability of the blood lipid levels. A subsequent 40-week
treadmill walking program using a similar population and protocol as
in the 20-week study likewise failed to increase the mean HDL
cholesterol concentration or significantly alter body weight or composition (126). The reasons for the gender difference in responsiveness of
HDL cholesterol levels to exercise are uncertain, but may reflect the
following: (a) a lower volume of exercise achievable in training studies

in sedentary women as compared to sedentary men, (b) the higher baseline concentrations of HDL cholesterol in sedentary women as compared to sedentary men, (c) greater resistance to body weight and composition changes during exercise training in women as compared to men, and (d) perhaps gender differences in body fat distribution and lipase activity (113).

A number of studies have reported that resistive or strength exercise training also may raise plasma HDL cholesterol levels as well as lower LDL cholesterol levels in nondiabetic men (112,127,128). These observations are contrary to what would be expected from lipid levels of weight lifters in cross-sectional observational studies (116). Moreover, these findings were not replicated in another resistive exercise training study (129).

It can be concluded that acute and chronic endurance exercise generally has beneficial effects on the blood lipid profile in sedentary men, but the effects are less likely to occur in women. Lipid changes with exercise include a marked improvement in both fasting and postprandial hypertriglyceridemia, which is related to an increase in lipoprotein lipase activity and associated accelerated catabolism of VLDL and chylomicrons, and a substantial increase in levels of the antiatherogenic lipoprotein, HDL, especially if training is accompanied by a significant weight loss. However, the volume of exercise needed for such improvements may prove excessive for most sedentary and usually overweight individuals. Work is needed to define the effects of resistive exercise on blood lipid levels as well as on other risk factors for CHD.

The effect of endurance exercise training on the blood lipid profile of diabetic men and women has not been extensively studied. Several studies in type I diabetic men have reported a favorable increase in the ratio of HDL cholesterol to total cholesterol with exercise training, but no significant changes in absolute concentrations of plasma HDL cholesterol, total cholesterol, or triglycerides (91,92). However, Wallberg-Henriksson et al. (93) failed to find any change from the preconditioning blood lipid profile in type I diabetic women. Similarly, type II diabetic patients in a study previously referred to from my laboratory showed no changes from baseline blood lipid levels following an exercise training program with body weight kept constant (94). Our findings are in agreement with those of Krotkiewski et al. (99). In contrast, Ruderman et al. (95) reported significant decreases in plasma total cholesterol and triglyceride levels with exercise training in type II diabetic patients in the absence of weight loss. Unfortunately, these investigators did not measure plasma HDL cholesterol

levels. The reader should keep in mind that improved control of diabetes alone by diet, weight loss, oral hypoglycemic agents, and/or
insulin administration, as well as smoking cessation, should all contribute to raising HDL cholesterol levels and normalizing of the blood
lipid profile (72,108). A great deal of work is needed to better establish
the role of exercise on the blood lipid profile of diabetic patients,
including the dose-response relationship and differentiation between
the acute and chronic effects of exercise.

Reduced Risk of CHD. There are other ways in which exercise can
potentially reduce the severity of atherosclerosis and the risk of CHD
in addition to its effects on body weight, adiposity, and blood lipids,
which are discussed above. These include an apparently blood
pressure–reducing effect demonstrated by both observational and
experimental research in nondiabetic subjects. Some, but not all, epidemiological studies have documented an inverse association between
physical activity or physical fitness and blood pressure levels (130–
134). Acute endurance exercise of 30 min or more duration also has
been shown to significantly increase both systolic and diastolic blood
pressures for several hours during recovery (133). This appears to primarily result from vasodilatation, although reduced cardiac output
may also be a contributing factor in older individuals. Hagberg (133)
recently received 33 published endurance exercise studies and found
that two-thirds of them reported reductions in mean systolic and diastolic blood pressure levels of about 10 mm Hg each.

From the available data, it appears that 30–60 min of low- to
moderate-intensity exercise training at 40–60% $\dot{V}O_{2\,max}$, at least every
other day, may be effective in reducing blood pressure levels in nondiabetic individuals (133). The resulting blood pressure reduction with
exercise may occur in the absence of wight loss, but an associated
weight loss undoubtedly provides an additive effect (108,134).
Whether similar changes occur in diabetic individuals remains to be
proven. Hypertensive patients have generally been advised to avoid
static and resistive exercises because of the potential for an accompanying marked increase in both systolic and diastolic blood pressures. However, recent reports suggest that resistive exercise training
may reduce blood pressure levels in both normotensive and hypertensive individuals, as well as possibly improving the blood lipid profile
(127,128,134). Additional research is needed to confirm these observations, including dose-response and safety issues.

The most plausible mechanism for the apparent antihypertensive
effect of exercise training, aside from a reduction in body fat, is
attenuation of sympathetic nervous system activity (131,133,134).

Reduced adrenergic activity is expected in turn to reduce renin-angiotensin system activity, to reset baroreflexes, and to result in arterial vasodilatation, and thereby a reduction in elevated peripheral vascular resistance commonly associated with essential hypertension. Furthermore, in adolescents with early or reactive hypertension, exercise training is believed to attenuate a hyperactive adrenergic system and reduce the associated elevation in the heart rate and cardiac output (133). Improved insulin sensitivity and the associated reduction in circulating insulin levels with exercise training also may contribute to blood pressure reduction by reducing insulin-mediated sodium reabsorption by the kidney tubules.

Another plausible mechanism by which exercise may reduce the risk of CHD in diabetic individuals is by reducing heightened platelet aggregability and associated hypercoagulability of the blood, thereby reducing the risk of coronary thrombosis. Endurance exercise conditioning attenuates increased coagulability of the blood associated with physical exertion by reducing platelet aggregability, apparently through an alternation in the prostaglandin balance between platelets and endothelial cells (135). In addition, fibrinolysis may be enhanced (136). However, these conclusions are based on observations in nondiabetic individuals and need to be confirmed in diabetic patients along with determination of the dose-response relationship.

There are other proposed mechanisms by which exercise may protect against major CHD events in both diabetic and nondiabetic individuals. These include an increase in myocardial vascularity (137–141), improved cardiovascular efficiency through a reduction in the heart rate and systolic blood pressure levels, thereby decreasing myocardial oxygen demands (137,141) and vulnerability to ventricular fibrillation and sudden death (137,142). Reduction in catecholamine secretions or increased rate of clearances may contribute to the reduced vulnerability to ventricular fibrillation (134,143).

Documentation of the apparent protective effects of regular physical activity or improved physical fitness has mainly come from large cohort studies, generally involving nondiabetic individuals (142,144–151). Over two-thirds of published observational studies show an inverse association between physical activity and CHD. The relative risk of CHD in the "better" studies reviewed by Powell et al. (146) for physically inactive people was almost twice the risk of active people. In a study involving over 12,000 middle-aged men at high risk of CHD (and thereby suspected advanced latent coronary atherosclerosis), our group found that 30 min or more daily of predominately moderate-intensity physical activity was associated with one-third fewer CHD deaths as compared to less active men (147). Statistical adjustments for other risk factors only slightly weakened the inverse association between physical activity and CHD in this and most other cohort studies, suggesting an independent protective effect of exercise against CHD. This study provides strong supporting evidence that exercise can reduce death from CHD even in the presence of advanced coronary atherosclerosis. This possibility is further substantiated by meta-analysis of pooled data on over 4000 patients who participated in controlled cardiac rehabilitation studies, which included an exercise component (152). Analysis of these pooled data revealed that active intervention participants had one-third fewer fatal recurrent coronary events as compared to control subjects. In addition, it has recently been demonstrated that an exercise program as part of a comprehensive lifestyle modification program can reduce the severity of severe angiographically documented coronary artery disease after only 1 year (153). Whether exercise conditioning can offer similar protection in diabetic individuals remains to be proven.

Psychosocial Benefits. It is widely believed among health professionals that regular exercise provides psychosocial benefits that improve the quality of life; however, this is difficult to substantiate by controlled studies (154). Improved feelings of well-being, health consciousness, self-confidence, self-control, and self-esteem provided by an exercise program are especially important for patients with a chronic disease such as diabetes. Exercise may also prove helpful in relieving muscular tension and mental depression, and in promoting sound sleep. In order to achieve such benefits, physical activities should be selected that are fun and enjoyable.

Exercise Hazards and Precautions

There are special problems and hazards associated with exercise for diabetic individuals, particularly for those requiring insulin for metabolic control. These are summarized in Table 8, and are discussed below in detail. Even detractors who feel that exercise is merely a "perturbation that makes treatment of diabetes difficult," agree that the "present knowledge and technology allow the well-informed and cooperative patients with IDDM to exercise and even to reach the elite level" (155).

Worsening of the Metabolic State. As was previously mentioned, individuals with DM should not perform vigorous or prolonged exercise if their fasting plasma glucose level exceeds 250–300 mg/dl, particularly if ketoacidosis is present, since this may result in a worsening of the metabolic state. Consequently, an exercise program should not be

Table 8 Potential Adverse Effects of Exercise in Diabetic Individuals

1. Worsening of the metabolic state
2. Hypoglycemia in patients receiving insulin or hypoglycemic drug therapy
3. Complications from proliferative retinopathy
4. Musculoskeletal or soft tissue injuries
5. Complications from superficial foot injuries
6. Myocardial infarction or sudden death

recommended until improved metabolic control is obtained by diet, and if necessary, by insulin or an oral hypoglycemic agent.

Hypoglycemia. For the diabetic individual receiving insulin therapy, an insulin reaction or hypoglycemia is a common problem associated with prolonged exercise. For example, one study reported hypoglycemic episodes related to exercise in 16% of 300 young people with IDDM over a 2-year period of observation (156). This problem also is of concern in patients on oral hypoglycemic drugs but is less common. The risk of hypoglycemia is most marked in exercisers receiving intensive, multidose insulin therapy or continuous insulin infusion delivery by pump. Even if hypoglycemia does not occur during the exercise itself, the possibility remains for a delayed episode of hypoglycemia for many hours after prolonged exercise owing to a common fall in blood glucose levels as depleted muscle and live glycogen stores are being replenished. In the study referred to above (156), hypoglycemia was most commonly reported 6–15 h after exercise and occurred up to 31 h postexercise. Therefore, the diabetic on insulin should avoid sports which place him or her or the public in jeopardy as a result of hypoglycemia; e.g., scuba diving, parachute jumping, hang gliding, or automobile racing. Certain guidelines and precautions are required to avoid or minimize hypoglycemic reactions during other forms of prolonged exercise. These have been discussed elsewhere (4,8,9,157), and are summarized in Table 9 and briefly reviewed below.

First, it is important for all diabetic individuals receiving insulin or oral hypoglycemic agents to try to maintain as much *consistency* in life habits as possible. This is particularly important for those who are participating in organized sports. The individual should keep as constant as possible the time of day for getting up and going to bed, for meals and snacks and their energy content, for the administration of insulin or a sulfonylurea drug, the dose(s) and form(s) of the medication, and the time of day for exercise and the volume and intensity of the exercise performed. Such consistency simplifies the process of

Table 9 General Precautions to Reduce Risk of Exercise-Induced Hypoglycemia in Diabetic on Insulin

1. Maintain consistency in life habits.
2. Careful self-monitoring of blood glucose levels.
3. Avoid using extremities involved in exercise as injection sites for insulin within an hour of exercise.
4. Avoid exercising during time of peak insulin or oral hypoglycemic agent activity.
5. Exercise following a light meal or after a carbohydrate snack.
6. Take carbohydrate snacks during and following prolonged exercise.
7. Inform others about diabetic condition, risk, and symptoms of hypoglycemia and proper response to hypoglycemic episodes.
8. Be alert for symptoms of hypoglycemia during and several hours after exercise.
9. Promptly cease exercise upon experiencing symptoms of hypoglycemia and take a carbohydrate snack.
10. Take sufficient fluid intake before, during, and after exercise to prevent dehydration.

regulating blood glucose levels. It also helps with the decision making for adjusting food intake and insulin or oral hypoglycemic medication dosage in response to changes in physical activity levels as the need arises. These adjustments have to be accomplished on an individualized basis because of the marked variability in responsiveness of the diabetic individual to exercise. Quantifiable or easily reproducible forms of exercise, such as walking, jogging, bicycling, and lap swimming, make blood glucose regulation easier to accomplish by adjustments in food intake and/or medication dosage to avoid hypoglycemia.

A major breakthrough for both improving metabolic control of DM and helping to avoid hypoglycemia related to exercise is the availability of simple self-monitoring techniques such as finger-stick methods for determining blood glucose levels. These techniques permit blood glucose levels to be checked by the patient with IDDM several times during the day; for example, upon arising, before meals, 90 min following meals, at bedtime, perhaps at 3 a.m. for those on intensive therapy, and before, during, and following prolonged exercise. For those participating in team sports, these techniques also make it possible to measure capillary blood glucose levels between periods of sporting events or whenever hypoglycemia is suspected.

When a type I diabetic individual first initiates an exercise program or sports participation, it is advisable, at least initially, to reduce the basal insulin requirements 10–40% to avoid hypoglycemia until a new balance between food intake, physical activity, and insulin levels is established. A conservative approach is to begin by decreasing the dose of the form of insulin with peak activity during the period of the day that the exercise is performed (157). For example, let's consider the hypothetical case of a patient with type I DM planning strenuous prolonged exercise in mid-morning. He is on a combination of regular and NPH insulin with divided doses administered before breakfast and before the evening meal for a total daily insulin requirement of 40 U/day. His usual morning breakfast dose of insulin consists of 8 U of regular insulin plus 12 U of NPH. The dose of his regular insulin should be reduced by at least 10% of his total daily insulin dose requirement, or in this case 4 U, since he is planning mid-morning exercise, at which time the pharmacological activity of regular insulin is at its peak. His adjusted morning insulin combination would then consist of 4 U of regular insulin plus 12 U of NPH. On the other hand, if the strenuous activity were planned for the afternoon, the 10% reduction in the 40-U daily insulin dosage, or −4 U would be applied to the morning NPH dose. The morning insulin combination would then still consist of 8 U of regular insulin, but the NPH dose would be reduced from 12 to 8 U, since the peak action of the NPH insulin is in the afternoon. If strenuous prolonged activities were planned for the entire day, such as backpacking or skiing, the morning dose of *both* types of insulin should be decreased by 10%. The morning insulin combination would then be 4 U of regular insulin (8 − 4) and 8 U of NPH (12 − 4). In this situation, it also would be particularly important for the diabetic individual to closely monitor blood glucose levels throughout the day, including during and following exercise. There is a strong possibility that it would be necessary based on blood glucose determinations for the individual to also decrease the dosage of evening insulins as well as to eat extra food. Additional adjustments of insulin dosages are based on records of self-monitoring glucose levels.

An alternative approach to reducing insulin dosage when initiating an exercise program if the DM is well controlled, is to consume extra food prior to, during, and following prolonged exercise. Requirements for extra food energy intake are based on the intensity and duration of the intended physical activity and the patients preexercise blood glucose level. Table 10 provides guidelines for increasing food intake based on these variables (157).

Another approach to determine the amount of extra food to consume in order to compensate for anticipated prolonged physical activity is to base the estimated needs for extra carbohydrate on the

Table 10 General Guidelines for Increasing Food Intake Prior to and During Exercise

Intensity (type exercise)	Blood glucose (mg/100 dl)	Quantity of extra carbohydrates	Food group exchange
Low-to-moderate (e.g., walking or leisurely cycling)	≤100	None before exercise if <30 min and 10–15 g/h during exercise	1 fruit or bread/cereal
	>100	None	
Moderate (e.g., tennis, swimming, jogging)	≤100	25–50 g before exercise and 10–15 g/h during exercise	1/2 meat sandwich + milk or fruit exchange
	100–180	None before exercise but 10–15 g/h during exercise	1 fruit or bread/cereal
	180–250	None	
	≤250	No exercise until blood glucose is under better control	
Strenuous (e.g., contact team sports basketball, competitive running, cycling, swimming, heavy physical labor)	≤100	50 g before exercise and subsequent amounts based on monitoring of blood glucose	1 meat sandwich + a milk and fruit exchange
	100–180	25–50 g before exercise and 10–15 g/h during exercise	1/2 meat sandwich + a milk or fruit exchange
	180–250	None before exercise and 10–15 g/ h during exercise	1 fruit or bread exchange
	>250	No exercise until blood glucose is under better control	

Source: Adapted from reference 157 with permission.

approximate energy cost of the activity. The energy cost is determined by the type of physical activity, its intensity and duration, and the body weight of the individual (158). For activities considered light or moderate (an intensity of 5 kcal/min or 300 kcal/h or less), no additional preexercise food is recommended unless the activity exceeds 30 min. A snack containing 5 g of carbohydrates is recommended for every 30 min of exercise. For heavier activities, one-half of the estimated caloric expenditure should be taken as a snack in advance of the exercise and 10 to 15 g/h during exercise. It is important to reiterate at this point the importance of the diabetic individual monitoring his or her blood glucose level at 1- or 2-h intervals following heavy exercise, and to make appropriate adjustments in insulin and food intake based on active unusual blood glucose levels. In addition, at least a small snack after prolonged strenuous exercise is usually necessary to prevent hypoglycemia.

It is commonly believed that insulin should not be administered subcutaneously in extremities directly participating in the activity, making the abdominal wall the preferred site of administration for the exerciser. This is because of the resulting accelerated rate of absorption from the active limbs. However, this only appears to be a cause of concern if exercise is performed within an hour of the insulin injection into an extremity involved in the exercise, in which case the abdominal area is the preferred site of insulin administration. Another reason for the habitual use of this site for insulin administration is the recent demonstration by Bantle et al. (75) that limiting insulin injections to the abdominal region rather than rotating anatomical regions, as is a common clinical practice, markedly reduces day-to-day variations in blood glucose levels. This fluctuation in blood glucose levels is probably due to variations in the rate at which insulin is absorbed from different subcutaneous anatomical sites. Such fluctuations in blood glucose levels expose patients to increased risks of both hypoglycemia and hyperglycemia.

The time of day selected for exercise also is an important consideration. If possible, heavy physical exertion should be avoided during the peak action of the form of insulin used; e.g., the peak action for NPH insulin is approximately 6–16 h after injection and is 2–4 h after administration of regular insulin. A particularly good time to exercise in terms of glycemic control is about 1–2 h after a meal, since postprandial blood glucose levels peak at this time. This is particularly true after breakfast when the blood glucose level tends to be at its peak for the day. This, of course, is not always practical. If exercise is performed in the afternoon, during the period of peak activity of intermediate-acting insulins, a blood glucose test should be performed prior to exercise and the guidelines previously discussed followed in terms of decision making on the need for extra food and/or adjustments in the morning dose of intermediate-acting insulin.

Type I diabetic individuals on divided doses of insulin, who exercise in the evening, should take their usual predinner insulin injection. They should then eat dinner and exercise an hour or so after eating. The blood glucose should then be tested after exercise and before their usual evening snack. If necessary, extra food should be added to the snack. It also is extremely important for diabetic individuals on insulin who exercies in the afternoon or evening to have a bedtime snack to compensate for the delayed fall in blood glucose level hours following prolonged or strenuous exercise.

In addition, it is important for diabetic individuals on insulin or oral hypoglycemic drugs who exercise regularly or are athletes to wear adequate medical identification, be aware of their usual early symptoms accompanying an insulin reaction, have available a source of easily ingested carbohydrates, and have a plan for aborting or treating a hypoglycemic reaction. During exercise, the following guidelines should be included in a plan of action:

1. Exercise should be promptly discontinued at the first suspicion of an insulin reaction.
2. Blood glucose should be promptly measured, if feasible.
3. A snack providing 10–15 g of simple carbohydrates should be consumed (Table 11).
4. The athlete should rest long enough to allow glucose absorption.
5. Blood glucose levels should be reassessed and exercise should only be resumed when the blood glucose level is above 100 mg/dl.

Furthermore, an athlete participating in team sports should make certain that his or her teammates, coaches, and trainer are aware of their diabetic state, usual symptoms and signs of hypoglycemia and the remedy provided for its management, and the location of the athlete's reserve carbohydrate supply.

Guidelines also are available for avoiding hypoglycemia during exercise for those with IDDM who use a portable continuous subcutaneous insulin injection system (158,160). It appears possible to regulate the rate of insulin administration using such a pump to provide excellent glycemic control during exercise. Nevertheless, prior to prolonged exercise, it is prudent to reduce both the basal insulin infusion rate as well as the usual premeal bolus of insulin. Another potential problem is that the catheter infusion sites are susceptible to disruption

Table 11 Commonly Available Sources of Simple
Carbohydrates for Management of Insulin or Oral
Hypoglycemic Drug-Induced Hypoglycemia

Source	Serving size to provide 10–15 g of carbohydrate
Fruit	
apple	3/4
(size 3/lb)	
orange	1
peach	2
pear	1/2
raisins	2 tsp
dried	1/4 cup
fruit roll-up	1
Beverages	
fruit juices	
apple	1/4 cup
cranberry	1/4 cup
grape	1/2 cup
lemonade	1/2 cup
orange	1/2 cup
milk	1 cup
soft drinks	
cola type	1/2 cup
gingerale	3/4 cup
Candy/sugar	
chocolate	1 oz.
corn syrup	2 tsp
glucose tablets	2–3
honey	2 tsp
life savers	7–8
sugar cubes	2 large or 5 small
table sugar	5 tsp

1 Cup = 8 fl. oz.

during exercise. Implantable pumps as they become more widely available should eliminate this problem. An alternative approach is to remove the portable pump prior to exercise and substitute a small dose of regular insulin for glycemic control. This approach is not feasible with the "closed loop" pumps, which have intravenous lines. This latter type of pump also is too large and cumbersome for use during vigorous exercise.

Finally, the concomitant use of β-adrenergic–blocking drugs is generally contraindicated in diabetic patients receiving insulin, particularly exercisers. These drugs may mask the symptoms of hypoglycemia, which are primarily related to the increased activity of the sympapathoadrenomedullary system. In addition, they interfere with the cardiovascular response to exercise by markedly reducing the heart rate, cardiac output, and functional capacity.

Complications from Proliferative Retinopathy. Simple or background retinopathy with microaneurysms of the small arteries of the retina and associated small retinal exudates or hemorrhages is not generally considered a contraindication to exercise, although contact sports or acceleration-deceleration trauma to the head and perhaps resistive or static exercise should be avoided. In a minority of diabetic individuals, this condition progresses to proliferative retinopathy with formation of new retinal vessels. These new vessels are friable and often easily rupture, causing large retinal and vitreous hemorrhages, retinal detachment, and sometimes blindness (14). Since blood flow and blood pressure acutely increase during exercise, there is concern that vigorous exercise may promote retinal hemorrhage in such individuals. Therefore, in addition to the precautions with simple retinopathy, strenuous exercise, resistive exercise, and exercises in which Valsalva-like maneuvers are used should be discouraged in patients with active proliferative retinopathy, at least until the condition has been controlled or treated with photocoagulation (161). Recent vitreous or major retinal hemorrhages are absolute contraindications to all types of exercise.

Musculoskeletal or Soft Tissue Injuries. There is no evidence that diabetic individuals are more prone to injuries of muscle and joints and their attaching structures, however to reduce the possibility of such injuries, similar precautions are advised as for nondiabetic individuals. These include warm-up and cool-down periods incorporating flexibility exercises; initiating a physical conditioning program at a relatively low intensity, duration, and frequency of exercise; and progressing gradually.

Contact sports were formerly prohibited for all diabetic individuals because of the fear that soft tissue injuries would not heal well. This is generally not true in diabetic persons whose diabetes is under reasonably good control, and such sports are now permitted for young diabetic individuals in the absence of significant retinopathy.

Complications from Superficial Foot Injuries. Proper foot care is extremely important for all diabetic individuals, and for those who are athletes in particular, since infections and ulcerations of the feet are a major cause of morbidity. Gangrene, amputation, and death may result from such foot problems. This is of particular concern to those over age 40 who are more likely to have coexisting circulatory problems. In general, serious foot problems in diabetic individuals who are exercising regularly are related to three factors: (a) neuropathy, which decreases the ability to perceive pressure and pain, making the diabetic individual unaware of repeated trauma; (b) impaired circulation in the feet due to peripheral vascular disease, which delays healing; and (c) poorly controlled DM, which increases susceptibility to infection.

It is especially important that the feet of diabetic individuals over the age of 40 and those who have had diabetes 20 years or more be examined regularly by a physician or podiatrist. Those with peripheral vascular insufficiency or insensitive feet should avoid high-impact activities such as running or aerobics. For such individuals walking, cycling, or swimming would be better-suited exercises. The presence of calluses and corns are other important signs of potential serious problems, since most foot ulcers start under these pressure areas. Such lesions should be pared off routinely by a podiatrist or physician. The source of the pressure causing their formation (e.g., ill-fitting shoes, foot deformities, or flat feet) also should be identified and corrective measures taken. Preventive measures may include softer or better-fitting shoes, prosthetic inserts for dress and sport shoes, and prophylactic surgery to correct foot defects.

Other important foot hygiene measures include careful trimming of the toenails, seeking professional help for ingrown or thickened toenails, proper care of the skin, including the use of talcum powder to remove excess moisture, and special medicated powders to treat fungal infections between the toes (athletes feet), and lanolin or other lubrication agents to lubricate dry skin.

Myocardial Infarction or Sudden Death. As previously indicated, coronary heart disease is the most common cause of death in diabetic adults. Even asymptomatic diabetic individuals over the age of 35 are likely to have significant underlying coronary atherosclerosis (including possible significant left main coronary artery disease), particularly if they have an abnormal blood lipid profile, elevated blood pressure, and/or smoke cigarettes (1,39). Medical evaluation before embarking on an exercise program, therefore, is imperative in diabetic individuals over age 35, or even for those who are younger who have significant coronary risk factors, or have had DM for 10 or more years. Selected clinical studies in such persons may help rule out silent myocardial ischemia and serve as a basis for prescribing safe levels of exercise.

This evaluation should include a standard multistage exercise ECG test and/or thallium scintigraphy using a treadmill or cycle ergometer protocol. In a study in our laboratory (95) involving 48 asymptomatic men aged 33–69 years with type II diabetes or glucose intolerance, 11 (23%) had ischemic ECG changes during a symptom-limited treadmill exercise test. Exercise test results, in addition to unmasking silent or latent ischemia, also provide objective information for prescription of exercise intensity and training heart rate levels. If ischemia is uncovered on an exercise ECG or a thallium scan, the training heart rate should be kept at least 15–20 beats/min below the level causing ischemic changes during the exercise test. All of the diabetic men in our study, referred to above, who had ischemic exercise ECG changes, were able to safely complete a 12-week supervised treadmill walking program by taking such precautions (94).

SUMMARY AND CONCLUSIONS REGARDING THE ROLE OF EXERCISE IN THE MANAGEMENT OF DIABETES AND BLOOD LIPID DISTURBANCES

There is growing evidence that regular exercise can reduce the risk of NIDDM, play a role in the management of type I and II diabetes, and perhaps reduce the risk of atherosclerotic complications. Both excess body weight and low levels of physical activity independently contribute to cell insulin resistance and are important risk factors for NIDDM, the most prevalent form of diabetes in the United States. Exercise has been proposed as therapy for diabetes mellitus since ancient times. Currently, it is widely used as an adjunct to dietary therapy and glucose-lowering drugs in diabetic management. Acute prolonged, rhythmic exercise involving large muscle groups lowers blood glucose levels and improves insulin sensitivity for up to 48 h postexercise in both diabetics and nondiabetic individuals. Endurance exercise and perhaps also resistive exercise training, if not compensated by excess energy intake, may further contribute to improvements in glycemic control, glucose intolerance, and insulin sensitivity in patients whose diabetes is at least under fair control by diet and/or medications. A minimum of 30–60 min of dynamic exercise at an intensity of 60% $\dot{V}O_{2\,max}$ or more for at least three or four times a week is required to maintain improved glucose-insulin dynamics. The value and dose-response relationship of resistive exercise training to improved glucose metabolism is less certain. Mechanisms for improved glycemic control with exercise training include the overlapping effects of the last exercise session, apparently related to the replenishment and augmentation of muscle glycogen stores, and improvements in skeletal muscle mass, blood supply, metabolic capacity, and insulin receptor activity. These adaptive changes, however, probably persist for less than 1 week after cessation of exercise.

Other potential beneficial effects of an exercise conditioning program to the diabetic individual are: (a) loss of excess fat, which can further substantially improve insulin sensitivity and glucose tolerance in individuals with NIDDM; (b) the reduced risk of atherosclerotic complications; and (c) improved quality of life.

A number of possible mechanisms exist by which exercise conditioning may reduce the severity of atherosclerosis and the risk of common cardiovascular complications often contributing to premature mortality in patients with long-term diabetes. These include a favorable effect on the blood lipid profile, particularly an increase in plasma levels of HDL cholesterol and a decrease in elevated levels of triglycerides and their principal lipoprotein carriers, VLDL and chylomicrons. Additional improvement in the blood lipid profile results from improving glycemic control by diabetic diet and drugs, loss of excess weight, and smoking cessation. Exercise training may also help correct elevated blood pressure levels and hypercoagulability of the blood, both often associated with diabetes, which should further reduce the severity of coronary atherosclerosis and help prevent thrombosis in narrowed coronary arteries. In addition, endurance exercise conditioning reduces adrenergic system activity, which in turn decreases the myocardial oxygen requirements by lowering the heart rate and systolic blood pressure levels. Animal research also strongly suggests that vigorous aerobic exercise training may increase the myocardial blood supply. These favorable effects of exercise conditioning on myocardial oxygen balance should reduce the vulnerability to ventricular fibrillation and sudden death. The quality of life also can be significantly enhanced by an exercise program through improved physical fitness and psychosocial benefits.

There are, however, potential risks accompanying strenuous exercise in diabetic individuals, which should be taken into consideration in planning an exercise program. These include aggravation of metabolic dysfunctions on exercising in the presence of severe uncontrolled insulin-dependent diabetes. On the other hand, in patients whose diabetes is well controlled by insulin or an oral hypoglycemic agent, hypoglycemia is a common problem during or following prolonged exercise. Frequent self-monitoring of blood glucose levels is crucial for the diabetic athlete or recreational exerciser to properly adjust insulin or oral hypoglycemic drug dosage with food intake to help avoid hypoglycemic episodes. Consistency in eating, exercise, administration of diabetic medications, and other habits is also important. A diabetic individual on insulin, when initiating a vigorous exercise program, must either reduce his or her insulin dose, increase food intake, or both. Insulin also should not be administered in an active extremity for at least an hour prior to exercise because of the associated increased rate of insulin absorption. An alternative is to use the abdominal wall as a site for insulin administration. Prolonged exercise should be preceded by a light meal or carbohydrate snack and supplementary carbohydrates should be administered regularly during and following exercise to prevent hypoglycemia based on self-monitored blood glucose levels.

Vigorous exercise, resistive exercise, and contact sports should be avoided in the presence of uncontrolled proliferative retinopathy because of the danger of retinal hemorrhage or separation. Proper fitting footwear and careful foot care and hygiene are crucial to the diabetic exerciser in order to avoid complications leading to gangrene and amputation, particularly in those with peripheral neuropathy and peripheral vascular disease.

In addition, careful cardiovascular screening, including exercise testing, is required in all diabetic individuals over age 35 or younger individuals with over a 10-year history of diabetes or other risk factors for CHD who wish to perform vigorous exercise in order to rule out latent manifestations of myocardial ischemia, as well as to establish a baseline fitness level for exercise prescriptive purposes. A prescribed exercise program should be commensurate with the severity of diabetes, fitness status, and recreational interests of the individual to minimize the risk of musculoskeletal and cardiovascular problems and promote compliance and psychosocial benefits. Exercise should be initiated at low-intensity and short-duration levels and progressed gradually to prescriptive levels. Warm-up and cool-down periods are of importance to minimize the risk of musculoskeletal injuries.

REFERENCES

1. West, K.M., *Epidemiology of Diabetes and Its Vascular Lesions.* Elsevier-North Holland, New York, pp. 1–579 (1978).
2. Anonymous, Diabetes in the 1980's: Challenges for the Future Report of the National Diabetes Advisory Board. U.S. Department of Health and

Human Services, Public Health Service, National Institute of Health, Washington, D.C., NIH Publication No. 82-2143, pp. 1-159 (1982).

3. American Diabetes Association 1990 Fact Sheet on Diabetes. American Diabetes Association, Alexandria, Virginia, pp. 1-12.

4. Kral, L.P., and Beaser, R.S., *Joslin Diabetes Manual.* 12th ed. Lea & Febiger, Philadelphia, pp. 1-406 (1989).

5. Bennett, P.H., in *Diabetes Mellitus Theory and Practice* 4th ed. Elsevier, New York, pp. 357-377 (1990).

6. World Health Organization Study Group, *Diabetes Mellitus, Report of a WHO Study Group.* WHO, Geneva, Technical Report Series 727, pp. 1-113 (1985).

7. Lilloja, S., Mott, D.M., Howard, V.B., Bennett, P.H., Yki-Jarvinen, H., Freymondy, D., Nyomba, B.L., Zurlo, F., Swinburn, B., and Bogardus, C., *N. Engl. J. Med., 318*: 1217-1224 (1988).

8. American Diabetic Association, *Physicians Guide to Insulin-Dependent (Type I) Diabetes. Diagnosis and Treatment*, American Diabetes Association, Alexandria, Virginia, pp. 1-150 (1988).

9. American Diabetic Association, *Physician's Guide to Non-Insulin-Dependent (Type II) Diabetes. Diagnosis and Treatment.* American Diabetic Association, Alexandria, Virginia, pp. 1-93 (1988).

10. Nerup, J., Mandrup-Poulsen, T., Molvig, J., Helquist, S., Wogensen, L., and Egeberg, J., *Diabetes Care* (Suppl. 1): 16-23 (1988).

11. Harold, K.C., and Rubenstein, A.H., *N. Engl. J. Med., 318*: 701-703 (1988).

12. Polonsky, K.S., Given, B.D., Hirsch, L.J., Tillil, H., Shapiro, E.T., Beebe, C., Frank, B.H., Galloway, J.A., and Van Cauter, E., *N. Engl. J. Med., 318*: 1231-1239 (1988).

13. Shulman, G.I., Rothman, D.L., Jue, T., Stein, P., DeFronzo, R.A., and Shulman, R.G., *N. Engl. J. Med., 322*: 223-228 (1989).

14. Rotwein, P.S., Chrigwin, J., Province, M., Knowler, W.C., Pettitt, D.J., Cordell, B., Goodman, M.H., and Permutt, M.A., *N. Engl. J. Med., 308*: 65-71 (1985).

15. Chen, M.K., and Lowenstein, F.W., *Am. J. Preven. Med., 2*: 14-19 (1986).

16. Ohlson, L.O., Larsson, B., Svardsudd, K., Wilhelmsen, L., Bjorntorp, P., and Tiblen, G., *Diabetes, 34*: 1055-1058 (1985).

17. Depres, J.P., Moorjani, S., Lupien, P.J., Tremblay, A., Nadeau, A., and Bouchard, C., *Atherosclerosis, 10*: 497-511 (1990).

18. Truglia, J.A., Livingston, J.N., and Lockwood, D.H., *Am. J. Med., 79* (Suppl.): 13-22 (1985).

19. Lipman, R.L., Schnure, J.J., Bradley, E.M., and LeCocq, F.R., *J. Lab. Clin. Med., 76*: 221-230 (1970).

20. Lipman, R.L., Raskin, P., Love, T., Triebwasser, L., LeCoq, F.R., and Schure, J.J., *Diabetes, 21*: 101-107 (1973).

21. Ahern, J.A., Kruger, D.F., Gatcomb, P., Petit, W.A., Jr., and Tamborlane, W.V., *Diabetic Education, 51*: 236-241 (1989).

22. Merimee, T.J., *N. Engl. J. Med., 322*: 978-983 (1990).

23. Klein, R., Moss, S.E., Klein, B.E.K., and DeMets, D.L., *Arch. Intern. Med.*, *149*: 266–272 (1989).

24. Marins, B.E., and Marins, R.G., *Diabetes Care*, *11*: 833–839 (1988).

25. Friedman, E.A., *Diabetes Mellitus. Theory and Practice*. 4th Ed. (H. Rifkin, D. Ponte, Jr., eds). Elsevier, New York, pp. 357–377 (1990).

26. Cowie, C.C., Port, F.K., Wolfe, R.A., Savage, P.J., Moll, P.P., and Hawthorne, V.M., *N. Engl. J. Med.*, *327*: 1074–1079 (1989).

27. Cerami, A., Vlassara, H., and Brownlee, M., *Diabetes Care*, *11*(Suppl. 1): 73–79 (1988).

28. Marre, M., LeBlanc, H., Suarez, L., Guyenne, F.T., Menard, J., Passa, P., *Br. Med. J.*, *294*: 1448–1452 (1987).

29. Anderson, S., and Barry, M.B., *Diabetes Care*, *11*: 846–849 (1988).

30. Greene, D.A., Sima, A.A.F., Albers, J.W., and Pfefer, M.A., in *Diabetes Mellitus. Theory and Practice*. 4th Ed. (H. Rifkin, D. Ponte, Jr., eds.). Elsevier, New York, pp. 710–755 (1990).

31. Brand, P.W., and Coleman, W.C., in *Diabetes Mellitus. Theory and Practice*. 4th Ed. (H. Rifkin, D. Ponte, Jr., eds.). Elsevier, New York, pp. 792–811 (1990).

32. Kannel, W.B., and McGee, D.L., *J.A.M.A.*, *241*: 2035–2038 (1979).

33. Davidson, M.B., *J. Chronic Dis.*, *34*: 5–10 (1981).

34. Jarrett, R.J., in *Metabolic Aspects of Cardiovascular Disease. Diabetes and Heart Disease* (R.J. Jarrett, ed.). Elsevier, New York, pp. 1–23 (1984).

35. Fein, F.S., and Scheuer, J., in *Diabetes Mellitus. Theory and Practice*. 4th Ed. (H. Rifkin and J. Porte, Jr., eds.). Elsevier, New York, pp. 812–823 (1990).

36. Smith, D.A., *Primary Cardiol.*, *16*: 67–70 (1990).

37. Zimmermann, B.R., Palumbo, P.J., O'Fallon, W.M., Osmundson, P.J., and Kazmier, F.J., *Mayo Clinic Proc.*, *56*: 217–253 (1981).

38. Beach, K.W., Bedford, G.R., Bergelin, R.O., Martin, D.C., Vandenberghe, N., Zaccardi, M., and Standness, D.E., Jr., *Diabetes Care*, *11*: 464–472 (1988).

39. Cowell, J.A., *J. Chronic Dis.*, *34*: 1–4 (1981).

40. Simonson, D.C., *Diabetes Care*, *11*: 821–827 (1988).

41. Nikkila, E.O., in *Metabolic Aspects of Cardiovascular Disease. Diabetes and Heart Disease* (R.J. Jarrett, ed.). Elsevier, New York, pp. 133–167 (1988).

42. Laker, M.F., in *The Diabetes Annual/3* (K.G. Alberti and L.P. Krall, eds.). Elsevier, New York, pp. 459–478 (1987).

43. Garg, A., and Grundry, S.M., *Diabetes Care*, *13*: 153–169 (1990).

44. Brunzell, J.D., and Chait, A., in *Diabetes Mellitus. Theory and Practice*. 4th Ed. (H. Rifkin and D. Ponte, Jr. eds.). Elsevier, New York, pp. 757–767 (1990).

45. Pekkanan, J., Linn, S., Heiss, G., Suchiandran, C.M., Leon, A., Rifkind, B.M., and Tyroler, H.A., *N. Engl. J. Med.*, *322*: 1700–1707 (1990).

46. Zilversmit, D.M., *Circulation, 60*: 473–485 (1979).
47. Greaves, M., and Preston, F.E., in *Metabolic Aspects of Cardiovascular Disease. Diabetes and Heart Disease* (R.J. Jarrett, ed.). Elsevier, New York, pp. 47–80 (1984).
48. Allexandrini, P., McRae, J., Feman, S., and Fitzgerald, G.A., *N. Engl. J. Med., 319*: 208–212 (1988).
49. Zeyman, F.J., and New, D.M., *Applications of Clinical Nutrition*. Prentice-Hall, Englewood Cliffs, New Jersey, pp. 222–256 (1988).
50. Kitabchi, A.E., Duckworth, W.C., and Stemz, F.B., in *Diabetes Mellitus. Theory and Practice*. 4th Ed. (H. Rifkin and D. Ponte, Jr. eds.). Elsevier, New York, pp. 71–88 (1990).
51. Vinik, A., and Wing, R.R., in *Diabetes Mellitus. Theory and Practice*. 4th Ed. (H. Rifkin and D. Ponte, Jr., eds.). Elsevier, New York, pp. 464–496 (1990).
52. Anonymous, *Arch. Intern. Med., 103*: 1073–1077 (1985).
53. Anonymous, *Build and Blood Pressure Study*. Vol. 1. Society of Actuaries, Chicago, pp. 1–530 (1959).
54. National Research Council, *Recommended Dietary Allowances*. 10th Ed., National Academy Press, Washington, D.C., pp. 10–38 (1989).
55. American Diabetic Association, *Diabetes Care, 10*: 126–132 (1987).
56. Shekelle, R.B., Shryock, A.M., Paul, O., Lepper, M., Stamler, J., Liu, S., and Raynor, W.J., *N. Engl. J. Med., 304*: 65–70 (1981).
57. Kushi, L.H., Lew, R.A., Stare, F.J., Ellison, C.R., Lozy, M. E., Bourke, G., Daly, L., Graham, I., Nickey, N., Mulcahy, R., and Kevaney, J., *N. Engl. J. Med., 312*: 811–818 (1985).
58. Keys, A., Menotti, A., Karvonen, M.J., Aravanis, C., Blackburn, H., Buzina, R., Keys, M.H., Kromhout, D., Nedeljkovic, S., Punsar, S., Seccareccia, F., and Toshimo, H., *Am. J. Epidemiol., 124*: 903–915 (1986).
59. Blackburn, H., in *Hypercholesterolemia and Atherosclerosis. Pathogenesis and Prevention* (D. Steinberg and J.M. Olefsky, eds.). Churchill Livingston, New York, pp. 53–98 (1987).
60. Abbott, W.G.H., Boyce, V.L., Grundy, S.M., and Howard, V.B., *Diabetes Care, 12*: 102–107 (1989).
61. Anderson, J.W., Story, L., Sieling, B., Chen, W.J.L., Petro, M.S., and Story, J., *Am. J. Clin. Nutri., 40*: 1146–1155 (1984).
62. Blackenhorn, D.H., Johnson, R.L., Mack, W.J., Elzein, H.A., and Valias, L.I., *J.A.M.A., 263*: 1646–1652 (1990).
63. Hollenbeck, C.B., Coulson, A.M., and Reaven, G.M., *Diabetes Care, 12*(Suppl. 1): 62–66 (1989).
64. National Cholesterol Education Program Expert Panels, *Arch. Intern. Med., 148*: 39–69 (1988).
65. Ginsberg, H.M., Barr, S.L., Gilbert, A., Karmally, W.M., Deckelbaum, R., Kaplan, K., Ramakrishnan, R., Holleran, S., and Dell, R.B., *N. Engl. J. Med., 322*: 574–579 (1990).

66. Herold, P.M., and Kinsella, J.E., *Am. J. Clin. Nutr., 43*: 566–598 (1986).
67. Kromhout, D., Bosschieter, E., and Coulander, A., *N. Engl. J. Med., 312*: 1205–1212 (1985).
68. Glauber, H., Wallace, P., Griver, K., and Brechtel, G., *Ann. Intern. Med., 108*: 663–668 (1988).
69. Bonaa, K.H., Bjerve, K.S., Straume, B., Gram, I.T., and Thelle, D., *N. Engl. J. Med., 322*: 795–801 (1990).
70. Jensen, T., Stender, S., Goldstein, K., Holmer, G., and Deckert, T., *N. Engl. J. Med., 321*: 1522–1527 (1989).
71. Hollenbeck, C.B., Leklem, J.E., Reddle, M.C., and Connor, W.E., *Am. J. Clin. Nutr., 38*: 41–51 (1983).
72. Calvert, G.D., Mannik, T., Graham, J.J., Wise, P.H., and Yeates, R.A., *Lancet, 2*: 66–68 (1978).
73. Kumar, D., in *Diabetes Mellitus for the House Officer* (P.M. Beigelman and K. Kumar, eds.). Williams & Wilkins, Baltimore, pp. 91–112 (1986).
74. Zinman, B., and Vramic, M., *Med. Clin. North Am., 69*: 145–157 (1985).
75. Bantle, J.P., Weber, M.S., Rao, S., Chattpadhyay, M.K., and Robertson, R.P., *J.A.M.A., 263*: 1802–1806 (1990).
76. Gerich, J.E., *N. Engl. J. Med., 321*: 1231–1245 (1989).
77. Anonymous, *Diabetes, 25*: 1129–1153 (1976).
78. Zinman, B., Zuniga-Guajardo, S., and Kelly, D., *Diabetes Care, 7*: 515–519 (1984).
79. Sutton, J.R., Farrell, P.A., and Harber, V.J., in *Exercise and Fitness. A Consensus of Current Knowledge* (C. Bouchard, R.J. Shephard, T., Stephens, J.H.R. Sutton, and B.D. McPherson, eds.). Human Kinetics, Champaign, Illinois, pp. 217–257 (1990).
80. Vranic, M., and Wassarman, D., in *Exercise and Fitness. A Consensus of Current Knowledge* (C. Bouchard, R.J. Shephard, T., Stephens, J.H.R. Sutton, and B.D. McPherson, eds.). Human Kinetics, Champaign, Illinois, 467–495 (1990).
81. Vranic, M., Wassarman, D., and Bukowiecki, L., in *Diabetes Mellitus. Theory and Practice.* 4th Ed. (H. Rifkin and D. Ponte, Jr. eds.). Elsevier, New York, pp. 198–219 (1990).
82. Schwartz, R.S., *Diabetes Care, 13*(Suppl. 2): 77–85 (1990).
83. Allen, F.M., *Boston Med. Surg. J., 173*: 743–744 (1915).
84. Lawrence, R.D., *Br. Med. J., 1*: 648–650 (1923).
85. Leon, A.S., Conrad, J., Hunninghake, D.B., Serfass, R., *Am. J. Clin. Nutr., 32*: 1776–1787 (1979).
86. Rauramaa, R., *Prevent. Med., 13*–46 (1984).
87. Reaven, G.M., *Clinicians Guide to Non-Insulin-Dependent Diabetes Mellitus. Pathogenesis and Treatment.* Marcel Dekker, New York, pp. 53–63 (1989).
88. Akerholm, K.H., Koivukangas, T., and Ikka, J., *Acta Paediatr. Scand., 293*(Suppl. 1): 50–52 (1979).
89. Campaigne, B.N., Gilliam, T.B., Spencer, M.L., Lampman, R.M., and Schork, M.A., *Diabetes Care, 7*: 57–62 (1984).

90. Landt, K.W., Campaigne, B.N., James, F.W., and Sperling, M.A., *Diabetes Care*, 8: 461–465 (1985).
91. Wallberg-Henriksson, H., Gunnarson, H., Henriksson, J., DeFronzo, R., Felig, P., Ostman, J., and Wahren, J., *Diabetes*, 31: 1044–1050 (1982).
92. Yski-Jarvinen, H., DeFronzo, R., and Koivisto, V.S., *Diabetes Care*, 7: 520–527 (1984).
93. Wallberg-Henriksson, H., Gunnarsson, R., Rossner, S., and Wahren, J., *Diabetologia*, 29: 53–57 (1986).
94. Leon, A.S., Conrad, J., Casal, D.E., Serfass, R., Bonnard, R.A., Goetz, F.C., and Blackburn, H., *J. Cardiac Rehabil.*, 4: 278–286 (1984).
95. Ruderman, N.B., Ganda, O.P., and Johansen, K., *Diabetes*, 28(Suppl.): 89–92 (1978).
96. Bogardus, C., Ravussin, E., Robbins, D.C., Wolfe, R.R., Horton, E.S., and Sims, E.A.H., *Diabetes*, 33: 311–318 (1984).
97. Kovisto, V.A., and DeFranzo, K.A., *Acta Endocrinol.*, 262(Suppl.): 107–111 (1984).
98. Salton, B., Lingarde, F., Houston, M., Horlin, R., Nygaard, E., and Gad, P., *Diabetes*, 28(Suppl.): 30–32 (1979).
99. Krotkiewski, M., Lonnroth, P., Mandroukas, K., Wroblewski, Z., and Reffe-Scrive, M., *Diabetologia*, 28: 881–890 (1985).
100. Holloszy, J.O., Schultz, J., Kusnierkiewicz, J., Hagberg, J.M., and Ehsani, A.A., *Acta Med. Scand.*, 71(Suppl.): 52–65 (1986).
101. Rodgers, M.A., *Med. Sci. Sports Exerc.*, 21: 362–368 (1989).
102. Trovati, M., Carta, Q., Cavalot, F., Vitali, S., Banaudi, C., Lucchina, P., Fiocchi, F., Emmanvelli, G., and Lenti, G., *Diabetes Care*, 17: 416–420 (1984).
103. Schneider, S.H., Amorosa, L.F., Khachadurian, A.K., and Ruderman, N.B., *Diabetologia*, 26: 355–360 (1984).
104. Reitman, J.S., Vasquez, B., Klimes, I., and Nagulespan, M., *Diabetes Care*, 7: 334–341 (1984).
105. National Institutes of Health, *Diabetes Care*, 10: 639–644 (1987).
106. Gwinup, G., *Arch. Intern. Med.*, 135: 6766–6800 (1975).
107. Krotkiewski, M., Mandroukas, K., Sjostrom, L., Sullivan, L., Wetterqvist, H., and Bjorntorp, P., *Metabolism*, 28: 650–658 (1979).
108. Leon, A.S., *Ann. Clin. Res.*, 20: 114–120 (1988).
109. Leon, A.S., in *Sports Medicine* (J.A. Ryan and F.L. Allman, Jr., eds.). 2nd ed. Academic Press, San Diego, pp. 593–617 (1989).
110. American College of Sports Medicine, *Med. Sci. Sports Exerc.*, 15: ix–xiii (1983).
111. Caspersen, C.J., Powell, K.E., and Christenson, G.M., *Publ. Health Rep.*, 100: 126–131 (1985).
112. Goldbert, L., and Elliot, D.L., *Med. Clin. North Am.*, 69: 41–59 (1985).
113. Haskell, W.L., *Acta Med. Scand.*, 711(Suppl.): 25–38 (1986).
114. Wood, P.D., and Stefanick, M.L., in *Exercise and Fitness. A Consensus of Current Knowledge* (C. Bouchard, R.J. Shephard, T. Stephens, J.R. Sut-

ton, and B.D. McPherson, eds.). Human Kinetics, Champaign, Illinois, pp. 409–424 (1990).

115. LaPorte, R., Brenes, G., and Dearwater, S., *Lancet, 1*: 1212–1213 (1983).

116. Ferrell, P.A., Maksud, M.G., Pollock, M.L., Foster, C., Anholm, J., Hare, J., and Leon, A.S., *Eur. J. Appl. Physiol., 48*: 77–82 (1982).

117. Haskell, W.L., Taylor, H.L., Wood, P.D., Schrott, H., and Heiss, G., *Circulation, 62*(Suppl. 4): 51–59 (1980).

118. Trsopanakis, A.D., Sgouraki, E.P., Pavlou, K.N., Nadel, E.R., and Bussolari, S.R., *Am. J. Clin. Nutr., 49*: 980–984 (1989).

119. Weintraub, M.S., Rosen, Y., Otto, R., Eisenberg, S., and Broslov, J.L., *Circulation, 79*: 1007–1014 (1989).

120. Wood, P.D., Haskell, W.L., Blair, S.N., Williams, P.T., Krauss, R.M., Lindgren, F.T., Alberts, J., Hot, P.H., and Farquhar, J.W., *Metabolism, 32*: 31–39 (1983).

121. Williams, P.T., Wood, P.D., Haskell, W.L., and Vranizan, K., *J.A.M.A., 247*: 2674–2679 (1982).

122. Sopko, G., Leon, A.S., Jacobs, D.R., Jr., Foster, N., Moy, J., Kuba, K., Anderson, J.T., Casal, D., McNally, C., and Frantz, I., *Metabolism, 39*: 227–236 (1985).

123. Schwartz, S., *Metabolism, 36*: 165–171 (1987).

124. Wood, P.O., Stefanick, M.L., Dreone, D.M., Frey-Hewitt, B., Garay, S.C., William, P.T., Superko, H.R., Fortmann, S.P., Alberts, J.J., Vranizan, K.M., Ellsworth, N.M., Terry, R.B., and Haskell, W.L., *N. Engl. J. Med., 319*: 1173–1179 (1988).

125. Santiago, M.C., Alexander, J.F., Stull, G.A., Serfass, R.C., Hayday, A.M., and Leon, A.S., *Scand. J. Sports Sci., 9*: 33–39 (1987).

126. Santiago, M.C., Effects of a 40-Week Walking Program of Twelve Miles per Week on Physical Fitness, Body Composition, and Blood Lipids and Lipoproteins in Sedentary Women. A thesis in partial fulfillment of the requirements for the Ph.D. degree, University of Minnesota, Minneapolis, pp. 1–208 (1990).

127. Hurley, B.V.F., Hagberg, J.M., Goldberg, A.P., Seals, D.R., Ehsani, A., Brenman, R.E., and Holloszy, J.O., *Med. Sci. Sports Exerc., 20*: 150–154 (1988).

128. Goldberg, J.A., *Med. Sci. Sports Exerc., 21*: 669–674 (1989).

129. Kokkinos, P.F., Hurley, B.F., Vaccaro, P., Patterson, J.C., Gardner, L.B., Ostrove, S.M., and Goldberg, A.P., *Med. Sci. Sports Exerc., 20*: 500–554 (1988).

130. Paffenbarger, R.S., Jr., Thome, M.C., and Wing, A.L., *Am. J. Epidemiol., 88*: 25–52 (1968).

131. Leon, A.S., and Blackburn, H., in *International Medical Review: Cardiology I. Hypertension* (P. Sleight and E. Fries, eds.). Butterworth, London, pp. 14–36 (1982).

132. Blair, S.N., Goodyear, M.N., Gibbon, S., and Cooper, K.H., *J.A.M.A., 252*: 487–490 (1984).

133. Hagberg, J.M., in *Exercise and Fitness. A Consensus of Current Knowledge* (C. Bouchard, R.J. Shephard, T. Stephens, J.R. Sutton, and B.D. McPherson, eds.). Human Kinetics, Champaign, IL: 455–466 (1990).
134. Jennings, G., Nielson, L., Nestel, P., Esler, M., Korner, P., Burton, D., and Bazelmans, J., *Circulation, 73*: 30–41 (1986).
135. Rauramaa, R., *Acta Med. Scand.*, (Suppl. 711): 37–42 (1986).
136. Stratton, J.R., Chandler, W.L., Cerqueira, M.D., Schwartz, R.S., Beard, J.C., Bradbury, V.L., and Abras, I.B., *Circulation, 80*(Suppl. II): 818 (1989) (Abst.).
137. Leon, A.S., in *Comparative Pathophysiology of Circulation Disorders* (C.M. Bloom, ed.). Plenum, New York, pp. 143–174 (1972).
138. Kramsch, D.M., Aspen, A.J., Abramowitz, B.M., Kreimendal, T., and Hood, W.B., Jr., *N. Engl. J. Med., 309*: 1483–1489 (1981).
139. Froelicher, V.L., *Eur. Heart J., 8*(Suppl. 6): 1–9 (1987).
140. Pelliccia, A., Spataro, A., Granata, M., Biffi, A., Caselli, G., and Alabiso, A., *Int. J. Sports Med., 2*: 120–126 (1990).
141. Forelicher, V.F., in *Exercise and Fitness. A Consensus of Current Knowledge* (C. Bouchard, R.J. Shephard, T. Stephens, J.R. Sutton, and B. D. McPherson, eds.). Human Kinetics, Champaign, IL: pp. 429–450 (1990).
142. Siscovick, D.S., Weiss, N.S., Fletcher, R.H., and Lasky, T., *N. Engl. J. Med., 311*: 874–877 (1984).
143. Cosineau, D., Ferguson, R.J., Gauthier, P., Cote, P., and Bourassaa, M., *J. Appl. Physiol., 43*: 801–806 (1977).
144. Leon, A.S., and Blackburn, H., *Ann. N.Y. Acad. Sci., 301*: 561–578 (1977).
145. Paffenbarger, R.S., Jr., and Hyde, R.T., *Prevent. Med., 13*: 3–22 (1984).
146. Powell, K.E., Thompson, P.D., Caspersen, C.J., and Kendrick, J.S., *Ann. Rev. Publ. Health, 8*: 253–287 (1987).
147. Leon, A.S., Connett, J., Jacobs, D.R., Jr., and Rauramaa, R., *J.A.M.A., 258*: 2388–2395 (1987).
148. Paffenbarger, R.S., Jr., and Hyde, R.T., *Prevent. Med., 13*: 3–22 (1984).
149. Slattery, M.L., and Jacobs, D.R., Jr., *Am. J. Epidemiol., 127*: 571–580 (1989).
150. Blair, S.N., Kohl, H.W., III, Paffenbarger, R.S., Jr., Clark, D.G., Cooper, K.H., and Gibbons, L.W., *J.A.M.A.*, 2395–2401 (1989).
151. Morris, J.N., Clayton, D.G., Everitt, M.G., Semmence, H., and Burgess, H., *Br. Heart J., 63*: 325–334 (1990).
152. O'Connor, G.T., Burlino, J.E., Yusaf, S., Goldhaber, S.Z., Olmstead, E.M., Paffenbarger, R.S., Jr., and Hennkens, D.H., *Circulation, 80*: 234–244 (1987).
153. Ornish, D., Brown, S.E., Schertwitz, L.W., Billings, J.H., Armstrong, W.T., Ponts, T.A., McClanahane, S.M., Icirkeeide, R.L., Brand, R.J., and Gould, K.L., *Lancet, 336*: 129–133 (1990).
154. Hughes, J.R., *Prevent. Med., 13*: 66–78 (1984).
155. Richter, E.A., and Galbo, H., *Sports Med. (N.Z.), 3*: 275–288 (1986).

156. McDonald, M.J., *Diabetes Care, 10*: 584–588 (1987).
157. Frantz, M.J., and Norstrom, J., *Your Game Plan for Diabetes and Exercise. Diabetes Actually Staying Healthy.* DCI Publishing, Wayzata, Minnesota, pp. 1–179 (1990).
158. McArdle, W.D., Katch, F.I., and Katch, V.L., *Exercise Physiology. Energy, Nutrition, and Human Performance.* 2nd Ed. Lea & Febiger, Philadelphia, pp. 642–649 (1986).
159. Trovati, M., Carta, Q., Cavalot, F., Vitali, S., Passarind, G., Rocca, G., and Emanuelli, G., *Diabetes Care, 7*: 327–330 (1984).
160. Rizza, R.A., *Mayo Clin, Proc., 61*: 796–805 (1986).
161. Jensen, M.D., *Mayo Clin. Proc., 61*: 813–819 (1986).

11

Exercise Therapy in Patients with Angina and Silent Ischemia

Gary J. Balady

*Boston University School of Medicine
and The University Hospital
Boston, Massachusetts*

INTRODUCTION

Ischemic heart disease, most commonly a result of atherosclerotic coronary artery disease, remains a formidable problem in contemporary society. It is estimated that over five million persons in the United States are afflicted with this condition, and its broad-based impact has important consequences even among those without coronary disease. Nearly half of all deaths in the United States are a result of atherosclerotic heart disease. Affected individuals are subject to a wide range of personal limitations leading to restricted activity in domestic, occupational, and recreational spheres. Such disability and ensuing health expenditures translate to major socioeconomic problems with annual costs estimated to be in billions of dollars (1).

Underlying coronary disease is most often expressed in episodes of ischemia. Until the past decade, attention has been focused on angina as the major clinical manifestation of this disease. Clinical decisions and management strategies were often based on the presence or absence of angina. A large and continuously growing body of recent data has focused attention on asymptomatic ischemia, with the realization that extensive coronary disease may, in fact, be painless, or "silent." Ischemia must then be considered as an entity composed of painful and painless episodes toward which diagnostic and therapeutic efforts are directed. The absence of angina no longer implies therapeutic success, and angina can no longer be considered a reliable gauge of ischemia.

A keen understanding of the pathophysiology of ischemia is necessary to affect its occurrence. A comprehensive familiarization with our current technologies to detect ischemia is essential to disclose the targets toward which our treatments are aimed. Contemporary therapeutic modalities continue to expand in every area. Revascularization techniques range from the conventional—coronary artery bypass surgery and coronary angioplasty—to the experimental (laser and athrectomy devices). Pharmacological agents encompass an ever-widening variety of drugs which affect β-adrenergic receptors, calcium channels, platelets, and numerous other receptor sites. Exercise, once felt to be proscribed among patients with coronary disease, is now being advocated (2) in the management of these patients.

An ever-increasing body of literature has yielded information regarding exercise and its affects on patients with atherosclerotic coronary artery disease. It is the purpose of this chapter to examine the role of exercise therapy among patients with ischemia—now realizing that manifestations of coronary disease can be both painful or completely silent.

ISCHEMIC HEART DISEASE

Pathophysiology

Myocardial ischemia occurs when the supply of oxygen to the myocardial cells is inadequate to meet its demands. This delicate balance of supply and demand for oxygenated blood can be affected by many factors. The variation in either supply or demand, or both, is an area of great and renewed interest (Fig. 1). Myocardial oxygen demand is related to heart rate, blood pressure, left ventricular contractility, and left ventricular wall stress (3). Left ventricular pressure, wall thickness, and cavity size will affect wall stress. Alterations in any of these factors—many of which are interdependent—can affect the myocardial need for oxygenated blood. Of these, the heart rate and blood pressure are the easiest parameters to measure and monitor. The product of the heart rate and systolic blood pressure, termed the rate-pressure product, has been found to be a very reliable index of myocardial oxygen demand (4), and therefore is the most widely used clinically.

Over the past 2 decades, much data have accumulated to challenge the traditional view that ischemia is due solely to an increase in

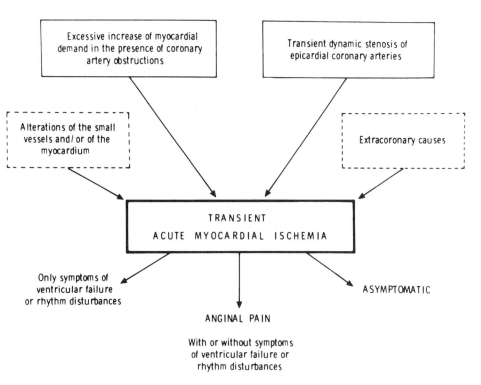

Figure 1 Possible pathophysiological mechanisms of ischemia and their clinical manifestations. See text for details. Extracoronary causes are typified by severe aortic stenosis. Alterations of the small vessels are represented by "syndrome X." (From Ref. 9; used with permission from The American Heart Association.)

myocardial oxygen demand. This is supported by observations that during ambulatory or intensive care unit monitoring ischemia can occur with little changes in the heart rate or systolic blood pressure (5). Therefore, transient reductions in coronary flow affecting regional myocardial oxygen supply must also be occurring. Nademanee (6) has found that exercise-induced ischemic parameters have a variability of 15–28% within any subject when compared to the 44–64% variability as measured during ambulatory Holter monitoring. This suggests that there is a fixed threshold for myocardial oxygen demand but a wide variation in oxygen supply (coronary flow). Most commonly, coronary flow is compromised as a result of an atherosclerotic plaque within the lumen of the coronary artery. Such a plaque may cause minimal stenosis or complete occlusion of the artery. Factors which influence the significance of a given luminal stenosis include: the degree of luminal obstruction; the length of the obstruction, the number and size of functioning collateral vessels, the magnitude of the supplied muscle mass, the shape and dynamic properties of the stenosis, and the autoregulatory capacity of the vascular bed (7).

Resistance to flow across a given stenosis is dependent upon the residual lumen area (relative to normal) and the length of the stenosis. Resistance increases as flow increases owing to local turbulence. Therefore, the transtenotic pressure gradient will increase with increased flow. However, a considerable degree of stenosis is necessary to impair flow. A 50–70% reduction in luminal diameter will impair peak reactive hyperemia, whereas a stenosis of $\geqslant 75\%$ will reduce resting flow (8).

Ninety percent of vascular resistance resides at the level of the arterioles, which can dilate four-fold. The pressure remaining to perfuse myocardium distal to a stenosis is inversely related to flow and directly proportional to both the lumen area at the stenosis and resistance in the distal vessel (5). The amount of smooth muscle within a given plaque may lead to variability in the affected lumen diameter. Local changes in vasomotor tone can influence the supply of oxygenated blood to the myocardium, thus affecting the ischemic threshold (8). This variable flow reserve is subject to the dynamic nature of coronary stenoses. Changes in coronary vasomotor tone may be due to neuromodulation as well as endothelial control. Additionally, local thrombosis may occur and be accompanied by changes in vasomotor tone, further reducing or completely obstructing flow (9).

The precise roles and interplay between neuromodulation and humeral control of vascular tone is yet to be determined. However, it appears that both of these factors are important in the regulation of flow, particularly at the site of a stenosis. In the normal coronary artery, α-adrenergic stimulation causes coronary vasoconstriction, whereas β-adrenergic activation produces direct coronary vasodilatation. Sympathetic stimulation in the normal coronary artery, however, produces a net vasodilatation. Conversely, in the presence of a coronary stenosis, the same level of sympathetic stimulation leads to a net coronary constriction (10). Acetylcholine when experimentally administered to coronary arteries leads to a vasodilatation, but in the presence of coronary stenosis causes vasoconstriction. This latter important observation was further developed by Furchgutt and Zawadski (11). They demonstrated that acetylcholine yielded a dilator response to isolated arterial strips if the endothelium was meticulously preserved during the preparation, although when endothelium was denuded, a constrictor response occurred. Since the time of these early experiments, much attention has been focused on the role of the endothelium in modulating vascular smooth muscle tone.

The endothelium is now recognized as a very important and complex structure which, through its release of various vasoactive substances, mediates the interaction between blood components, neural factors, and vascular smooth muscle. Among these substances is endothelium-derived relaxing factor (EDRF), which is thought to be nitric oxide or a ready source of it (12). This acts to stimulate guanylate cyclase to increase cyclic guanosine monophosphate (cGMP) in vascular smooth muscle and platelets, which has both relaxant and anti-aggregatory effects. Many stimuli can affect the release of EDRF, which with its very short half-life, acts locally in vivo (Fig. 2). Acety-

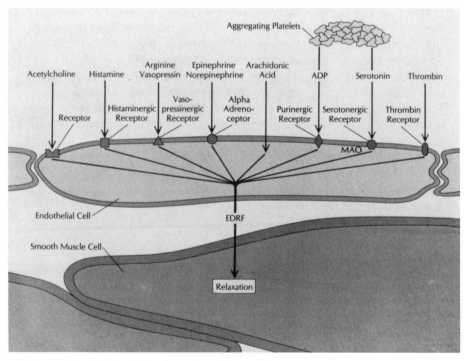

Figure 2 Endothelial cells mediate coronary artery smooth muscle relaxation in response to a wide variety of stimuli. Endothelium-derived relaxing factor (EDRF) is central to this process. (From Vanhautte, P., Hosp. Pract., 22(5):78 [1988]; used with permission. Illustration by Ilil Arbel.)

choline, epinephrine, adenosine diphosphate (ADP) from aggregating platelets, and thrombin are a few of the increasing number of substances found to trigger EDRF release. Increases in shear stress, such as that due to a sudden increase in blood velocity during exercise can increase EDRF and induce vascular smooth muscle relaxation. An interesting relationship exists between platelets and EDRF. Platelet aggregation in normal endothelium can cause release of EDRF, which in turn causes vasodilatation. Consequently, there is an increase in blood velocity, which then flushes away clot before it endangers circulation and compromises flow (13).

Damaged and diseased endothelium cannot release EDRF. Thus, underlying vascular smooth muscle is exposed to direct vasoconstrictor substances such as seratonin and thromboxane A_2 from aggregating platelets. Moreover, other substances released by the endothelium, termed endothelium-derived contracting factor and endothelium-derived hyperpolarizing factors, may lead to vasoconstriction in the absence of EDRF. Acetylcholine has been demonstrated to stimulate these constricting factors as well. This may account, at least in part, to the seemingly paradoxical constriction which occurs after acetylcholine administration in diseased coronary arteries (12). Endothelium-dependent contraction appears to become prominent in pathological conditions such as hypoxia, hypertension, and atherosclerosis. Endothelium-derived relaxing factor has been found to decrease with age (14), although the clinical consequences of this occurrence remain to be elucidated.

The pathophysiology of ischemia involves a complicated scheme of events. As exercise can affect many of the variables involved in the occurrence of ischemia, as will be discussed below, it is important to understand some of these underlying mechanisms.

Ischemia—Painful and Silent

The clinical manifestations of ischemia are quite variable. Ischemia may produce symptoms of typical angina, or appear in a more vague presentation as dyspnea or fatigue. It is now widely accepted that the occurrence of angina is late in the sequence of observed pathophysiological consequences of ischemia. Inadequate perfusion of the myocardium due to alterations in either supply and/or demand will lead to diminished regional contractility, followed by electrocardiographic changes, and finally the occurrence of angina (15). However, as early as the 1930s, it was recognized that ischemia can manifest as ST-segment changes during exercise testing without accompanying angina

(16). More recent data from the Framingham Heart Study demonstrates that greater than 25% of the myocardial infarctions which occurred over a 30-year period were initially discovered by the presence of new diagnostic electrocardiographic changes on routine follow-up examination. Of these, more than half were completely silent, whereas the remainder were symptomatically atypical (17). Large trials which evaluated exercise testing among patients with angiographically documented coronary artery disease have yielded remarkable findings. Weiner et al. (18) report that among the 2982 patients in the Coronary Artery Surgery Study (CASS) Registry, 424 demonstrated ischemic ST depression during exercise testing without angina. Mark et al. (19) found that among 1698 consecutive symptomatic patients who underwent exercise testing at Duke University Medical Center, 242 had painless exercise ST deviation. These data confirm that ischemia without angina is not uncommon. Furthermore, Campbell et al. (20) observed the characteristics of ischemic occurrences in seven asymptomatic subjects with documented coronary artery disease. Notably, 35% of all episodes of ischemic ST depression detected by ambulatory monitoring were not associated with a change in the heart rate. Fifty-four percent of ischemic episodes occurred at rest or with light physical activity, 38% during exercise, and 8% during sleep. Fourteen percent of all episodes occurred during periods of mental stress. Additionally, nearly 60% of all episodes occurred in the morning between 6 and 12 o'clock.

An important question remains: Why is ischemia sometimes silent and sometimes painful? The answer is not yet clear, although several hypotheses exist: (a) Silent myocardial ischemia represents a less severe ischemia which is not sufficient to reach pain thresholds (15). There are several studies which would argue against this point. Cabin and Roberts (21) have demonstrated no difference in the extent or severity of coronary disease between patients with and without angina prior to sudden death. Moreover, radionuclide studies confirm that major perfusion or wall motion abnormalities can occur during ischemia without associated pain (22,23). (b) There are differences in pain thresholds or pain perception among individuals with coronary artery disease (24). Whether or not these differences are due to variation in endorphin levels remains controversial. (c) Patterns of disturbed flow during silent and painful ischemia may be different (15).

Both painful and painless ischemia have been categorized into several types. Angina is grouped into functional classes, primarily based on the individual's ability to perform a given level of activity without the occurrence of angina. The most commonly used classification schemes are outlined in Table 1, with class I representing the least symptomatic patients and class IV representing the most limited group (25). Silent ischemia, however, has been classified into three different types by Cohn (26). These subtypes are not functional, since silent ischemia may occur in a wide variety of activity settings within a given patient. They are employed to define prevalence, and include: (a) type I—totally asymptomatic persons in whom ischemia is detected on routine screening. Cohn estimates that approximately 1–2 million middle-aged men in the United States are currently within this group; (b) type II—silent myocardial ischemia in the postinfarction patient. Based on exercise test data, this group appears to comprise 50,000 newly detected cases per year; and (c) type III—individuals with both angina and silent ischemia. In the United States alone, it is estimated that there are approximately 4 million such patients.

Ischemia—Methods for Detection

Exercising Testing

The realization that ischemia may be present among individuals with or without symptoms has generated an additional importance to the diagnostic methods used to detect ischemia. Foremost among these is the exercise test, which has for many decades yielded valuable information in the management in persons with either proven or suspected coronary artery disease. As the exercise test plays a key role in exercise therapy and exercise prescription, it is important to review several issues with particular reference to patients with both painful and silent ischemia.

Although there are various exercise test protocols available, all share the common goal of creating a gradual increase in muscular activity which will, in turn, increase myocardial oxygen demand. This increase in demand may provoke a supply/demand imbalance for oxygenated blood to the myocardium, and thus precipitate ischemia. The treadmill and bicycle are the most commonly used exercise modalities. The presence or absence of symptoms is noted as well as the heart rate and blood pressure response to each given level of exercise. The electrocardiographic analysis of the ST-segment response to exercise remains the most widely accepted and employed marker of exercise-induced ischemia. Interpretation of the ST-segment shift during exercise testing involves a familiarity with the sensitivity, specificity, and predictive value of this test in detecting coronary artery disease.

Bayesian analysis of test interpretation emphasizes the importance of the prevalence of disease in the population being tested. Consideration of the patient's age, sex, symptoms, and coronary risk factors will influence the pretest risk, and thus affect how a "positive" or "negative" outcome is viewed. Thus, the likelihood that coronary artery disease is either present or absent will depend both on the outcome of the test and the pretest likelihood of coronary disease for the individual being tested (27,28). When such an analysis is applied to the exercise test results of patients in the Coronary Artery Surgery Study (CASS), all of whom underwent coronary angiography as well, this point becomes clear. A positive test among subjects with a high pretest likelihood of disease (e.g., older men with definite angina) was highly predictive of coronary disease, whereas a negative test in this group was more likely to be a false negative. Alternately, a negative test among subjects with a low pretest likelihood of coronary disease (e.g., young women with atypical chest pain) was highly predictive of the absence of coronary disease, whereas a positive test in this group usually represented a false-positive response (29). However, a test should not be considered negative unless the patient reaches an adequate level of exercise—usually considered to be at 85% of maximum predicted heart rate for age. Moreover, underlying resting electrocardiographic abnormalities due to digitalis, hyperventilation, hypokalemia, left ventricular hypertrophy, or intraventricular conduction defects decrease the specificity of the ST-segment response to exercise. This increases the false-positive rate and weakens the validity of the test results. In such cases, or when the ST-segment response is equivocal, exercise radionuclide testing with thallium (30,31) or with echocardiography (32–34) will provide additional sensitivity and specificity for diagnostic interpretation.

The use of exercise testing in the detection of ischemia (as a manifestation of underlying coronary artery disease) in completely asymptomatic patients is discussed in detail in a separate chapter of this text. However, as the issue of silent ischemia is here being addressed, the following points will be made. Exercise testing when used for screening completely asymptomatic patients is problematic. Several investigators have addressed this complex issue. Piepgrass et al. (35) evaluated 771 healthy asymptomatic air crew men with exercise testing. Of the 20 men with an abnormal ST-segment response, only two demonstrated significant angiographic coronary disease. Froelicher et al. (36) performed cardiac catheterization of 138 asymptomatic men with an abnormal treadmill test and found that less than one-third of subjects had a coronary stenosis of $\geq 50\%$. The predictive value of a positive test in this group for coronary disease was only 26%. The Seattle Heart Watch Study (37) assessed the value of exercise testing in

Table 1 Three Methods of Cardiovascular Functional Classification

Class	New York Heart Association classification	Canadian Cardiovascular Society classification	Specific activity scale
I	Patients with cardiac disease but without resulting limitations of physical activity. Ordinary physical activity does not cause undue fatigue, papiltation, dyspnea, or anginal pain.	Ordinary physical activity such as walking and climbing stairs does not cause angina. Angina with strenuous or rapid or prolonged exertion at work or recreation.	Patients can perform to completion any activity requiring $\geqslant 7$ METs.
II	Patients with cardiac disease resulting in slight limitation of physical activity. They are comfortable at rest. Ordinary physical activity results in fatigue, palpitations, dyspnea, or anginal pain.	Slight limitation of ordinary activity. Walking or climbing stairs rapidly, walking uphill, walking or stair climbing after meals, in cold, in wind, or when under emotional stress, or only during the few hours after awakening. Walking more than two blocks on the level and climbing more than one flight of ordinary stairs at a normal pace and in normal conditions.	Patients can perform to completion any activity requiring $\geqslant 5$ METs but cannot and do not perform to completion activities requiring $\geqslant 7$ METs.

| III | Patients with cardiac disease resulting in marked limitation of physical activity. They are comfortable at rest. Less than ordinary physical activity causes fatigue, palpitation, dyspnea, or anginal pain. | Marked limitation of ordinary physical activity. Walking 1–2 blocks on the level and climbing more than one flight in normal conditions. | Patients can perform to completion any activity requiring ≥2 METs but cannot and do perform to completion any activities requiring ≥5 METs. |
| IV | Patients with cardiac disease resulting in inability to carry on any physical activity without discomfort. Symptoms of cardiac insufficiency or of the anginal syndrome may be present even at rest. If any physical activity is undertaken, discomfort is increased. | Inability to carry on any physical activity without discomfort—anginal syndrome may be present at rest. | Patients cannot or do not perform to completion activities requiring ≥2 METs. |

METs = metabolic equivalents.
Source: Adapted from Ref. 25; used with permission from The American Heart Association.

2365 asymptomatic men without prior cardiac history or diabetes. Only individuals with two or more conventional coronary risk factors and a positive exercise test were found to have a greater incidence of subsequent coronary events. Finally, Uhl et al. (38) studied 225 asymptomatic men with positive exercise test for ST depression. They found that the predictive value of the ST-segment response increased as the number of risk factors increased.

Epstein et al. (16) has theorized the practical implication for screening a large cohort of asymptomatic individuals (Fig. 3). In this provocative analysis, he concludes that there would be a greater abso-

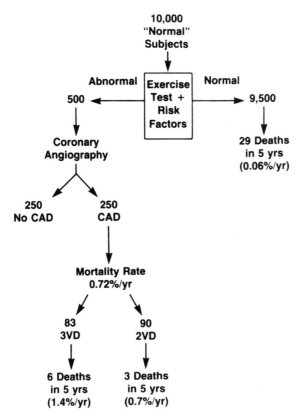

Figure 3 Implications of screening 10,000 subjects for asymptomatic coronary artery disease using exercise testing in risk factor assessment. (From *N. Engl. J. Med.*, 318:1041 [1988]; used with permission.)

lute number of estimated deaths per year in the group with a normal exercise test than among "high-risk" individuals with both abnormal exercise test and conventional risk factors. However, the death rate among the high-risk subgroup is greater (but still low). It appears that routine exercise screening to identify asymptomatic individuals prone to sudden death is of limited utility. However, exercise testing in asymptomatic individuals with conventional risk factors is more likely to identify underlying coronary artery disease, particularly among men over 35 years of age who also have: (a) an abnormal exercise thallium scan; (b) a reduced exercise capacity; (c) ≥ 2 mm ST-segment depression during exercise testing or (d) a decreased systolic arterial pressure with increasing workloads during exercise (39,40).

Among patients with known coronary artery disease, the exercise testing data is less ambiguous. Mark et al. (19) found that patients with exercise-induced angina exercised for a shorter duration, reached lower peak heart rates, and developed more ST depression at a lower workload than those with silent ischemia during exercise. Among 4083 medically treated patients with symtomatic coronary artery disease (41), individuals were stratified into low-risk and high-risk groups based on coronary anatomy, left ventricular systolic function, and exercise test variables. Those at greater risk with an annual mortality of greater than 5% included patients with congestive heart failure, or ≥ 1 mm ST-segment depression and a final stage I or less (using the Bruce treadmill protocol). Low-risk individuals with an annual mortality of less than 1% included patients who demonstrated <1 mm ST depression exercising into Bruce stage III or greater. Additionally, the ischemic response can be used to assess the severity of underlying coronary disease. Weiner et al. (42) evaluated 436 consecutive patients referred for diagnostic coronary arteriography for suspected coronary artery disease who also underwent exercise testing. A combination of factors, including 2 mm of downsloping ST-segment depression in five leads during stage I of a Bruce protocol treadmill test, lasting 6 min into recovery, was highly predictive of significant three-vessel (74%) or left main (32%) coronary artery disease.

Several studies have addressed the issue of exercise-induced silent ischemia with regard to prognosis. Callaham et al. (43) evaluated 1747 patients referred for exercise testing at a Veterans Administration Hospital. Sixty percent of individuals with abnormal exercise-induced ST depression had no accompanying pain. Ischemic ST depression conferred an adverse 2-year prognosis among those with or without exercise-induced angina. The prevalence of exercise-induced silent ischemia was found to increase with age. Bonow et al. (44) and Weiner et al. (18) have also reported that patients with exercise-induced ischemia share the same adverse prognosis whether or not angina was present. Figure 4 well illustrates the 7-year prognosis among patients with exercise-induced ST depression without angina when stratified according to severity of coronary artery disease. These survival rates were similar to those patients who experienced both angina and ST-segment depression during exercise testing. Mark et al. (19) also found that exercise-induced silent ischemia conferred a worse prognosis, although the survival rates among these patients were better than those with exercise-induced angina.

Finally, analysis of exercise-induced silent ischemia in the Coronary Artery Surgery Study demonstrates that patients with either silent or symptomatic ischemia during exercise testing among medically treated patients with documented coronary artery disease have a similar 7-year risk of developing acute myocardial infarction or sudden death (45). Moreover, among patients with exercise-induced silent ischemia with three-vessel disease and left ventricular dysfunction, survival was enhanced by coronary artery bypass surgery. This survival benefit is similar to that observed among patients in similar sub-

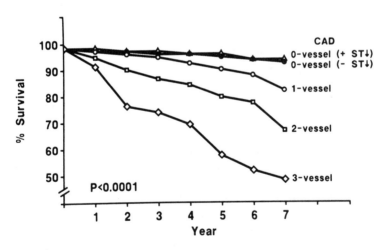

Figure 4 Seven years survival rates among coronary artery study (CASS) registry patients with silent ischemia on exercise testing (+ST↓) stratified according to number of diseased coronary vessels; 0-vessel (−ST↓) represents a control group of 1117 patients without coronary artery disease or ST-segment depression during exercise testing. (From Ref. 18; used with permission from the *American Journal of Cardiology*.)

groups who have symptomatic exercise-induced ischemia. Therefore, it is the presence or absence of ischemia during exercise testing which influences prognosis—whether ischemia is silent or not.

The reproducibility of the exercise ischemic threshold is of particular interest, especially when exercise tests are used to formulate an exercise prescription for exercise training. Several studies have addressed this issue, and most agree that the heart rate–blood pressure product at onset ischemic ST depression is fairly constant when serial testing using the same protocol is performed (50,51). Importantly, when differing protocols are used, the exercise-induced ischemic threshold may vary. Differences in exercising limbs (52), exercise position (53), and whether or not a warm-up precedes the exercise (50) all appear to influence the heart rate–blood pressure product at onset ischemia. Opasich et al. (54) have shown that among patients with exertional ischemia at a low workload, the heart rate–blood pressure product at onset ischemia varied in 55% of patients tested. Thus, reproducibility of the exercise-induced ischemic threshold depends upon subjects being tested and the type of test being performed.

Ambulatory Monitoring

The application of ambulatory monitoring for the detection of myocardial ischemia has been an area of growing interest. Advances in instrumentation have enhanced the detection of ST-segment shifts and have enabled the determination and measurement of these shifts with increased accuracy and reliability. However, it is important to realize that the predictive values of ambulatory ECG for the detection of ischemia (like exercise testing) are dependent upon the sensitivity and specificity of the test as well as the prevalence of disease in the population being tested. Currently, ambulatory monitoring is not recommended as a diagnostic procedure to detect underlying atherosclerotic coronary artery disease when the diagnosis is otherwise uncertain (47). Among patients with known atherosclerotic coronary disease, ambulatory monitoring is a technique with evolving applications. Campbell et al. (20) performed ambulatory monitoring and exercise testing in 309 patients with coronary artery disease. None of the patients without ischemia during an exercise test demonstrated ischemic ST-segment shifts on ambulatory monitoring. Of those with a positive exercise, 67% had silent ischemia on ambulatory monitoring. Patients who developed ischemic ST changes before 6 min of a Bruce protocol treadmill test, or at a heart rate of <150 beats/min, or whose ST-segment depression persisted greater than 5 min after exercise were found to have episodes of ischemia with greater frequency and longer duration.

Mulcahy et al. (48) evaluated 277 patients with angiographically documented coronary artery disease using exercise testing and 48-h ambulatory monitoring. In this study, >90% of all ischemic episodes detected by ambulatory electrocardiography occurred in patients with positive exercise tests. If only exercise testing had been utilized, <10% of patients with ischemia would have been missed. When patients with coronary spasm were excluded from analysis, ischemia on ambulatory ECG among the patients with a negative exercise test was found to be very infrequent and of brief duration. These authors conclude that ambulatory monitoring adds little to the results of exercise testing in detecting ischemia, except in patients who have a history of coronary artery spasm. Whether ischemia on ambulatory monitoring is an independent predictor of those with an adverse prognosis is yet to be determined. However, Rocco et al. (49) have found that this is so among patients with coronary disease and a positive exercise test. To summarize the relationship of ischemia on ambulatory monitoring and exercise testing, the following statements can be made:

1. Ischemia demonstrated on ambulatory monitoring is almost always evoked during exercise testing.
2. Only patients with ischemia at low levels during exercise testing demonstrate prolonged and frequent episodes on ambulatory electrocardiography.
3. Patients who demonstrate ischemia at high levels of exercise rarely have silent ischemia during ambulatory monitoring.
4. The patient with true coronary vasospasm will usually be diagnosed by history. Ambulatory monitoring may be of additional help in establishing the diagnosis in this setting (16,47).

Additionally, ambulatory monitoring can be used to document episodes of ischemia among patients with documented coronary disease during the performance of routine daily activities. The precise role for such monitoring is yet to be defined, but may have application in cardiac rehabilitation.

EFFECTS OF EXERCISE ON MYOCARDIAL OXYGEN SUPPLY/DEMAND RELATIONSHIPS

The physiological responses to exercise are detailed in a separate chapter in this text; however, the specific effects of acute and chronic exercise on myocardial oxygen supply and demand relationships will be addressed here.

Acute Affects of Exercise

During acute endurance exercise the cardiac output rises in response to the metabolic needs of the exercising muscles. Factors which influence this rise in cardiac output include an increase in sympathetic tone, which increases the heart rate and left ventricular contractility—both indices of myocardial oxygen consumption. Stroke volume rises due to increases in venous return of blood from exercising muscles. During exercise, blood flow is redistributed from the renal, splanchnic, and cutaneous circulation to the exercising muscles. The accumulation of metabolites in the actively contracting muscles causes a vasodilatation in muscle arterioles. This increases skeletal muscle blood flow up to four times that of the resting level, whereas reducing the overall aortic outflow impedance. This reduction in impedance allows for a more complete systolic ejection, thereby further increasing stroke volume. Systolic blood pressure increases primarily owing to the augmentation of the cardiac output, whereas diastolic blood pressure either remains constant or falls (55,56). The size and location of the exercising muscle group may affect hemodynamic responses to exercise. Dynamic arm exercise elicits greater heart rate and systolic and diastolic blood pressure responses during any given workload compared to leg exercise. Differences in sympathetic output, peripheral vasodilatation, venous return, and metabolic requirements of the exercising muscle mass may account for the greater heart rate–blood pressure product during arm work compared to leg work (55-57).

Isometric work (heavy resistance, low repetition) generates an increased sympathetic response with a resulting increase in the heart rate. Venous return, especially during straining, may decrease. Therefore, the rise in the cardiac output (relatively small compared to dynamic exercise) is primarily due to increases in the heart rate. External compressive forces on muscle capillaries during isometric exercise leads to an elevated peripheral resistance. This rise in resistance and the cardiac output yields an increase in both the systolic and diastolic pressures. Elevations in the systolic blood pressure from rest to exercise are usually proportionally greater than those in the heart rate (55,58). Therefore, during both dynamic and isometric exercise myocardial oxygen demand increases owing to rises in the heart rate, blood pressure, contractility, and left ventricular wall stress.

Coronary blood flow increases during exercise in response to neurohumoral stimulation (primarily sympathetic β-receptor) and possibly endothelial substances which are released (e.g., EDRF). Thus, during acute exercise, coronary blood flow is augmented in response to the increases in the myocardial oxygen demand. Among patients with atherosclerotic coronary artery disease, the demand may exceed the supply, and thus ischemia ensues. Moreover, Brown et al. (59) have shown that diseased coronary arteries may inappropriately vaso-constrict during exercise. This is possibly due to increases in α-adrenergic stimulation, although endothelial factors may also play a role. Such a response further compromises the supply/demand relationship and therefore promotes ischemia.

Chronic Effects of Exercise

A regular program of exercise training yields a number of physiological adaptations which affect the oxygen supply/demand relationship. Consistent observations among individuals with and without coronary artery disease include changes in autonomic tone at rest and during exercise; central cardiac adaptations; and peripheral changes in muscle capillary density, myocyte mitochondrial number, and enzymes involved with the metabolism of glycogen and fat. A complex interrelationship among these factors leads to:

1. Resting bradycardia.
2. Decreased heart rate and systolic blood pressure response at any submaximal workload.
3. Increases in exercise capacity (maximal oxygen consumption).
4. Increase in maximal cardiac output—mostly observed in normal healthy persons.
5. More rapid return to recovery hemodynamics after exercise.
6. Decrease in lactic acid concentration during submaximal exercise.
7. Increase in blood flow in exercising skeletal muscles.
8. Increased artieral-venous oxygen differences due to greater extraction of oxygen by the exercising muscles. This enables an increased oxidative metabolism of muscle fuels and the generation of more high-energy phosphates for muscle contraction (61).

The major product of these adaptations is the resulting increased functional capacity which can be employed in numerous domestic, occupational, and leisure/recreational/athletic activities. However, intuitive analysis would also argue that reduction in the heart rate–blood pressure product (an index of myocardial oxygen demand) at submaximal exercise levels translates to an improvement in the myocardial oxygen/supply demand relationship at that workload. Indeed, this appears to be the case, as many investigators have demonstrated a diminution of the ischemic response at a given submaximal workload in cardiac patients after training (60,62–65,67–69). However, several provocative studies have reported a decrease in the ischemic response—angina (65), ST-segment depression (63,66,68), thallium perfusion defects (64)—at a given heart rate–blood pressure product after training compared to the pretrained state. These findings suggest that there is an improvement in myocardial oxygen supply (i.e., coronary blood flow) at a given level of myocardial oxygen demand. There are many mechanisms or combinations thereof which may explain these findings. Pathological studies in animals reveal that endurance training causes an increase in the size of the superficial coronary arteries, and an increased myocardial capillary density. However, angiographic studies to date have not confirmed this finding in humans (70). Schuler et al. (71) demonstrated that of 28 patients who revealed increased myocardial perfusion on thallium scanning after 12 months of training, only five displayed regression of coronary stenoses on coronary angiography. However, blood viscosity in the 28 patients was found to decrease significantly after training. It is possible that alterations in blood rheology may be one of several factors to account for increased perfusion. Ernst et al. (72) have shown that various rheological parameters are affected by exercise training among patients with peripheral vascular disease. These include a decrease in blood and plasma viscosity, a decrease in red cell aggregability, and an increase in blood cell filterability. Another possible mechanism for improved myocardial profusion includes changes in coronary vasomotor reactivity. Various parameters which regulate coronary vascular smooth muscle may be affected by exercise training as well. Bove et al. (73) have documented a blunting of the α-adrenergic constrictor response in coronary arteries of dogs after training. Exercise training may thus effect several of the factors which influence coronary blood flow. Further work is needed to elucidate the role of exercise training in this complex paradigm.

Effects of Cardiac Medications on Training

Many patients with documented ischemic coronary artery disease take medications which influence autonomic tone, vascular smooth muscle tone, myocardial contractility, and many other parameters involved with physiological responses to acute exercise. It is clearly the purpose of these medications to reduce or eliminate the occurrence of myocardial ischemia. However, do these medications affect the beneficial responses to long-term exercise training by interfering with mechanisms involved with the attainment of a training effect? This topic will be addressed in detail in a separate chapter of this text; however, a few points here need to be made. β-Adrenergic blockers have been the most widely evaluated in this regard. It appears that these agents, in reducing exercise-induced ischemia, allow the patient to work at higher levels than they would have achieved without medications. Moreover, exercise capacity has been shown to increase in individuals who have completed an exercise training program and are taking β-blocking agents. However, this improvement appears to be relatively attenuated compared to those individuals taking placebo (74–76). The influence of calcium channel blocking agents on training has been less well evaluated, although studies to date have demonstrated no negative effects on the training response when compared to placebo (77,78).

RECOMMENDATIONS FOR EXERCISE TRAINING OF PATIENTS WITH ISCHEMIC HEART DISEASE

Exercise therapy among patients with ischemic heart disease should be prescribed as one would for any form of treatment, such that the effectiveness of therapy is optimized and the risks are minimized. The goals of exercise therapy, when used as such, should be individualized to meet the patient's needs in domestic, occupational, and leisure time activity. One must also take into account the limitations which they may incur from their cardiac and other preexisting diseases.

Medical Screening

Any patient with ischemic heart disease who is considering or being considered for an exercise program should undergo medical evaluation by a qualified physician. The medical history, with particular reference to cardiovascular status, is essential. Symptoms of angina, dyspnea, palpitations, and syncope should be sought. The patient should be questioned regarding the previous occurrence of myocardial infarction, coronary angioplasty, or bypass surgery. A complete list of medications and dosing intervals must be reviewed, as these may affect the responses to exercise. Patients taking insulin or oral hypoglycemics will require particular attention and monitoring for signs and symptoms of hypo- or hyperglycemia. Associated illnesses, including pulmonary, neurological, and musculoskeletal conditions, must also be considered in the evaluation. Social and detailed occupational history will yield valuable information such that program training and goals are tailored to meet individual needs.

Physical examination should focus at least on the heart rate, blood pressure, and pulmonary, cardiac, vascular, and musculoskeletal areas. Signs of congestive heart failure and valvular disease should be evaluated with further work-up if deemed appropriate.

Prior to beginning each exercise session, the patient should be questioned regarding new or worsening symptoms suggesting cardiovascular instability. Patients should also be instructed, when exercising in a supervised or unsupervised setting to be aware of these issues and address them to the appropriate medical personnel. Any changes in medications should be reported as these may affect the exercise prescription. A resting electrocardiogram and physician-supervised exercise test are integral to the medical evaluation and the exercise prescription itself. Exercise testing can be used to detect ischemia—whether symptomatic or silent—with particular reference to the workload and heart rate–blood pressure product at which ischemia begins. Risk stratification using these parameters will greatly assist in determining the adequacy of current therapy as well as the level of supervision and monitoring necessary in a given patient. Serial exercise testing is quite useful to monitor functional capacity, evaluate the training effect, and assess changes in the ischemic threshold. Such follow-up testing should be done every 3 months initially, and then every 6 months to 1 year thereafter. Should medication changes occur which may effect training parameters, it is prudent to repeat the exercise test such that the exercise prescription can be adjusted accordingly. Exercise testing is also useful in the evaluation of new or changing symptoms of chest pain or dyspnea, particularly when the etiology is not clear.

The role of ambulatory monitoring in evaluating patients before, during, or after exercise therapy is as yet undefined. From the preceding discussion, it appears that high-risk patients and those with silent ischemic will be identified using standard exercise testing methods. A potential use for ambulatory monitoring might be in evaluating a patient with silent ischemia who wishes to perform an activity at home or at work, in which the cardiovascular response cannot be well predicted (an example might be the various duties required of an auto mechanic).

The Training Program

The exercise prescription is formulated based on the evaluation as detailed above. Important components should include the type of exercise; limbs being used; and intensity, duration, and frequency of exercise sessions. Optimal training effects will occur when exercise is performed three to four times per week, for 20–40 min duration, at a specified heart rate. The training heart rate should be determined from the results of the exercise test. Using the peak heart rate achieved on the exercise test, at least two methods of target range formulation can be used:

1. 70–85% of maximum heart rate achieved
2. [{peak heart rate − resting heart rate} × 60%] + resting heart rate to [{peak heart rate − resting heart rate} × 80%] + resting heart rate (Karvonen method).

If angina or ischemic ST depression occurs during testing, then the heart rate at which this occurs should be substituted for the peak heart rate in the formulation (79). It is important to note that the use of the Karvonen method generates the target heart range, which is usually not far from the peak heart rate. This occurs particularly among patients taking medications which blunt the peak heart rate response. If the heart rate at ischemia is employed as the peak heart rate in this situation, patients may be exercising at a rate range near the ischemic threshold. Careful monitoring and caution should be used here, particularly among patients who demonstrate ischemia at a low heart rate and low workload. Serious consideration for optimization of medical therapy and/or revascularization should be entertained in this high-risk patient group prior to exercise therapy. Exercise training at lower intensity would be appropriate in this group.

As the physiological and ischemic responses to different types of exercise vary according to limbs used, body position, and relative amounts of dynamic and isometric work (52,53,57,58), one must consider that the ischemic threshold and functional capacity measured during one type of exercise testing may not translate to another type of exercise. Exercise prescription should be formulated using a testing protocol which reflects the major type of exercise modality which will be used during exercise therapy sessions. When modalities are altered, particularly among patients with silent ischemia, exercise testing using that specific type of exercise (e.g., arm ergometry/rowing) should be considered. Alternatively, more careful monitoring, including telemetry, might be used during the initial phases of the new modalities. It appears that during arm ergometry (52) and isometric exercise (58), the ischemic threshold is higher than when measured during treadmill testing. Therefore, it is unlikely that individuals will exceed their ischemic threshold when performing either arm ergometry or weight training within a given target heart rate range as determined from treadmill testing.

Alternate methods of training should be incorporated into exercise therapy. Specifically, arm ergometry (79) and circuit weight training (80) have been shown to yield benefits of both strength and endurance in patients with cardiac disease, whereas being relatively safe modalities of training. Patients with ischemic heart disease whose occupations or activities involve upper extremity and/or isometric (lifting) work would particularly benefit from such a program. Stretching exercises and low resistance warm-up and cool-down should be employed at each exercise session.

Safety of Exercise Therapy in Patient with Ischemic Heart Disease

Exercise training among patients with cardiac disease has been found to be relatively safe. VanCamp and Peterson (81) have accumulated important data from 167 outpatient cardiac rehabilitation programs involving a total of 51,000 patients. In this survey: The incidence of cardiac arrest was 1/112,000 person-h, with 86% of patients being successfully resuscitated; the incidence of myocardial infarction was 1/294,000 person-h—all myocardial infarctions were nonfatal; and the incidence of death was 1/784,000 person-h. No difference in event rate was found between programs which employed continuous electrocardiographic (telemetry) monitoring versus those who used intermittent monitoring.

Continous telemetry monitoring would be most appropriate among individuals who are designated as high risk based on their exercise test results, low ejection fraction, symptom class, history of syncope, malignant arrhythmias, or sudden death. Telemetry monitoring would also be useful among patients who are unable to monitor their own pulse. However, application of the Borg scale of perceived exertion (82) can be very useful and effective in this group. Among patients with asymptomatic ischemia, the scale of perceived exertion should be emphasized to maintain exercise training intensity, as well as outside unmonitored activities, below the exercise-induced ischemic threshold.

Is exercise therapy among patients with purely silent ischemia safe? To date, this has not been specifically addressed in a separate study. However, there are a few points which can be derived from the existing literature, as presented earlier:

1. Individuals with atherosclerotic coronary artery disease who demonstrate long and frequent episodes of silent ischemia are usually those who manifest ischemia at low heart rates and low workloads during exercise testing.
2. Individuals in whom silent ischemia has been shown to impart an adverse prognosis will be among those to manifest ischemia at a low level on exercise testing, especially when associated with low ejection fraction or multivessel coronary disease.
3. These individuals can be identified through the initial screening process such that appropriate monitoring can be arranged.
4. Among VanCamp and Peterson's (81) population of patients enrolled in cardiac rehabilitation, it is highly likely (considering Cohen's [26] prevalence data) that there were many patients with asymptomatic ischemia.

As the reported overall complication rates were low, it is likely that with appropriate screening and monitoring, the incidence of complications of exercise therapy among patients with silent ischemia would also be low.

Clearly, further study in this newly recognized important subgroup of patients needs to be performed. DeBusk et al. (83) addressed the safety of home exercise performed using heart rate monitors and transtelephonic ECG transmission. Although these investigators found that this method was safe and effective, the population enrolled in this study represents a very low–risk group. These patients would be a small fraction of those with ischemic coronary artery disease referred for exercise therapy, as they were: ≤70 years of age and without congestive heart failure, unstable angina, valvular heart disease, atrial fibrillation, bundle branch block, previous cerebrovascular accident, limiting orthopedic abnormalities, chronic obstructive lung disease, history of coronary bypass surgery, peripheral vascular disease, or intercurrent noncardiac illness.

CONCLUSIONS

Recent years have witnessed an impressive growth in the understanding of ischemic heart disease and in the area of exercise therapy. These knowledge bases intersect on many levels, including pathophysiology, clinical testing, and therapeutic application. Exercise therapy among individuals with ischemia should be prescribed with a full understanding of the methodologies available to maximize outcome and minimize risk. Now realizing that significant ischemia can occur without presenting symptoms, medical personnel responsible for prescribing and administering exercise therapy must be even more astute in their management of patients with coronary artery disease. Familiarity with the methods of detecting ischemia and appraising risk in these patients provides essential information necessary to guide treatment. Exercise therapy among patients with coronary artery disease appears to be effective in reducing exercise-induced ischemia. Effects on the total ischemic burden (all episodes of ischemia) are still unknown, but remain a challenge for further investigation.

REFERENCES

1. Rutherford, J.D., Braunwald, E., and Cohn, P.F., in *Heart Disease: A Textbook of Cardiovascular Medicine* (E. Braunwald, ed.). Saunders, Philadelphia, p. 1314 (1988).
2. American College of Sports Medicine, *Guidelines for Exercise Testing and Prescription.* 3rd Ed. (S.N. Blair, L.W. Gibbons, P. Painter, R.R. Pate, C.B. Taylor, and J. Will, eds.). Lea & Febiger, Philadelphia, pp. 53–71 (1986).
3. Braunwald, E., and Sobel, B.E., in *Heart Disease: A Textbook of Cardiovascular Medicine* (E. Braunwald, ed.). Saunders, Philadelphia, pp. 1191–1193 (1988).
4. Kitamura, K., Jorgensen, C.R., Gobel, F.L., Taylor, H.L., and Wang, Y., *J. Appl. Physiol., 32:* 516–522 (1972).
5. Brown, B.G., and Smith, B.H., in *Silent Myocardial Ischemia and Angina* (B.N. Singh, ed.). Pergamon Press, New York, pp. 16–27 (1988).
6. Nademanee, K., in *Silent Myocardial Ischemia and Angina* (B.N. Singh, ed.). Pergamon Press, New York, pp. 223–233 (1988).
7. Herzil, H.O., Leutwyler, R., and Krayenbuehl, H.P., *J. Am. Coll. Cardiol., 6:* 275–284 (1985).
8. Maseri, A., Davies, G., and Hackett, D., in *Silent Myocardial Ischemia and Angina* (B.N. Singh, ed.). Pergamon Press, New York, pp. 28–33 (1988).
9. Maseri, A., *J. Am. Coll. Cardiol., 9:* 249–262 (1987).
10. Marcus, M., *Hosp. Pract., 22:* 105–132 (1988).
11. Furchgott, R.F., and Zawadski, J.V., *Nature, 288:* 373–376 (1980).
12. Griffith, T.M., Lewis, M.J., Newby, A.C., and Henderson, A.H., *J. Am. Coll. Cardiol., 12:* 797–806 (1988).
13. Vanhoutte, P.M., *N. Engl. J. Med., 319:* 512–513 (1989).
14. Shiraski, Y., Su, C., Lee, T.J., Kolm, P., Cline, W.H., and Nickols, G.A., *J. Pharmacol. Exp. Ther., 239:*861–866 (1986).
15. Rozanski, A., and Berman, D.S., *Am. Heart J., 114:* 615–626 (1987).
16. Epstein, S.E., Quyyumi, A.A., and Bonow, R.O., *N. Engl. J. Med., 318:* 1038–1043 (1988).
17. Kannel, W.B., *Circulation, 75:* II4–II5 (1900).
18. Weiner, D.A., Ryan, T.J., McCabe, C.H., Luk, S., Chaitman, B.R.,

Sheffield, L.T., Tristani, F., and Fisher, L.D., *Am. J. Cardiol.*, 59: 725–729 (1987).

19. Mark, D.B., Hlahtky, M.A., Califf, R.M., Morris, J.J., Sisson, S.D., McCants, C.B., Lee, K.L., Harrel, F.E., and Pryor, D.B., *J. Am. Coll. Cardiol.*, 14: 885–892 (1989).

20. Campbell, S., Barry, J., Rebecca, G.S., Rocco, M.B., Nabel, E.G., Wayne, R.R., and Selwyn, A.P., *Am. J. Cardiol.*, 57: 1010–1016 (1986).

21. Cabin, H., and Roberts, W., *Am. J. Cardiol.*, 50:677–681 (1982).

22. Deanfield, J.E., Shea, M., Ribiero, P., DeLandsheer, C.M., Wilson, R.A., Horlock, P., and Selwyn, A.P., *Am. J. Cardiol.*, 54: 1195–1200 (1984).

23. Cohn, P.F., Brown, E.J., Wynn, J., Holmon, B.L., and Adkins, H.L., *J. Am. Coll. Cardiol.*, 1: 931–933 (1983).

24. Glazier, J.J., Chierchia, S., Brown, M.J., and Maseri, A., *Am. J. Cardiol.*, 58: 667–672 (1986).

25. Goldman, L., Hashimoto, B., Cook, E.F., and Loscalzo, A., *Circulation*, 64: 1227–1234 (1981).

26. Cohn, P.F., *Cardiol. Board Rev.*, 4: 25–27 (1987).

27. Epstein, S., *Am. J. Cardiol.*, 46: 491–499 (1980).

28. Rifkin, R.D., and Hood, W.B., *N. Engl. J. Med.*, 297: 681–686 (1977).

29. Weiner, D.A., Ryan, T.J., McCabe, C.H., Kennedy, J.W., Schloss, M., Tristani, F., Chaitman, B.R., and Fisher, L.D., *N. Engl. J. Med.*, 302: 230–235 (1979).

30. Iskandrian, A.S., and Hakki, A.H., *Am. Heart J.*, 109: 113–128 (1985).

31. ACC/AHA Task Force on Assessment of Cardiovascular Procedures (Subcommittee in Nuclear Imaging), *J. Am. Coll. Cardiol.*, 8: 1471–1483 (1986).

32. Robertson, W.S., Feigenbaum, H., Armstrong, W.F., Dillon, J.C., O'Donnell, J., and McHenry, P.W., *J. Am. Coll. Cardiol.*, 2: 1085–1091 (1983).

33. Berberich, S.N., Zager, J.R.S., Plotnick, G.D., and Fisher, M.L., *J. Am. Coll. Cardiol.*, 3: 284–290 (1984).

34. Ryan, T., Vasey, C.G., Presti, C.F., O'Donnell, J.A., Feigenbaum, H., and Armstrong, W.F., *J. Am. Coll. Cardiol.*, 11: 993–999 (1988).

35. Piepgrass, S.R., Uhl, G.S., Hickman, J.R., Hopkirk, J.A.C., and Plowman, K., *Aviat. Environ. Med.*, 53: 379–382 (1982).

36. Froelicher, V.F., Thompson, A.J., Wothlius, S., Fuchs, R., Balusek, R., Longo, M., Triebwater, J.H., and Lancaster, M.L., *Am. J. Cardiol.*, 39: 32–38 (1977).

37. Bruce, R.A., DeRouen, T.A., and Hossack, K.F., *Am. J. Cardiol.*, 46: 371–378 (1980).

38. Uhl, G.S., and Froelicher, V., *J. Am. Coll. Cardiol.*, 1: 946–955 (1983).

39. ACC/AHA Task Force on Assessment of Cardiovascular Procedures (Subcommittee on Exercise Testing), *J. Am. Coll. Cardiol.*, 8: 725–738 (1987).

40. ACC/AHA Task Force on Assessment of Cardiovascular Procedures (Subcommittee on Nuclear Imaging), *J. Am. Coll. Cardiol.*, 8: 1471–1483 (1986).

41. Weiner, D.A., Ryan, T.J., McCabe, C.H., Chaitman, B.R., Sheffield, L.T.,

Ferguson, J.C., Fisher, L.D., and Tristani, F., *J. Am. Coll. Cardiol.*, 3: 772–779 (1984).

42. Winer, D.A., McCabe, C.H., and Ryan, T.J., *Am. J. Cardiol.*, 46: 21–27 (1980).

43. Callaham, P.R., Froelicher, V.F., Klein, J., Risch, M., Dubach, P., and Friis, R., *J. Am. Coll. Cardiol.*, 14:1175–1180 (1989).

44. Bonow, R.O., Bacharach, S.L., Green, M.V., LaFreniere, R.L., and Epstein, S.E., *Am. J. Cardiol.*, 60:778–783 (1987).

45. Weiner, D.A., Ryan, T.J., McCabe, C.H., Ng, G., Chaitman, B.R., Sheffield, L.T., Tristani, F.E., and Fisher, L.D., *Am. J. Cardiol.*, 62: 1155–1158 (1988).

46. Weiner, D.A., Ryan, T.J., McCabe, C.H., Chaitman, B., Sheffield, L.T., Ng, G., Fisher, L.D., Tristani, F.E., and the CASS Investigators, *J. Am. Coll. Cardiol.*, 12:595–599 (1988).

47. ACC/AHA Task Force on Assessment of Diagnostic and Therapeutic Cardiovascular Procedures (Subcommitee on Ambulatory Electrocardiography), *Circulation, 79*: 206–215 (1989).

48. Mulcahy, D., Keegan, J., Sparrow, J., Park, A., Wright, C., and Fox, K., *J. Am. Coll. Cardiol.*, 14: 1166–1172 (1989).

49. Rocco, M.B., Nabel, E.G., Campbell, S., Goldman, L., Barry, J., Mead, K., and Selwyn, A.P., *Circulation, 78*:877–884 (1988).

50. Pupita, G., Kaski, J.C., Galassi, A.R., Vejar, M., Crea, F., and Maseri, A., *Am. Heart J.*, 118: 539–544 (1989).

51. Waters, D., McCans, J.L., and Crean, P.A., *J. Am. Coll. Cardiol.*, 6: 1011–1015 (1985).

52. Balady, G.J., Weiner, D.A., McCabe, C.H., and Ryan, T.J., *Am. J. Cardiol.*, 55: 37–39 (1985).

53. Whetherbe, J.N., Banrah, V.S., Ptacin, N.J., and Kalbfleish, J.H., *J. Am. Coll. Cardiol.*, 11: 330–337 (1988).

54. Opasich, C., Falcone, C., Cobelli, F., Assandri, J., LaRovere, M.T., Riccardi, G., Tramarin, R., Ardissino, D., and Speechia, G., *Eur. Heart J.*, 8: 402–408 (1987).

55. Balady, G.J., and Weiner, D.A., *Comprehen. Ther.*, 11: 15–18 (1985).

56. Clausen, J.P., *Prog. Cardiovasc. Dis.*, 18: 459–495 (1976).

57. Pendergast, D.R., *Med. Sci. Sports Exerc.*, 21:S121–S125 (1989).

58. Wilke, N.A., Sheldahl, L.M., Tristani, F.E., Hughes, C.V., and Kalbfleish, J.H., *Am. Heart J.*, 110: 542–545 (1985).

59. Brown, B.G., Lee, A.B., Bolson, E.L., and Dodge, H.T., *Circulation, 70*: 18–24 (1984).

60. Ehsani, A., *Cardio, 5*: 95–97 (1988).

61. Froelicher, V.F., in *Exercise and the Heart.* Year Book Chicago, pp. 341–385 (1987).

62. Ehsani, A.A., Heath, G.W., Hagberg, J.M., Sobel, B.E., and Holloszy, J.O., *Circulation, 64*: 1116–1124 (1981).

63. Rogers, M.A., Yamamoto, C., Hagberg, J.M., Holloszy, J.O., and Ehsani,

A.A., *J. Am. Coll. Cardiol.*, 10: 321–326 (1987).
64. Schuler, G., Schierf, G., Wirth, A., Mautner, H.P., Scheurlen, H., Thomm, M., Roth, H., Schwartz, F., Kohlemeier, M., Mehmel, H.C., and Kubler, W., *Circulation*, 77: 172–181 (1988).
65. Ben-Ari, E., Kellermann, J.J., Rothbaum, D.A., Fisman, E., and Pines, A., *Am. J. Cardiol.*, 59: 231–234 (1987).
66. Ades, P.A., Grunvald, M.H., Weiss, R.M., and Hanson, J.S., *Am. J. Cardiol.*, 63: 1032–1036 (1989).
67. Myers, J., Ahnve, S., Froelicher, V.F., Livingston, M., Jensen, D., Abramson, I., Sullivan, M., and Mortara, D., *J. Am. Coll. Cardiol.*, 4: 1094–1102 (1984).
68. Raffo, J.A., Luksic, I.Y., Kappagoda, C.T., Mary, D., Whitaker, W., and Linden, R.J., *Br. Heart J.*, 43:262–269 (1980).
69. Detry, J., and Bruce, R.A., *Circulation*, 44: 390–397 (1971).
70. Scheuer, J., *Circulation*, 66: 491–495 (1982).
71. Schuler, G., Hambercht, R., Neumann, J., Schweizer, M., Scheffler, E., and Schlierf, G., *Circulation*, 80: II610 (1989) (Abst.).
72. Enrst, E.E.W., and Matrai, A., *Circulation*, 76: 1110–1114 (1987).
73. Bove, A.A., and Dewey, J.D., *Circulation*, 71:620–625 (1985).
74. Ewy, G.A., Wilmore, J.H., Morton, A.R., Stanforth, P.R., Constable, S.H., Buono, M.J., Conrad, K.A., Miller, H., and Gatewood, C.F., *J. Cardiac. Rehabil.*, 3: 25–29 (1983).
75. Sable, D.L., Brammell, H.L., Sheehan, M.W., Nies, A.S., Gerber, J., and Horwitz, L.D., *Circulation*, 65:679–684 (1982).
76. Pratt, C.M., Welton, D.E., Squires, W.G., Kirby, D.E., Hartung, G.H., and Miller, R.R., *Circulation*, 64: 1125–1129 (1981).
77. Duffey, D.J., Horwitz, L.D., and Brammell, H.L., *Am. J. Cardiol.*, 53: 908–911 (1984).
78. Kelemen, M.H., Effron, M.B., Valenti, S.A., and Stewart, K., *J. Am. Coll. Cardiol.*, 13: 241A (1989) (Abst.).
79. Franklin, B.A., Hellerstein, H.K., Gordon, S., and Timmis, G.C., in *Exercise in Modern Medicine* (B.A. Franklin, S. Gordon, and G.C. Timmis, eds.). Williams & Wilkens, Baltimore, pp. 44–80 (1989).
80. Kelemen, M.H., Stewart, K.G., Gillilan, R.E., Ewart, C.K., Valenti, S.A., Manley, J.D., and Keleman, M.D., *J. Am. Coll. Cardiol.*, 7: 38–42 (1986).
81. VanCamp, S.P., and Peterson, R.A., *J.A.M.A.*, 256: 1160–1163 (1986).
82. Borg, G., *Scand. J. Rehabil. Med.*, 2: 92–98 (1970).
83. DeBusk, R.F., Haskell, W.L., Miller, N.H., Berra, K., and Taylor, C.B., *Am. J. Cardiol.*, 55: 251–257 (1985).

12

Exercise in Patients with Heart Failure

L. Kent Smith

Arizona Heart Institute
Pheonix, Arizona

INTRODUCTION

A patient presenting with the clinical syndrome of dyspnea and/or fatigue may be manifesting heart failure. However, these two symptoms may indeed be from a variety of causes other than heart failure. It is essential that there be adequate documentation of an abnormality in cardiac function in a patient presenting with the potential clinical symptoms of heart failure (dyspnea and/or fatigue). More precisely, the failure of the heart to perform its function of pumping blood adequately to meet the needs of the body (right ventricular pumping of unoxygenated blood to the lungs and left ventricular pumping of oxygenated blood to body tissue) is a failure of the systolic function of the heart (myocardial failure). Heart failure is a somewhat broader term which also encompasses abnormal function in the filling of the heart (diastolic dysfunction). Newer technologies (specifically radionuclide angiography and two-dimensional [2D] echocardiography) allow for the determination of the relative contributions of systolic and/or diastolic dysfunction in a patient manifesting heart failure. Circulatory failure is yet a broader term. This term encompasses all of the components of the circulation; the heart, the blood volume, the arterial and venous circulatory beds and the releasing capacity of hemoglobin as potential causes for the clinical manifestation of "failure."

In cardiovascular disease in adults in this country, myocardial failure is far and away the most common cause for circulatory failure.

Specifically, various disorders which reduce the heart's systolic function account for the vast majority of cases where patients present with the clinical syndrome of circulatory failure. Based upon the emerging technologies of radionuclide studies and 2D echocardiography, however, cases of diastolic dysfunction are more frequently being documented. Very early manifestations of coronary artery disease can manifest as diastolic dysfunction only, unaccompanied by systolic dysfunction. Certain infiltrative disorders of the heart muscle (amyloidosis) also manifest as diastolic dysfunction. Mitral valvular stenosis also produces left ventricular diastolic dysfunction. Since none of these entities are generally dealt with in patients presenting for cardiac rehabilitation, they will not be discussed. Furthermore, the extracardiac causes of circulatory failure shall also not be discussed. Nevertheless, it is important for the cardiac rehabilitation professional to be certain that these extracardiac causes are not present in their patient. For instance, diminished blood volume in patients with excessive diuretic therapy or patients manifesting a low hemoglobin concentration need to be recognized and corrected.

In the last 5 years, significant new information has become available dealing with the important issues of exercise assessment and exercise training in patients with heart failure. The scientific basis for this information is well founded and has clarified our understanding of the alterations in physiology in patients with heart failure. Such understanding has in turn lead to the capability of assessing the altered physiological state in patients with heart failure and formulating an appropriate management strategy.

DEFINITION, CLASSIFICATION, AND PATHOPHYSIOLOGY

Cardiac failure is defined by Braunwald (1) as "the pathophysiological state in which an abnormality of cardiac function is responsible for failure of the heart to pump blood at a rate commensurate with the requirements of the metabolizing tissues, or to do so only from elevated filling pressure." As discussed in the introduction to this chapter, this definition requires documentation of cardiac or myocardial dysfunction itself. Although the clinical examination findings of an S3 gallop and the often accompanying finding of an abnormally enlarged cardiac silhouette on chest x-ray were sufficient evidence of myocardial dysfunction in earlier times, more objective criteria are now required. These objective criteria are most often met with a noninvasive assessment of myocardial systolic and diastolic functions.

Specifically, two-dimensional echocardiography and/or radionuclide ventriculography form the objective basis for documenting myocardial failure.

The traditional clinical classification of heart failure has been long established (2). This is the familiar delineation of four separate classes of heart failure enumerated using Roman numerals. This is a purely clinical classification scheme based upon the symptomatic status of patients. The least symptomatic status forms class I in which the patient has no limitation with ordinary physical activity, but fatigue or dyspnea with extraordinary activity. Functional class II encompasses patients who are comfortable at rest, but show slight limitation from symptoms of shortness of breath or fatigue with physical activity. Functional class III comprises the more disabled patients, who are markedly limited with even ordinary physical activity producing the symptoms. In functional class IV are the most severely limited patients, who are unable to carry on any physical activity without shortness of breath or fatigue and are symptomatic even at rest.

Obviously, this purely subjective clinical classification of heart failure patients implies that the cardiovascular system is not able to sufficiently carry out its function of delivering oxygen to metabolizing tissue. This inability presents as symptoms. However, only assessing myocardial performance (by means of the noninvasive techniques mentioned above) accounts for the cardiac contribution to the circulatory demands of the body. Very important peripheral compensatory mechanisms are present with congestive heart failure and, of course, these need to be assessed and measured as well. Not surprisingly, therefore, the clinical classification of heart failure as defined by the subjective or symptomatic presentation of a patient does not correlate very accurately with measured degrees of left ventricular function (degrees of impairment of left ventricular ejection fraction). Considerable overlap is seen between the various clinical classifications of heart failure and degrees of left ventricular ejection fraction impairment.

Cardiac failure can be acute or chronic. In the context of this chapter, only the exercise capacity and exercise conditioning of patients with chronic cardiac failure will be addressed. In chronic heart failure, both cardiac and peripheral compensatory mechanisms occur. These compensatory mechanisms tend to restore partially the impaired left ventricular systolic function. Dilatation of the left ventricle can occur which, through the Frank-Starling mechanism, tends to maintain stroke volume. Left ventricular hypertrophy can also be seen, particularly when heart failure is based upon systemic hypertension or aortic valvular stenosis, and such hypertrophy increases left ventricular wall thickness in an attempt to increase wall stress. This compensatory mechanism has the adverse consequences, however, of producing left ventricular diastolic dysfunction. In addition, peripheral mechanisms are activated. The adrenergic nervous system produces vasoconstriction, which increases total peripheral resistance that, unfortunately, then feeds back into the stress on the ventricle by increasing afterload. A vicious cycle feedback system is thereby established. In addition, stimulation of the renin-angiotensin-vasopressin system occurs, which in turn leads to potent vasoconstriction. As a consequence of these peripheral adaptations, blood flow to the kidneys, gut, and periphery are reduced, but coronary and cerebral blood flow tend to be preserved. With diminished blood flow to the kidneys, salt and water retention occur, leading to the congestive symptoms and physical examination findings (peripheral edema as well as hepatic and pulmonary congestion). Reversal of the adverse consequences of the adrenergic and renin-angiotensin system is the basis for the treatment of the patient with heart failure with angiotensin-converting enzyme inhibitor medications (Captopril and Enalapril).

EPIDEMIOLOGY AND ETIOLOGY

In contrast to the steady decline in mortality from stroke and coronary heart disease seen in this country over the last 20 years (stroke mortality declining nearly 50% and coronary heart disease mortality by 33%), no such mortality reduction has been documented in patients with congestive heart failure. The prevalence as well as mortality from congestive heart failure has remained unaltered. Approximately 400,000 patients die annually in the United States from heart failure, and congestive heart failure is one of the most common diagnoses for hospital admissions of patients aged 65 and greater in this country. A large proportion of patients dying from heart failure die suddenly (35–45%). This annual fatality occurs in a pool of approximately 3 million patients who have the diagnosis of heart failure. Furthermore, heart failure is a disease seen with increasing age. Data from the Framingham Heart Study showed the annual incidence of heart failure to be three per 1000 subjects prior to age 65, but 10 or more per 1000 after age 65.

The etiology of heart failure is various. The leading underlying condition is, of course, coronary artery disease. In various series, between 50 and 75% of patients with heart failure have coronary artery disease as the underlying cause (3). Hypertension still accounts for a large number of cases with congestive heart failure. In fact, in a 1988 report from the Framingham Heart Study, a 30-year review of heart failure occurring in the Framingham population documented prior hypertension was seen in fully 70% of the cases, whereas 50% had prior coronary artery disease (4). Primary cardiomyopathy accounts for a small but tragic proportion of patients with heart failure, often occurring at a young age and from a viral etiology.

NATURAL HISTORY

Congestive heart failure is an ominous disease. Even when first diagnosed in the outpatient setting, the prognosis is poor. Data from the Framingham Heart Study (4) show that fully 60% of men and 40% of women are dead within 4 years of the initial diagnosis of congestive heart failure, even when the diagnosis was made in the outpatient setting in the Framingham population. This mortality is six to seven times greater than an age-matched cohort in the general population without heart failure. Between 40 and 50% of the deaths were sudden. In the Framingham database, 70% of the heart failure patients who died suddenly also had concomitant coronary artery disease.

In the patient suffering an acute myocardial infarction who manifests heart failure, the prognosis is also poor. Nine hundred seventy-two survivors of an acute myocardial infarction who demonstrated clinical evidence of heart failure while in the coronary care unit (S3 gallop, rales, x-ray findings, or ejection fraction less than 40%) showed a poor outcome (5). Specifically, patients showing clinical signs of heart failure and having a left ventricular ejection fraction of less than 0.4 had a 26% 1-year mortality compared to only 3% of patients showing more normal left ventricular ejection fraction and no clinical findings of heart failure during the coronary care unit stay. Additionally, if a patient also showed x-ray findings of congestive heart failure during the acute myocardial infarction period, the 1-year mortality increased to 36%. Review of the coronary care unit clinical records as well as x-ray findings and radionuclide assessment of left ventricular ejection fraction (if available) serve as important risk stratification markers for a patient entering a cardiac rehabilitation program after an acute myocardial infarction. Ventricular ectopy is frequently seen in the congestive heart failure patient. Several studies have documented the presence of couplets and multiform ventricular extra beats as well as nonsustained ventricular tachycardia in as high as 70–95% of patients having 24-h

Holter monitoring. The finding of complex ventricular arrhythmia in patients with heart failure defines a risk of sudden death of at least 50%. No effective medication regimen for rhythm control has been established.

MEDICAL MANAGEMENT

The medical management of the patient with congestive heart failure is multifaceted. Nonpharmacological approaches are both important and effective. Patient education as well as education of the patient's family should seek to establish an understanding of the disease and its impact on daily living. Dietary measures which clearly restrict sodium as well as optimize weight when appropriate should take place. Avoidance of undue emotional and/or physical stress is beneficial. Depression is commonly seen in patients who have limitation on their lifestyle. Care should be given to this problem, which can interfere with the successful outcome of other therapeutic approaches.

A wide array of medications is also available in the management of the patient with heart failure. When appropriate, antianginal medication may be necessary. Additionally, adequate control of hypertension needs to be addressed. The symptoms of heart failure themselves very often require the judicious use of a diuretic. However, when diuretics do not sufficiently alleviate symptoms, other classes of medication are available.

Digitalis has been long used in patients with heart failure. Very recent clinical trials have documented the beneficial role of digitalis. It is of considerable benefit in the patient who is not in normal sinus rhythm in order to control the ventricular response to atrial dysrhythmia. In addition, digitalis has shown to be effective in patients in normal sinus rhythm. This appears to be particularly the case in patients with the more severe classes of heart failure. In these patients, digitalis improves symptoms as well as improves the objective measures of ventricular performance (enhancing left ventricular ejection fraction).

Drugs which competitively inhibit angiotensin-converting enzyme (ACE) have a well-established beneficial role in patients with heart failure. Two of these drugs, Captopril and Enalapril, are approved for use in patients with heart failure. These drugs not only improve the signs and symptoms of heart failure, but have been shown to reduce mortality in placebo-controlled trials. Specifically, patients with functional classes III and IV heart failure patients assigned to Captopril treatment had a 96% survival at 90 days com-

Table 1   Causes of Death

	Enalapril	Placebo	p
Progression of CHF	22	44	0.001
New cardiac event			
within 24 h	20	19	ns
within 1 h	14	14	ns

pared with a 79% survival in the placebo-assigned group (6). Enalapril has been studied in 253 patients with functional class IV heart failure. This double-blind placebo-controlled study documented 75% 6-month survival in Enalapril-treated patients compared to 55% 6-month survival in placebo-assigned patients (Table 1). In addition, 72% of the survivors in the Enalapril treatment group improved their functional capacity compared with only 47% in the placebo-treated group (7) (Table 2). The usefulness of ACE inhibition in patients recovering from an acute myocardial infarction has also been documented in two studies (8,9). Both of these placebo-controlled trials showed a significant improvement in ventricular function as assessed by echocardiography in a Captopril-treated group compared to placebo up to 1 year following acute myocardial infarction. The untreated group showed a progressive increase in end-diastolic and end-systolic volume as measured by echocardiography, whereas the ACE inhibitor–treated group showed improvement in these parameters as well as in increment in ejection fraction over 1 year. Also, the Captopril-treated patients showed increased exercise performance on quarterly treadmill testing throughout the 1-year trial. This trial did not include exercise training. The absence of deterioration of ventricular function noted in the ACE inhibitor–treated patients may have considerable importance in

Table 2   Functional Class of Survivors

Class	Enalapril	Placebo
I	3	0
II	13	2
III	38	25
IV	21	30
Deaths	50	68

considering strategies for exercise therapy in patients having survived myocardial infarction but showing diminished ventricular performance following the heart attack (see rehabilitation discussion to follow).

EXERCISE CAPACITY AND PERFORMANCE TESTING

No correlation exists between measures of exercise capacity in a patient with heart failure and concomitant measures of ventricular performance. Studies have shown that echocardiographic or radionuclide measurements of left ventricular ejection fraction at rest or with exercise show no relationship to bicycle or treadmill exercise duration (10). The patient's ability to perform exercise cannot be predicted from assessment of either a resting left ventricular ejection fraction or a change in ejection fraction with exercise. The prognostic value of exercise capacity evaluation has been established. In a study of 115 patients with a myocardial infarction and a resting left ventricular ejection fraction less than a 35% treadmill exercise capacity was assessed (11). When the patients were stratified by MET (metabolic equivalent) level the patients with the lowest level (<4) had a 3.5-fold greater risk of subsequent fatality than patients with the highest MET level performance (>7). This exercise capacity prognostic marker was independent of low left ventricular ejection fraction measurement.

Since the exercise capacity has clinical prognostic meaning, the ability to predict the response to exercise training is an important issue to the patient contemplating an exercise training or rehabilitation program. Specifically, are there any parameters that would predict a successful outcome in an exercise program in patients with heart failure? This important issue has been well studied in the work from Duke University (12,13). The classic measure of a training response (increase in peak VO_2) to a 4- to 6-month conditioning program showed no correlation to any of the baseline pretraining measurements. These baseline measurements included the resting left ventricular ejection fraction as well as the response of the left ventricular ejection fraction to exercise testing. These direct measures of ventricular performance did not predict an increase in VO_2 as a result of the exercise training regimen. Furthermore, baseline determination of VO_2 did not predict the response to the exercise training program. This study did establish that exercise training in patients with impaired left ventricular performance can be safely carried out and achieve the beneficial training effect.

REHABILITATION

As recently as 1982, conservative recommendations regarding exercise in the patient with congestive heart failure was standard teaching (14). In fact, rest was called "a traditional mainstay of therapy." The teaching also included the fact that "rest is sometimes overlooked as an effective instrument for decreasing the cardiac burden." This traditional and conservative teaching has more recently given way to a more enlightened regard for the role of physical activity in patients with heart failure. In the 1988 Third Edition of Braunwald's *Heart Disease. A Textbook of Cardiovascular Medicine* (1), the recommendation was given to "tailor the degree of physical activity depending on the symptoms" in the patient with congestive failure. Furthermore, "the patient is urged to remain active, short of becoming symptomatic." Also, Cohn, in a review of the therapies for patients with heart failure, gave the following advice regarding exercise (15):

> traditional advice to the patient with heart failure has been to avoid exercise and maintain a sedentary existence. It is now clear that such striking restriction of exercise leads to deconditioning that may adversely affect exercise tolerance. Careful exercise training in patients with heart failure can augment peak exercise capacity and improve the comfort with which submaximum exercise can be carried out.

However, in a cautionary note, this same author went on to state "what is not yet proved is whether this improvement in exercise capacity can be accomplished without having an adverse effect on the prognosis of the syndrome by virtue of some aggravation of ventricular dysfunction by chronic increases in workload" (15).

Recent studies have documented the role of exercise training in patients with chronic heart failure. No large-scale multicenter study involving hundreds of patients, however, has been carried out specifically in patients with heart failure. Nevertheless, enough evidence is now in hand to help the health care profession involved in cardiac rehabilitation formulate a program for patients with heart failure. The generally poor prognosis of the heart failure patient compared with patients participating in a rehabilitation program with normal ventricular performance should be emphasized. The natural history of the heart failure patient is not good. Therefore, complications and even death in patients with heart failure participating in a rehabilitation program are to be expected. Tailoring of the program to meet the unique needs of the heart failure patient is essential. Careful documentation of each patient's performance as they participate in a training program will be required. Even more than other patients entering a rehabilitation program, documentation of the clinical stature of the heart failure patient is essential. Specifically, information regarding the function of the ventricle (assessed by invasive techniques at cardiac catheterization or noninvasive echocardiographic or radionuclide studies) should be made available to the cardiac rehabilitation professional. Furthermore, the assessment of ventricular irritability by 24-h Holter monitoring should be sought. Additionally, this patient group, by definition, is at high risk and telemetered monitoring of each exercise session seems advisable. In addition, as will be evident from review of the study by Jugdutt (17), a certain group of patients needs to be approached cautiously for cardiac conditioning following acute myocardial infarction.

The most extensive physiological measurement of the impact of exercise training in patients with heart failure comes from the investigators at Duke University (12,13). These studies were carried out in 16 patients with chronic heart failure as evidenced by a baseline left ventricular ejection fraction averaging only 24%. Functional classification I was seen in two patients, class II in eight, and class III in six. Nine of the patients had underlying coronary artery disease, and in seven patients the heart failure was due to idiopathic cardiomyopathy. Patients were invited to participate in a traditional phase II cardiac rehabilitation program lasting 16–24 weeks. Exercise sessions were carried out three times per week at an intensity of 75% of the peak effort at the baseline graded exercise test evaluation. Although 16 patients entered the program, four patients (25%) dropped out prior to completion. One drop out occurred because of an orthopedic injury, but the other three were for cardiovascular concerns. Two of the patients had increasing heart failure symptoms and could not complete the program. In one patient, sudden death occurred. Therefore, in three of 16 patients with chronic heart failure, cardiovascular problems prevented completion of a phase II rehabilitation program.

Twelve patients completed the program with significant improvement occurring. Specifically, $VO_{2\,max}$ increased on average 26%. Peak workload increased by 18%, and exercise duration also showed an 18% increment. In addition, in this small number of patients, a trend toward an increased peak cardiac output of 11% was also documented ($p = 0.13$) (Table 3). As with patients undergoing cardiac rehabilitation not manifesting congestive heart failure, these patients showed improved peripheral adaptation to exercise training. There was a sta-

Table 3 Results

	Baseline	Training	Change	p
$VO_{2\,max}$ (ml/kg/min)	1.11	1.40	+26	0.01
Peak workload (kpm/min)	520	613	+18	0.02
Exercise time (s)	582	690	+18	0.03
CO peak exercise (L/min)	8.9	9.9	+11	0.13

tistically significant increase in peak leg blood flow as well as peak leg VO_2 differences (Table 4). The correlation between an increase in the maximum cardiac output and an increase in exercise training $VO_{2\,max}$ was strong (R = 0.6). An even stronger correlation (R = 0.67) was seen between the hours of exercise training and increased VO_2. The increase in peak exercise VO_2 did not, however, develop until 75 or more days of training had occurred and then showed persistent improvement through the 165 days of the training study. Central or cardiac adaptations to exercise training were also measured using direct hemodynamic measurement as well as radionuclide techniques. No change in rest or exercise measurements of the left ventricular performance occurred. The authors (12,13) also measured the ventilatory anaerobic threshold and found it to be delayed to a statistically significant degree as a result of training. A measure of submaximum workload using a constant protocol also showed a significant increase in the exercise duration from 938 s at baseline to 1429 s at the end of

Table 4 Results

	Baseline	Training	Change	p
Leg PVO_{2diff}, peak	14.5	16.1	+11	0.07
Systemic AVO_2, peak (ml/dl)	13.1	14.6	+11	0.05
Peak leg blood flow (L/min)	2.5	3.0	+20	0.01

the training period. In addition, the pulmonary capillary wedge pressures did not change in the trained patients.

These elegant studies establish that a training effect can indeed occur in patients with limited left ventricular performance as a result of exercise training. The authors conclude that

> exercise training improved maximum exercise tolerance in ambulatory patients with chronic heart failure attributed to left ventricular systolic dysfunction. A major element of the training response involved peripheral adaptations. In some patients, increased peak cardiac output also contributed to improved exercise performance.

These studies also help to clarify the important question as to why patients with heart failure are limited by their symptoms. The authors (12,13) conclude "skeletal muscle anaerobic metabolism, and not increased pulmonary capillary wedge pressure, is the major limiting factor during submaximum endurance exercise in stable patients with chronic heart failure."

Investigators at the University of Pittsburgh have recently studied 65 patients with chronic heart failure in a phase II rehabilitation program (16). Patients participated in a 12-week outpatient program three sessions per week. The initial intensity of effort was between 50 and 75% of peak VO_2 and in the final 10 weeks the intensity increased to 75–80%. Twenty-five of the 65 subjects had impaired left ventricular ejection fraction defined as resting <0.4. Eleven of these 25 patients also showed ischemic ST-segment depression during the initial preexercise treadmill test. Interestingly, the subjects with an impaired ejection fraction and a concurrent positive treadmill ischemic ST-segment change at baseline did not show statistically significant $VO_{2\,max}$ improvement as a result of their participation in the phase II cardiac rehabilitation program. However, the low left ventricular ejection fraction group showing no ischemic ST-segment change on initial treadmill testing did document a statistically significant improvement in peak VO_2 levels (44% increase). The 1-year follow-up data report also showed five deaths occurred, all in the patients with an ejection fraction under 40% (five of 25 patients, or 20% 1-year mortality). It would appear from this study that the value of exercise training in the post–myocardial infarction patient having both impaired left ventricular performance and ischemia as evidenced by ST-segment depression on initial treadmill testing may not show a training effect from cardiac rehabilitation.

Jugdutt's study of exercise training in patients with congestive failure is instructive as well (17). This was a study of 13 patients surviving an anterior wall myocardial infarction. They participated in a standard phase II 12-week cardiac rehabilitation program. An additional group of 24 patients having had an anterior Q-wave myocardial infarction served as a nonrandomized control group. The exercise program was conducted three times per week for 12 weeks. At baseline, all patients had a measurement of asynergy of the left ventricular using a two-dimensional echocardiography. The patients showing >18% asynergy at baseline echocardiogram were compared with patients showing lesser degrees of asynergy. The patients also had radionuclide measurement of the resting left ventricular ejection fraction (LVEF). The patients with greater degrees of asynergy had a mean LVEF of 0.42 compared with 0.56 in those showing less asynergy. Also, the patients with greater asynergy had considerably higher peak creatinine phophokinase levels at the time of infarction compared with those showing less asynergy (2200 versus 900) (Table 5). The peak exercise duration increased in both groups. Specifically, the group with less asynergy showed a 91% increase in the peak exercise duration after 12 weeks of training and the group with greater asynergy had a 100% increase. However, echocardiographic and left ventricular ejection fraction measurements at the end of training showed disturbing results. Specifically, the group with greater asynergy at baseline increased the percent of asynergy from 32 to 40% as measured at the end of 12 weeks of phase II cardiac rehabilitation training. Corresponding with this increase in echocardiographic asynergy was a deterioration of radionuclide resting LVEF from 43 to 30%. Both of these measures of deterioration of ventricular function achieves statistical significance ($p < 0.05$) (Table 6). In the control group of patients with

Table 5 2-D echo Determined Baseline Asynergy (Akinesia and/or Dyskinesia), Resulting in 4 groups (Asynergy <18 or ≥18%)

	Exercise groups		Control groups	
	1	2	3	4
% asynergy	6 ± 6	32 ± 6	9 ± 6	26 ± 5
LVEF	59 ± 4	43 ± 7	54 ± 7	40 ± 4
Peak CK	747 ± 344	2305 ± 1230	1295 ± 1160	2071 ± 863

Table 6 Changes

	Exercise groups		Control groups	
	1	2	3	4
Total work During GXT (W)	378 → 725[a]	350 → 700[a]	Not done	
% asynergy	none	32 → 40%	None	None
LVEF	none	43 → 30%	None	None

[a] p < 0.05.

greater degrees of asynergy at baseline, no deterioration by echocardiographic or radionuclide measurement was seen. Specifically, even in patients who showed diminished LVEF and asynergy of >18% at baseline showed no further deterioration of these two measurements of ventricular performance when measured 12 weeks later without the intervening exercise program (the control group). Furthermore, patients showing less asynergy and having an average ejection fraction of 0.56 at baseline showed no deterioration of ventricular performance with 12 weeks of exercise training. The authors (17) of this important paper conclude

> the results support the view that exercise training might be injurious in patients with extensive transmural infarction that is not healed completely. Equally important, echocardiographic measures identify those patients in whom low level exercise training did not have an adverse effect on left ventricular function and topography.

This was the first study to carefully assess and measure the impact of exercise training in patients following a transmural anterior myocardial infarction and placed in a standard phase II exercise training cardiac rehabilitation program within 15 weeks of the infarction. The cardiac rehabilitation professional must be aware of this important single study on this critical issue pertaining to the timing and intensity of cardiac rehabilitation training in patients surviving acute myocardial infarction, but with diminished left ventricular performance and high degrees of ventricular asynergy.

CONCLUSIONS

Congestive heart failure is an important and multifaceted cardiovascular challenge. Its prevalence has not diminished over the last 20 years as has been the case for coronary artery disease mortality and stroke mortality. Three million or more individuals manifest congestive heart failure annually in the United States, from which over 400,000 deaths occur. As our population ages and as acute myocardial infarction management keeps people from dying from cardiogenic shock, the number of patients with congestive heart failure may very well increase in the decade ahead. The emerging understanding of alterations in physiology in the patient with heart failure and the various therapeutic options to limit the sequelae of this disease will be essential in the management of this growing clinical problem. Pharmacological and nonpharmacological treatment measures need to be specifically tailored to the individual patient's pathophysiological status. Furthermore, documentation of the impact of the therapeutic endeavors needs to occur and serve as a guide to alteration of the therapeutic plan. Rehabilitation of patients with congestive heart failure has gone from an overly cautious avoidance of this important parameter of therapy to a carefully administered and documented use of exercise training in this high-risk patient group. Studies over the next decade should bring about increasing information to help guide the cardiac rehabilitation professional in the optimum management of the patient with congestive heart failure.

REFERENCES

1. Braunwald, E., *Heart Disease. A Textbook of Cardiovascular Medicine.* Saunders, Philadelphia (1988).
2. Criteria Committee, New York Heart Association, *Diseases of the Heart and Blood Vessels. Nomenclature and Criteria for Diagnosis.* 6th Ed. (1964).
3. Franciosa, J.A., Wilen, M., Ziesches, et al., *Am. J. Cardiol.,* 51: 831–836 (1983).
4. Kannel, W.B., Plehn, J.F., and Cupples, L.A., *Am. Heart J.,* 115: 869–875 (1988).
5. Nicod, T., et al., *Cardiol.,* 61: 1165–1171 (1988).
6. Dennick, L.G., et al. *N. Engl. J. Med.,* 317: 1350 (1987).
7. The CONSENSUS Trial Study Group, *N. Engl. J. Med.,* 316: 1429–1435 (1987).

8. Pfeffer, M.A., et al., *N. Engl. J. Med., 319*: 80–87 (1988).
9. Sharpe, N., et al., *Lancet, 8550*: 255–259 (1988).
10. Port, S., et al., *Circulation, 63*: 856–863 (1981).
11. Pilote, L., et al., *Circulation, 80*: 1636–1641 (1989).
12. Sullivan, M.J., et al., *Circulation, 78*: 506–515 (1988).
13. Sullivan, M.J., et al., *Circulation, 79*: 324–329 (1989).
14. Wyngaarden, J.B., and Smith, L.H., *Cecil Textbook of Medicine.* Saunders, Philadelphia (1982).
15. Cohn, J.N., *Circulation, 78*: 1099–1107 (1988).
16. Arvan, S., *Am. J. Cardiol., 62*: 197–201 (1988).
17. Jugdutt, B.I., et al., *J. Am. Coll. Cardiol., 12*: 362–372 (1988).

13

Exercise and Children with Congenital Heart Disease

David S. Braden

Portsmouth Naval Hospital
Porstmouth, Virginia

William B. Strong

Medical College of Georgia and Georgia Prevention Institute
Augusta, Georgia

INTRODUCTION AND PURPOSE

Children differ from adults in their responses to exercise.
Children with congenital heart disease (CHD) differ from healthy children in their responses to exercise.

The purpose of this chapter will be fourfold:

To review the effects of CHD on the responses to both acute and chronic exercise
To summarize the mechanisms by which exercise performance is altered in children with CHD
To review accepted recommendations for preparticipation evaluation and athletic participation in these children
To briefly discuss the effectiveness of rehabilitation of children with "corrected" CHD

REVIEW OF NORMAL CARDIOVASCULAR RESPONSES TO UPRIGHT EXERCISE IN CHILDREN

In healthy children, dynamic upright exercise causes a predictable increase in oxygen consumption (VO_2) with increasing intensity of exercise—increasing 10- to 12-fold from rest to maximum exercise. This is accompanied by a three- to fourfold increase in cardiac output from rest to maximum. Heart rate increases steadily two- to threefold from rest to maximum (1,2). Stroke volume increases during the first one-third to one-half of a graded maximum exercise test (GXT), and plateaus thereafter (3). Figure 1 summarizes the normal cardiovascular responses to exercise in healthy children.

Peripheral vasodilatation occurs with dynamic exercise, causing a fall in systemic vascular resistance (SVR). Although the systolic blood pressure increases in response to dynamic exercise, the falling SVR causes the diastolic blood pressure to change minimally. As a result, excessive increases in mean arterial pressure are prevented. Figure 2 summarizes the blood pressure and systemic vascular resistance responses to exercise in healthy children.

In contrast, isometric exercise causes an increase in the systemic vascular resistance with less marked increases in cardiac output. The mean arterial pressure increases to a much greater degree with isometric exercise compared to dynamic exercise (4,5).

MECHANISMS OF DIMINISHED EXERCISE PERFORMANCE IN CHILDREN WITH CONGENITAL HEART DISEASE

The "international gold standard" for the determination of the maximal aerobic capacity or exercise capacity is the maximum oxygen consumption ($\dot{V}O_{2\,max}$). The relationship between the $\dot{V}O_{2\,max}$ and the cardiovascular responses to exercise is summarized by the following

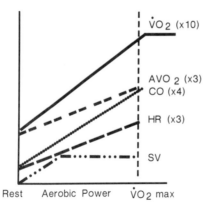

Figure 1   Normal cardiovascular responses to exercise in healthy children.

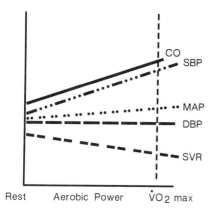

Figure 2 Blood pressure and systemic vascular resistance responses to exercise in healthy children.

equation: $\dot{V}O_{2\,max} = SV_{max} \times HR_{max} \times (C\bar{a}O_2 - C\bar{v}O_2)_{max}$. Owing to abnormalities of one or more of these variables, children with congenital heart disease (CHD) may have diminished exercise performance (6).

A subnormal maximal *stroke volume* (SV_{max}) response may occur for various reasons. The SV_{max} may be hindered by altered ventricular geometry or by outflow obstruction (arotic stenosis, pulmonic stenosis, tetralogy of Fallot). Children with aortic stenosis or insufficiency may have impaired coronary perfusion. Deficient contractility may be the cause of a subnormal SV_{max} in children with cardiomyopathies or deconditioning. In children with ventricular septal defects (VSDs), the "forward" SV_{max} may be deficient due to left-to-right shunting. Residual defects after surgery may also alter the SV_{max} by any of the above mechanisms.

The maximum cardiac output (CO_{max}) and, therefore, the $\dot{V}O_{2\,max}$ may also be diminished secondary to chronotropic insufficiency. This diminished maximal heart rate (HR_{max}) response to exercise may either be primary in nature or secondary to medication. In children with congenital complete heart block (CHB), the ventricular rate response to exercise may be inadequate, thereby hindering exercise performance. Chronotropic insufficiency may also be present in children with cyanotic or admixture lesions. Hypoxemia has been implicated as a common etiology for this blunted HR_{max}, but this does not explain the persistence of this blunted response after surgical repair. Other possible causes for the persistently diminished HR_{max} include: intrinsic abnormalities of autonomic control of the heart rate, sinus node dysfunction after cardiopulmonary bypass, conduction disturbances such as bundle branch blocks, and persistent abnormalities of ventilation and pulmonary function. Children on β-blockers for ventricular dysrhythmias for the prevention of hypercyonotic episodes in tetralogy of Fallot may also have diminished exercise performance secondary to chronotropic insufficiency.

A diminished arterial oxygen content ($C\bar{a}O_2$) may also limit exercise performance. Children with cyanotic CHD will exhibit resting cyanosis and/or desaturation with exercise. Accompanying respiratory or chest wall abnormalities may also lower the $C\bar{a}O_2$ and limit the $\dot{V}O_{2\,max}$. Oxygen transport may also be hindered by anemia or hyperviscosity secondary to polycythemia. Table 1 summarizes these mechanisms of altered exercise performance.

Table 1 Mechanisms of Altered Exercise Performance in Children with Congenital Heart Disease

SV_{max}[a]	HR_{max}[b]	$CaO_{2\,max}$[c]
Altered ventricular geometry	Medications (β-blockers)	Cyanotic lesions
Outflow obstruction	Complete heart block with inadequate ventricular rate	Respiratory of chest wall abnormalities
Impaired coronary perfusion	Hypoxemia	Polycythemia
Deficient contractility	Autonomic dysfunction	Anemia
Left-to-right shunting	Sinus node dysfunction	
	Conduction abnormalities	

Comparison of death by specific cause in patients treated with Enalapril versus placebo in the double-blind study of patients with class IV heart failure. The reduction in death favoring the Enalapril-treated group resulted entirely from diminished death due to progression of congestive heart failure (7).

[a] Maximal stroke volume.

[b] Maximal heart rate.

[c] Arterial oxygen content.

RESPONSES TO ACUTE EXERCISE

The typical responses to acute exercise will now be considered—both prior to and after surgical repair.

Pressure Overload Lesions

Table 2 summarizes the characteristic exercise responses in children with pressure overload lesions—both preoperatively and postoperatively.

Aortic Stenosis

Aortic stenosis (AS) is one of the few pediatric lesions in which physical exertion may be detrimental. However, the occurrence of detrimental events is related to the severity of the lesion and is strongly associated with the symptomatic complaints of dyspnea on exertion (DOE) and easy fatigability (7,8). Effort-induced syncope in children with AS is not completely understood, but it is presumably secondary to cerebral ischemia due to low CO. Children who can increase their CO and systolic blood pressure (SBP) at low exertional levels may have an abrupt decrease in both these variables at higher levels of exertion (9). This may be secondary to a sudden decrease in peripheral vascular resistance in nonexercising muscles due to a reflex response to the activation of baroreceptors in the left ventricle (10).

Chest pain has been reported in 5–10% of children with aortic stenosis associated with ST-T–wave changes of subendocardial ischemia. This is most likely secondary to an inequality of myocardial oxygen supply and demand. Sudden death in aortic stenosis is rare, but it has been reported in 1–7% of young people with AS. Although most cases have occurred at rest, in some there has been a temporal connection between exertion and sudden death (7,11). Most of these have been associated with a history of symptoms; i.e., fatigability, DOE, syncope, and exertional chest pain. These represent the severe end of the spectrum of the lesion and virtually all have had ST-T–wave changes of subendocardial ischemia on resting ECGs.

In spite of these risks, exercise testing is being used with increasing frequency in the pediatric population with AS (12). The risk of exercise is much less than in adults, in whom AS is considered a relative contraindication to exercise. Catheterization has long been considered the best method of determining the severity of AS—by the measurement of the pressure gradient and the calculation of aortic valve area. However, exercise testing together with Doppler echocar-

Table 2 Characteristic Exercise Responses in Children with Pressure Overload Lesions

	Aortic stenosis		Coarctation		Pulmonic stenosis	
	preop	postop	preop	postop	preop	postop
HR	Normal; increase with increasing severity	Normal to slightly decreased	Normal	Normal	Normal	Normal
SBP	Very high	High	Very high	High	Normal	Normal
DBP	Normal	Normal	Normal	Normal	Normal	Normal
PP	Very high	High	Very high	High	Normal	Normal
Pressure gradient	Very high	Minimally increased	Very high	Variable	High	Minimally increased
SV	Low	Normal to minimally decreased			Low	Normal to minimally decreased
CO	Low	Normal to minimally decreased			Low	Normal to minimally decreased
PWCI	Normal; increases with increasing severity	Normal to slightly decreased	Normal to slightly decreased	Normal	Normal	Normal to slightly decreased
Ischemia, Occasional	Common; increases with increasing severity	Frequent	Occasional	Occasional	Occasional	
Dysthythmia, Occasional	Rare	Occasional	Rare	Rare	Rare	

Change in functional status of survivors at 6 months after random double-blind assignment to Enalapril versus placebo. All patients started as functional class IV. Seventy-two percent of survivors in the Enalapril group improved their functional status compared with only 47% in the placebo group (7).
Abbreviations: HR = heart rate, SBP = systolic blood pressure, DBP = diastolic blood pressure, PP = pulse pressure, SV = stroke volume, CO = cardiac ouput, PWCI = physical work capacity index (all values at maximum exercise).

diography is helpful in determining which patients need catheterization and as an adjunct to catheterization in determining the functional severity of AS. Exercise is helpful, primarily by identifying abnormalities of hemodynamic function and detecting the presence of myocardial ischemia.

The classic triad of abnormalities seen in response to exercise testing in children with AS include (13):

Subnormal blood pressure response; i.e., <35-torr rise of SBP
"Ischemic" response on electrocardiogram
Decreased working capacity

These findings have both a high specificity and sensitivity for identifying those children who need surgery as well as identifying those who may be at risk for syncope and sudden death.

The systolic blood pressure normally increases with dynamic exercise parallel to the increase in CO. In children with significant AS, SBP may increase subnormally, by as much as 50 torr less than expected (12,14–18). Occasionally, there may be no change or even a fall in SBP with increasing intensity of exercise. Any of these findings are an indication for catheterization even if the child is asymptomatic. Because the diastolic blood pressure changes little or increases slightly, exercise may also yield a low pulse pressure.

The left ventricular systolic pressure (LVSP) may be exceedingly high with exercise in severe AS. Because of the increase in LVSP and the subnormal or falling SBP, the left ventricular outflow tract (LVOT) gradient is exceedingly high—as much as 20–25 torr higher than that observed at rest (15,19). The maximum LVOT gradient may reflect the degree of AS more than any other physiological function. The left ventricular end-diastolic pressure (LVEDP) may increase greater than 3 torr from rest (19).

Figure 3 graphically demonstrates the left ventricular and aortic pressure responses to acute exercise in children with AS.

Children with significant AS often have a low resting SV which can barely increase with exercise (10). Therefore, any increase in CO with exercise is almost entirely dependent upon an increase in HR. Cardiac output at submaximal and maximal exercise is low (20). The low CO_{max} is the major cause of the low maximal aerobic power seen in children with significant AS. Other causes for a diminished working capacity included a low myocardial oxygen supply as well as detraining secondary to parental and patient overprotection. However, most children with mild and even moderate AS have working capacities which are well within the range of normal (20–22).

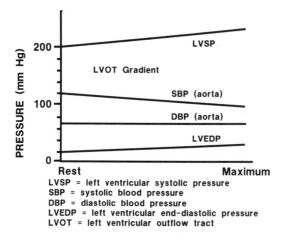

Figure 3   Left ventricular (LV) and aortic pressure responses to acute exercise in children with aortic stenosis.

The exercise ECG is more sensitive than the resting ECG for the identification of ST depression in children with AS. The pathological nature of ST depression during exercise has been correlated with measurements of the LV oxygen supply/demand ratio in the catheterization laboratory (23,24). Figure 4 demonstrates the P-R method of measuring J-point depression during exercise testing.

Demand increases with increasing exercise intensity, with the supply limited by the increased LVEDP and the shortened diastolic filling time. Chandramouli observed that ST changes are generally indicative of an LVOT gradient ≥50 torr (25). Lewis et al. observed that prolonged subendocardial ischemia may result in permanent

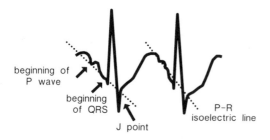

Figure 4   The P-R method of measuring J-point depression during exercise testing.

fibrotic replacement of LV muscle (24). Therefore, those children with ST depression indicative of subendocardial ischemia should strongly be considered as surgical candidates.

Postoperative exercise testing is useful for the longitudinal follow-up of residual impairment. Generally, if there is adequate relief of the LVOT obstruction, the signs of myocardial ischemia resolve (12) and the SBP (19) and the physical working capacity index (PWCI) increase progressively toward normal. The degree of improvement is often related to the severity of obstruction preoperatively (13). Although the postoperative exercise-induced ST depression is not as reliable as preoperative changes in predicting the LVOT gradient, the exercise test may help identify those with residual LV dysfunction as evidenced by:

Decreased PWCI
Subnormal SBP_{max}
Submaximal HR_{max}

Coarctation of the Aorta

Exercise-related complaints observed in children and adolescents with coarctation (COA) include calf pain during intense jumping or running and exertional dyspnea and fatigability—especially in those with comcomitant left-to-right shunts (6). Most children with COA should have surgery. Exercise testing is helpful in deciding the urgency of surgical repair (26). The SBP in the arm may be extremely high in the unoperated patient performing strenuous activity with levels of 250–300 torr not being uncommon (26–28). The higher the SBP_{max}, the greater the urgency of surgery. The DBP response to exercise is generally normal, producing a markedly increased pulse pressure and mean arterial pressure in the arteries proximal to the coarctation.

Concomitant upper and lower extremity blood pressures can be used to predict the pressure gradient across the coarctation. This gradient may increase markedly with exercise, exceeding 120 torr (26). The LVEDP may also increase during exercise. There may also be evidence of subendocardial ischemia (6,13).

Exercise testing is probably more valuable postoperatively. Surgery generally abolishes the gradient across the coarctation site. However, surgery is no guarantee against the subsequent development of hypertension. Exercise testing may help identify hypertension in postoperative patients with or without resting hypertension (13). This may be an indication for antihypertensive medication. Exercise testing may also help identify those patients with residual coartation. ST depression may be observed in patients with residual obstruction or exercise-induced hypertension (29). Although further study is needed, adolescents and young adults with ST depression after coarctectomy may be at increased risk for the development of coronary artery disease (30).

Pulmonic Stenosis

Exercise testing is a valuable diagnostic tool in children with pulmonary stenosis (PS) as an indicator of the need for valvotomy and a tool for the functional evaluation of the child after surgical repair. Although not as commonly as with AS, children with significant PS may complain of exertional dyspnea and easy fatigability.

The most consistent pressure-related abnormality ́in children with PS is an increased RV peak systolic pressure at rest and especially during exercise. This occurs secondary to valvar narrowing and compensatory RV hypertrophy. There is a weak relationship between the degree of valvar narrowing and the magnitude of the exercise-induced increase in the RV peak systolic pressure. The RVOT gradient also increases with exercise, inversely proportional to the cross-sectional area of the valve (31–33).

The RV end-diastolic pressure (RVEDP) increases with exercise in proportion to the degree of stenosis (33–36). Normally, there is no change in RVEDP with exercise. This increase in RVEDP may reflect decreased RV myocardial compliance secondary to RV hypertrophy. Figure 5 graphically summarizes the changes in right ventricular pressures with acute exercise in children with PS.

The increase in SV and CO with increasing exercise intensity are subnormal, especially in severe PS. At submaximal work loads, there

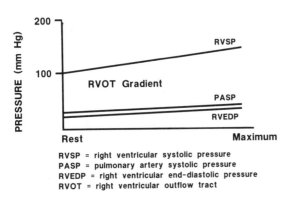

RVSP = right ventricular systolic pressure
PASP = pulmonary artery systolic pressure
RVEDP = right ventricular end-diastolic pressure
RVOT = right ventricular outflow tract

Figure 5   Right ventricular and pulmonary arterial pressures changes observed with exercise in children with pulmonic stenosis.

may be a compensatory increase in O_2 extraction and the arterio-venous O_2 difference (AVO_{2diff}), with resultant normal submaximal working capacity. At maximal workloads, HR and O_2 extraction can no longer increase, and maximal aerobic power is diminished. A sub-normal CO_{max} and a VO_{2max} indicate the need for surgery or valvulo-plasty, especially when associated with an increased RVEDP.

Exercise responses consistent with successful valvotomy or val-vuloplasty include the following (32,36,38):

A decreased exercise RVOT gradient
A normal RV peak systolic pressure
Normal RVEDP (32,36)
Adequate increases in SV and CO

The ability to increase SV in response to exercise determines the improvement in the working capacity after repair (38). The earlier the repair, the more encouraging are the exercise responses. The above-favorable responses are not always seen in those repaired as adults, possibly secondary to decreased RV compliance from long-term myo-cardial fibrosis (39). Table 3 summarizes the cardiovascular responses to exercise in children with volume overload lesions.

Volume Overload Lesions

Left-to-Right Shunts

Functional severity in a child with a ventricular septal defect (VSD) is dependent upon the size of the defect and the presence or absence of pulmonary artery hypertension (40,41). Most children with significant defects have surgery prior to 2 years of age. Therefore, there is limited information regarding the exercise responses in these children. Chil-dren with small shunts and no pulmonary hypertension have no symptoms at rest or with exercise. They have normal HR and blood pressure responses to exercise with no ischemia or dysrhythmias. The PWCI is usually normal (41). Those children with larger shunts more often have exercise-induced complaints; e.g., exertional dyspnea and easy fatigability. The PWCI in these children is seldom > 25th percen-tile for age (40). Exercise may also increase the magnitude of the left-to-right shunt (42).

In the child with associated pulmonary hypertension, there is often a marked increase in mean pulmonary artery pressure with exer-cise, often to suprasystemic levels. There is a decrease or even a rever-sal in the left-to-right shunt (43), with a marked increase in the ratio of pulmonary to systemic vascular resistance.

Table 3 Characteristic Exercise Responses in Children with Volume Overload Lesions

	VSD		ASD		Aortic[a] insufficiency	Aortic[a] insufficiency
	preop	postop	preop	postop		
HR	Normal	Normal	Normal	Normal	Variable; decreased with increasing severity	Variable; decreased with increasing severity
BP	Normal	Normal	Normal	Normal	Greater than normal	Normal to accentuated
PWCI	Usually normal	Normal to slightly decreased	Normal	Normal to slightly decreased	Decreased with increasing severity	Decreased with increasing severity
Ischemia	Rare	Rare	Rare	Rare	Common	Occasional
Dysthythmia	Rare	Occasional	Rare	Occasional	Rare	Occasional

Outcome of a 16- to 24-week Phase II cardiac rehabilitation program in patients with heart failure. Improvement in exercise capacity was statistically significant and a positive upward trend in cardiac output at peak exercise was also noted (12,13).
Abbreviations: HR = heart rate, BP = blood pressure, PWCI = physical work capacity index (all values at maximum exercise).

[a] Preoperative data only

Postoperative exercise assessment in the child with a VSD is valuable for the evaluation of inappropriately low CO_{max}, elevated pulmonary artery pressures, and rare dysrhythmias. The PWCI generally normalizes in the child with a large defect and subnormal aerobic power preoperatively. There is an inverse relationship between the age of repair and the degree of improvement in hemodynamic function. In general, children who are repaired prior to age 10 years have better myocardial function and respond to intense exercise with less intense increases in pulmonary artery pressure (42).

Responses to exercise are similar in children with atrial septal defects (ASDs). Most children are asymptomatic with a few with larger defects complaining of fatigability during exercise and play. Responses to acute exercise are generally normal in children with small defects (40,41,45). With increasing magnitude of the left-to-right shunt, there is an increasing likelihood of diminished aerobic power. In one study, 33% of children with a large ASD performed ⩽ the 10th percentile for age on a Bruce treadmill test (40). Although data varies, some children will have an increase in the magnitude of the left-to-right shunt with exercise (42,45).

Older children with an ASD and associated pulmonary hypertension are especially handicapped when exercising. In these patients, the magnitude of the intracardiac shunt does not seem to affect the responses to exercise.

Postoperative assessment of the child with an ASD typically reveals a normal PWCI (40). If surgical repair is postponed until adulthood, the CO_{max} and PWCI may be subnormal after repair. Postoperative exercise assessment may help identify those children and young adults with inappropriately low CO_{max} and PWCI as well as help in the evaluation of the rare child with a postoperative dysrhythmia.

Regurgitant Lesions

Exercise testing can be useful as a management tool in children with mitral or aortic insufficiency—as an aid in determining the time of surgical intervention. Especially with aortic insufficiency, there are few clear-cut hemodynamic measurements to use as markers for intervention. The possibility exists that myocardial injury may be sustained while the clinician awaits "signs" that the valve should be replaced. With increasing hemodynamic severity of the regurgitant lesions, the child has a progressive decrease in maximal aerobic power. The child has a lower heart rate at each workload. This lower HR allows for an increased regurgitant fraction. Especially worrisome is the appearance of ST depression suggestive of diminished coronary flow. ST charges herald the possible development of degenerative changes of the myocardium and signify the need for strong consideration of surgical intervention (46).

Cyanotic/Admixture Lesions

Virtually all children with cyanotic congenital heart disease have diminished exercise performance. Children with complex cyanotic defects, e.g., univentricular heart, Ebstein's anomaly, and tricuspid atresia, respond to exercise testing with diminished maximal aerobic power, progressive hypoxemia, and subnormal heart rate and blood pressure responses (47–50). Exercise electrocardiography reveals ischemia and dysrhythmias. After Fontan and Mustard procedures, the PWCI improves significantly but it is still less than normal (50–58). Blood pressure and chronotrapic responses may remain subnormal; electrocardiographic abnormalities may persist. Similar abnormalities are seen in children with Ebstein's anomaly, with the exception that ischemia is less frequently observed.

Both cardiovascular and pulmonary factors contribute to decreased exercise tolerance in children with tetralogy of Fallot. The high RVOT gradient and right-to-left shunt lead to decreased pulmonary blood flow (PBF) and progressive hypoxemia with exercise. Although many of these children have a decreased response to hypoxemia at rest, most respond to exercise-related desaturation with hyperventilation (59). The increased pulmonary ventilation combined with a diminished PBF leads to a large physiological dead space.

These children respond to exercise with increases in RV peak systolic pressure, RVEDP, and the RVOT pressure gradient (20,60). Exercise causes increased contractility of both ventricle with a decrease in forward flow through the RVOT. Pulmonary blood flow decreases because of a decrease in systemic vascular resistance and a fixed or increasing obstruction of the RVOT and increased right-to-left shunting (68). Progressive arterial desaturation results secondary to the increased right-to-left shunt and progressively less saturated venous blood.

Palliative surgery (Blalock-Taussig shunt) leads to increased lung perfusion, but the exercise responses remain abnormal (61). The saturation of the venous blood decreases because of increased peripheral extraction caused by the demands of exercise. Figure 6 graphically summarizes these responses in a child with tricuspid atresia and a Blalock-Taussig shunt. Total correction produces a reduction in the

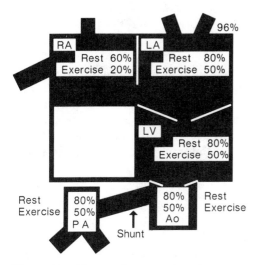

Figure 6   Changes in saturations in response to acute exercise in a child with tricuspid atresia and a Blalock-Taussig shunt.

RVOT gradient, the RV peak systolic pressure, and the RVEDP; an increase in pulmonary blood flow; and an abolition of the intracardiac shunt. Exercise testing in the postoperative patient generally serves two purposes:

Determination of physical working capacity (functional improvement)
Prediction of the potential for developing ventricular dysrhythmias

Following repair of tetralogy of Fallot, most children have a marked improvement in maximal aerobic power with PWCI values approaching normal (40,62–68). There is an inverse relationship between maximal aerobic power and age of repair (62,67,68). In those who have persistently diminished maximal aerobic power, there are several possible reasons for the lack of normalization, including (6):

Residual pulmonic stenosis and/or insufficiency
Decreased myocardial compliance secondary to hypertrophy and scar-
    ring, resulting in an increase of RVEDP with exercise
Persistent desaturation secondary to a residual right-to-left shunt, pul-
    monary vascular obstructive disease from a previous systemic-to-
    pulmonary shunt, or deficient gas exchange
Anatomical defects such as RVOT aneurysm or the incision itself
Sedentary lifestyle and detraining

These residual defects may be more apparent during exercise. The HR_{max}, SV_{max}, and CO_{max} may be persistently subnormal, further limiting the $\dot{V}O_2$max.

Twenty to 30% of postoperative children with tetralogy may have ventricular dysrhythmias (64), and may be at risk for sudden death. Exercise testing in conjunction with Holter monitoring performed intermittently may help to identify some children at risk for sudden death. It may also serve as a guide for the need of antiarrhythmic therapy and help delineate which children should avoid strenous activity.

Mitral Valve Prolapse

Exercise testing may be useful in the child with mitral valve prolapse (MVP) to identify any relationship between chest pain and increased cardiac output. It may also serve to induce associated dysrhythmias. Schwartz observed frequent premature ventricular contractions (PVCs) in three of 30 8- to 12-year-old children with MVP (70). Six of 30 of these children had PVCs during recovery.

Ischemic changes are also observed, but many of these may be false-positive responses. Otherwise, children with MVP had normal exercise parameters. At times, maximal aerobic power may be limited by the child and/or the parent. Performing a GXT_{max} in the presence of the parents may be psychologically therapeutic.

Dysrhythmias

Congenital Complete Heart Block

In children with complete heart block (CHB), the atrial rate is normal at rest and increases normally in the response to submaximal and maximal exercise. The ventricular rate is low at rest and often rises little with exertion. It increases in proportion to the workload, but independently of the atrial rate (71,72); seldom exceeding 100-120 beats/min. There is poor correlation between the resting ventricular rate and the ability of the ventricular rate to increase with exercise (71–74). Figure 7 demonstrates a typical chronotropic response to exercise in a child with CHB.

The stroke volume is usually greater than normal both at rest and during exercise (73,74). The cardiac output may be low normal at rest because of the slow ventricular rate, and may increase subnormally in response to exercise (74,75). The ability of these children to increase $\dot{V}O_2$ in response to exercise is highly dependent upon their ability to

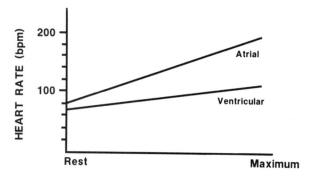

Figure 7 Typical chronotropic response to exercise in a child with complete heart block.

increase oxygen extraction from capillary blood, thereby increasing their $AVO_{2\,diff}$. Those who can increase neither their $AVO_{2\,diff}$ or CO become highly fatigued with exercise (74). Low physical working capacity is now appreciated as an indication for pacemaker implantation.

Premature ventricular contractions and other ventricular ectopy are also frequent (30–70%) (71,72,74) with exercise, but rare at rest. The occurrence of ventricular ectopy is positively related to age and the level of exercise, but negatively related to working capacity (78). Exercise testing may help identify those patients at risk for life-threatening dyshythmias or syncopal attacks. It also may help measure the potential of the child to increase CO and cope with the metabolic demands of even daily activities. In those children who are obviously incapacitated, pacemaker placement is indicated without the need of exercise testing. Children who complain of mild fatigue, exertional dyspnea, or dizziness should undergo a submaximal exercise test that would increase the HR to 160–170 beats/min in a healthy child. If the ventricular rate increases <50% over resting values, pacemaker placement is probably indicated.

Tachydysrhythmias/Extrasytoles

Exercise testing may also be useful in the provocation, characterization, and therapeutic evaluation of cardiac dysrhythmias. It is most commonly used in the evaluation of ventricular ectopy. Children with benign premature ventricular contractions (PVCs) have structurally normal hearts and PVCs at rest that decrease or disappear with exercise—often reappearing in the immediate recovery period (1,78). On the other hand, ventricular ectopy induced or exacerbated by exercise may be the first indication of an underlying cardiac abnormality such as subclinical cardiomyopathy, arrhythmogenic right ventricular dysplasia, coronary anomalies, or mitral valve prolapse (1,79,80).

Supraventricular tachycardia (SVT) may also be unmasked by exercise testing (78). The rate response of SVT may be enhanced by exercise stress. Exercise testing may help predict the antegrade effective refractory period in Wolff-Parkinson-White syndrome (81), and help to identify those children requiring electrophysiological testing. It has also been reported to uncover the existence of multiple accessory pathways (82).

Exercise testing may also help in evaluating the response to pharmacological therapy in children with tachydysrhythmias (78–80). It is a useful adjunct for athletic preparticipation evaluation in such individuals (83).

ATHLETIC PARTICIPATION

What level of activity can the child with CHD tolerate? What about the child with "repaired" CHD—what intensity level can he or she tolerate? These are frequently asked questions of the pediatric cardiologist.

Before being allowed to participate in competitive athletics, the child with CHD needs a recent history and physical examination. A recent electrocardiogram (ECG) and chest radiograph (CxR) are recommended and are generally helpful. Other tests that may be needed prior to participation include: echocardiographic (Echo) and Doppler assessment; graded exercise test (GXT); 24-h ambulatory electrocardiography (Holter); and, infrequently, a cardiac catheterization with angiography. A child with CHD should not be excluded from sports participation by anyone other than their pediatric cardiologist. The pediatric cardiologist best understands the individuals defect, the demands of the sport, and the psychological profile of the child.

The Bethesda Task Force Report (1984) (84) delineated general and specific recommendations regarding athletic participation in children with CHD. In general, all sports, including high physical-intensity sports, are usually permissible in children with mild disease (84). Moderate physical intensity sports are usually safe in children with moderate disease, but individual evaluation is generally required (84). In children with severe CHD, strenuous exercise might be detrimental, leading to irreversible worsening of their cardiovascular status or possibly sudden death (84). Table 4 presents a classification of sports based on aerobic and isometric intensity as well as the potential for collisions.

Pressure Overload Lesions

Aortic Stenosis

In children with aortic stenosis (AS), permissible activities are determined by the type of the activity and the severity of the lesion as evidenced by the left ventricular outflow tract (LVOT) gradient. In the asymptomatic child, all low-intensity or recreational activities are permitted unless there is LV strain on the resting ECG or ST depression or ventricular dysrhythmias during GXT.

In the child with mild AS (LVOT gradient ≤20 torr), participation is allowed in high-intensity or competitive activities if the following are present (84):

Normal resting ECG
Normal PWCI, blood pressure, and rhythm responses to GXT without ischemia
No cardiomegaly
Normal LV function (echocardiogram, angiogram, or nuclear assessment)
No arrhythmia at rest, with exercise or Holter (Lown grade ≤2)

The child with moderate AS (LVOT gradient 21–39 torr) should be allowed to participate in low-intensity sports (84). High-intensity sports with moderate static and low dynamic demands are permissible if the following are present:

Mild or no LVH and no LV strain on resting ECG
Normal GXT
No arrhythmias at rest, with exercise, on a Holter

Such a child should have a yearly assessment that includes echocardiographic assessment of LV pressure and function, a continuous wave Doppler estimate of the LVOT gradient, and a GXT. If this evaluation indicates progression of disease, repeat catheterization is indicated. Catheterization is also generally repeated past a child's rapid growth spurt in adolescence. Participation in competitive sports is not allowed in the child with severe AS (LVOT gradient ≥40 torr) (84).

In the symptomatic child with AS, the guidelines are not as clear cut. Activity should be limited if the child relates a history of syncope or chest pain (6). In the child with dyspnea on exertion or fatigability, if there is a normal ECG and no other objective evidence of advanced

Table 4 Classification of Sports

I. Intensity and type of exercise performed
  A. High to moderate intensity
    1. High to moderate dynamic and static demands
        Boxing
        Crew/rowing
        Cross-country skiing
        Cycling
        Downhill skiing
        Fencing
        Football
        Ice hockey
        Rugby
        Running (spring)
        Speed skating
        Water polo
        Wrestling

    2. High to moderate dynamic and low static demands
        Badmiton
        Baseball
        Basketball
        Field hockey
        Lacrosse
        Orienteering
        Ping-pong
        Race walking
        Racquetball
        Running (distance)
        Soccer
        Squash
        Swimming
        Tennis
        Volleyball

    3. High to moderate static and low dynamic demands
        Archery
        Auto racing
        Diving
        Equestrian
        Field events (jumping)
        Field events (throwing)
        Gynmastics
        Karate or judo
        Motorcycling
        Rodeoing
        Sailing
        Ski jumping
        Water skiing
        Weight lifting

432

Table 4   (continued)

 B. Low intensity (low dynamic and low static demands)
    Bowling
    Cricket
    Curling
    Golf
    Riflery

II. Danger of body collision
    Auto racing[a]
    Bicycling[a]
    Boxing
    Diving
    Downhill skiing[a]
    Equestrian[a]
    Football
    Gynmastics[a]
    Ice hockey
    Karate or judo
    Lacrosse
    Motorcycling[a]
    Polo[a]
    Rodeoing[a]
    Rugby
    Ski jumping[a]
    Soccer
    Water polo[a]
    Water skiing[a]
    Weight lifting[a]
    Wrestling

Statistically significant improvement in measures of peripheral adaptation with exercise training in congestive heart failure patients as a result of a 16- to 24-week Phase II cardiac rehabilitation program (12,13).

[a] Increased risk if syncope occurs.

Source: From Ref. 84; used with permission.

obstruction, deconditioning may be the cause of low maximal aerobic power (6). In such a child, moderate-intensity activity may be helpful in conditioning.

Postoperatively, the predictive value of diagnostic exercise testing is less than preoperatively (85). Such children should undergo a periodic noninvasive assessment every 1–2 years with CxR, ECG,

GXT, echo, and Holter. The child with a trivial resting LVOT gradient can engage in all competitive sports based upon the criteria used preoperatively for mild AS (84). The child with moderate residual AS may engage in low-intensity sports as well as some high-intensity sports (moderate static/low dynamic) if the following are present (84):

Normal to minimally increased heart size
No to mildly increased LV function on echo or angiogram
Normal to mild aortic insufficiency
Normal exercise test
No ventricular arrhythmias at rest, during GXT, or on Holter

Coarctation of the Aorta

In the child or adolescent with unoperated coarctation, the risk of aortic rupture from the trauma of athletics must be taken into consideration (86). Likewise, the clinician has to consider the long-term effects of hypertension in these patients on ventricular function and the risk of cerebrovascular accidents (87,88). If the degree of obstruction is mild and there is no evidence of collaterals or aortic root dilatation, low-intensity activity is allowed if exercise testing is normal (normal PWCI, rhythm, and HR response, and normal maximal upper extremity blood pressure) (84). In selected cases, participation is allowed in some high-intensity (moderate dynamic/low static) activities. *No collision sports are allowed* (84). Participation is not allowed in competitive sports if there is evidence of hypertension at rest or with exercise.

Minimal evaluation in the operated patient includes CxR, ECG, GXT, and assessment of LV function by echo, angiogram, or nuclear imaging. Participation is allowed in competitive sports 6 months postrepair, and in collision sports 12 months postrepair if the following are present (89,90):

No resting blood pressure (BP) gradient between upper and lower extremities
Normal BP at maximal exercise
Minimal or no hypertrophy on ECG or echo
Normal LV function

Pulmonic Stenosis

Recommendations for participation in sports in the child with pulmonic stenosis (PS) are based upon the severity of the obstruction. The child with mild PS is typically asymptomatic with a typical auscultatory complex (ejection sound, short systolic ejection murmur), a normal ECG or mild right ventricular (RV) enlargement, and a normal CxR except mild pulmonary artery dilatation. Minimal evaluation in these children is an annual or biannual history and physical examination. In the child with clinical evidence of more severe PS, the minimal evaluation includes the following (84):

Hemodynamic assessment of the right ventricular outflow tract (RVOT) gradient in the catheterization laboratory
Assessment of RV function by echo, angiogram, or nuclear imaging
Continuous wave Doppler estimation of the RVOT gradient

If the peak systolic RVOT gradient is less than 50 torr and the RV function is normal, participation is allowed in all competitive sports (84). If the gradient is equal to or greater than 50 torr and there is evidence of RV dysfunction, surgical or balloon intervention is likely. However, participation in some low-intensity sports may be allowed in more moderate cases (84).

Minimal evaluation is the same in the postoperative patient. Participation in all competitive sports is allowed 6 months postrepair if there is noninvasive evidence of mild residual PS (84). This interval may be even shorter if balloon valvuloplasty is utilized for relief of the obstruction. If there is moderate to severe residual PS (RVOT gradient $\geqslant 50$ torr), low intensity sports alone are allowed (84).

Volume Overload Lesions

In the child with a ventricular septal defect (VSD), decisions regarding athletic participation are based upon the size of the defect and the presence or absence of pulmonary arterial hypertension. In the child with a small VSD (Qp/Qs < 1.5) participation is allowed in all competitive sports (84). Participation is allowed in all low-intensity sports in the child with a moderate VSD (Qp/QS = 1.5–2.0) and normal pulmonary vascular resistance (PVR). If the defect is large (Qp/Qs > 2) and the PVR is normal, participation is allowed in some low-intensity sports (84). In moderate or large VSDs with elevated PVR, participation in competitive sports is not recommended (84).

In the postoperative patient, minimal preparticipation evaluation should include CxR, ECG, GXT, and Holter. A repeat catheterization is needed if pulmonary hypertension is present preoperatively. In those children without residual VSDs, participation in all competitive sports is allowed 6 months postoperatively if the following are present:

Normal pulmonary artery pressures
Normal Holter (Lown grade $\leqslant 2$)
Normal GXT (no ventricular arrhythmias and normal PWCI)
Minimal or no hypertrophy on ECG

Low-intensity activity alone is allowed if there is evidence of a moderate or large residual VSD. If there is persistent pulmonary hypertension, participation in competitive sports is not recommended (84).

Most children with an atrial septal defect (ASD) will have repair before they are old enough for competitive sports. However, this is not always true owing to increasing participation by younger children in youth sports programs. If there is no evidence of pulmonary hypertension, participation is allowed in all competitive sports (84). If pulmonary hypertension is suggested by examination or ECG, catheterization is recommended prior to any decision regarding activity (84). If pulmonary hypertension (mean pulmonary artery pressure >20 torr) is present, low-intensity sports alone are recommended.

Postoperatively, minimal evaluation includes CxR, ECG, and Holter. A catheterization is also required if there was preoperative pulmonary hypertension. Competition is allowed 6 months postrepair if the sternotomy is well healed and *none* of the following are present:

Mean pulmonary artery pressure >20 torr
Sinus node dysfunction as evidenced by symptomatic bradycardia/ tachycardia syndrome at rest or on Holter
Complete AV block
Cardiomegaly on CxR (Cardiothoracic ratio >0.55)

If any of these are present, the child can still participate in low-intensity sports (84).

In the child with a small patent ductus arteriosus, i.e., no symptoms, normal heart size, and normal ECG, participation is allowed in all competitive sports (84). If the examination, CxR, and ECG suggest a moderate or large patent ductus arteriosus (PDA, GXT, Holter, echo and possibly catheterization may be needed prior to allowing the child to participate in low-intensity sports) . Ligation of the PDA is required prior to unrestricted competitive participation.

The postoperative patient with no symptoms and normal examination, CxR, and ECG may participate in all competitive sports 6 months postoperatively (84). If there was pulmonary artery hypertension preoperatively, catheterization will be required with restricted activity if there is persistent pulmonary hypertension.

Cyanotic/Admixture Lesions

The child with unrepaired cyanotic congenital heart disease often limits his or her own activity because of dyspnea and easy fatigability.

Therefore, recommendations are less necessary regarding athletic participation in this group of children. The discussion will, therefore, be limited primarily to the child or adolescent who has undergone palliation or correction of his or her heart disease. For those children with uncorrected and unpalliated defects who desire to do so, participation in low-intensity sports alone is recommended (84,91–93).

Palliative surgery often provides significant relief of symptoms at rest. However, these children may still experience arterial desaturation during sports activities (49,92,93). Therefore, participation should generally be limited to low-intensity sports. More moderate activities may be included in selected cases if the following are present (84):

Arterial saturation >80% with exercise
No arrhythmia at rest, with exercise, or on Holter
Mild or no chamber dilatation on CxR or echo
Nearly normal PWCI

Recommendations regarding activity after corrective surgery are dependent upon the type of defect and the surgery. The child with corrected tetralogy of Fallot may have persistent abnormalities without obvious symptoms, including:

Residual RV/PA gradient
Fibrotic RV
Persistent VSD

Such children may be at risk for sudden death with exercise (64). Minimal evaluation in these children should include CxR, ECG, GXT, and Holter. Catheterization is indicated if there is any suggestion of persistent RV hypertension. Yearly reevaluation is recommended with special attention to the late development of dysrhythmias.

In general, participation in low-intensity activity is allowed 6 months postoperatively with participation in all competitive sports if the following are present (84):

Almost normal RV pressure (peak RV systolic ⩽40 torr) at rest and
    ⩽70 torr with supine exercise to a HR of 120 beats/min; RV end-
    diastolic pressure ⩽8 torr at rest
No persistent right-to-left shunt
No or very small VSD with Qp/Qs <1.5
No ventricular dysrhythmia at rest or with exercise; Lown grade 0 or 1
    on Holter
Minimal or no cardiac enlargement on CxR
Normal ventricular function by echo, angiogram, or nuclear imaging

If the RV is *mildly* dilated or has *mildly* diminished function, low-intensity sports alone are recommended (84). However, in selected cases, more moderate-intensity sports are allowed if the following are present (84):

Normal or nearly normal exercise duration
No ventricular dysrhythmia at rest, with exercise, or on Holter

Some work has been done regarding habitual activity in adolescents with corrected tetralogy. Lambert, using a 6-month recall of physical activity, found no difference between postrepair males and healthy male controls (66). Female patients attended fewer physical education classes with significant correlations with lower $VO_{2\,max}$ values. In another study, only 50% of adolescents postrepair participated in physical activities at school (73).

Children and adolescents who have undergone the Fontan procedure for correction of tricuspid atresia or a univentricular heart may feel well, but are likely to have limited exercise capacity. Participation in competitive athletics is, therefore, not likely to be an issue. Minimal evaluation prior to participation in any activity should include CxR, ECG, GXT, and an evaluation of LV function. If there is no evidence of cardiomegaly or dysrhythmia, participation is allowed in low-intensity sports (84). Participation is allowed in less-intensity sports in selected cases if the following are present (84):

Nearly normal PWCI
No ventricular or supraventricular (SVT) dysrhythmia at rest or during
    GXT
No ventricular dysrhythmia (Lown grade >1), SVT, or severe sinus
    bradycardia on Holter
No signs of congestive heart failure
No arterial desaturation <80% with exercise
Normal or nearly normal LV function

The adolescent or young adult who has undergone a Mustard or Senning procedure for transposition of the great vessel (d-TGA) may feel healthy and wish to compete in sports. However, several persistent abnormalities and concerns are present, including (84):

Abnormal systemic (RV) function
Limited cardiac output with exercise
The risk of sudden death from atrial dysrhythmias or sinus node dys-
    function
The possibility of deterioration in RV function with training

Increased vagal tone with training and the possible deleterious effect
   of sinus bradycardia
Unknown effect of dilatation and hypertrophy from conditioning

Because of these concerns, no high physical–intensity isometric or
aerobic sports are recommended (84).
   Minimal preparticipation evaluation in this group should include
CxR, ECG, echo, GXT, Holter, and catheterization. These should be
repeated yearly with the exception of catheterization, with special
attention paid to the late development of arrhythmias (84). Almost all
of these patients should be allowed to participate in moderate- and
low-intensity sports. They can engage in high to moderate dynamic
and low-static activities if the following are present (84):

No cardiac enlargement on CxR
Normal ECG except for low-voltage P-waves and RVH; no conduction
   disturbances, junctional rhythm, or atrial dysrhythmias
Normal or nearly normal RV size and function
No SVT or severe sinus bradycardia on Holter
No ventricular dysrhythmia, SVT, or bradycardia during GXT

   Included in this section are those children with pulmonary vascular obstructive disease (PVOD) secondary to Eisenmenger's syndrome
or primary pulmonary hypertension. These children are at particularly
high risk of sudden death during sports activities. Children with progressive PVOD experience resting cyanosis and intense cyanosis with
exercise. Exertion may also produce symptoms of right-sided heart
failure and complex ventricular dysrhythmias. Therefore, these children *should not* participate in competitive sports because of the greatly
increased chance of sudden death even without physical activity.

Mitral Valve Prolapse

Sudden death has been reported in mitral valve prolapse (MVP), but it
is exceedingly rare (94–99). As of 1985, only three cases of sudden
death with exercise had been reported (94,96,96)—only one of these
was a trained athlete (97). Therefore, a child or adolescent with MVP
should be allowed to participate in all competitive sports if none of the
following are present (84):

History of syncope
Family history of sudden death secondary to MVP
Chest pain exacerbated by exercise

Repetitive ventricular ectopy or sustained SVT, particularly if worsened by exercise

Moderate or marked mitral insufficiency

Associated dilatation of the ascending aorta in those rare instances when Marfan's syndrome is also present

If any of the above are present, participation in low-intensity sports may be allowed.

Congenital Complete Heart Block

Habitual activity in the child with complete heart block (CHB) may be self-determined or may be limited by the ventricular response to exercise. A sedentary lifestyle may also be imposed by the parent(s) (74).

Exercise testing is useful as a guide to determine participation in activities. In general, to participate in normal daily activities, a doubling of the ventricular HR with maximal exercise is needed. There are numerous descriptions of young people with CHB who have been able to *compete* in athletics (100–102). Other factors that may affect physical activity include:

The presence or absence of additional cardiac defects

The presence of ventricular ectopy with exercise

The child's ability to increase cardiac output or peripheral oxygen extraction during exercise

The child's motivation

REHABILITATION OF CHILDREN WITH CONGENITAL HEART DISEASE

Although data are limited, many authors have shown the children with CHD may be able to improve their aerobic power through rehabilitative training. Goldberg et al. evaluated the effect of physical training on exercise performance following surgical repair in 16 patients with tetralogy of Fallot and 10 patients with ventricular septal defects (103). They observed a 25% improvement in maximum work capacity after a 6-week training program without a significant increase in $\dot{V}O_2$. James et al. demonstrated normal exercise tolerance in postoperative tetralogy patients who actively engaged in competitive athletics (104). Ruttenberg et al. observed a significant improvement in maximal treadmill performance (time and stage) in patients with postoperative tetralogy, AS, and transposition of the great arteries (d-TGA) and atrioventricular canal (105). Similar to the results of Goldberg et al.,

Table 5 Effect of Rehabilitation on Exercise Performance in Children with CHD

Ref.	Lesion	Surgery	Work capacity	VO_{2max}
103	Tetralogy of Fallot	Complete repair	25%	No Change
	Ventricular septal defect	Complete repair	Increase	No Change
104	Tetralogy of Fallot	Complete repair	Improved	——
105	Tetralogy, AS, TGA, AVC	Complete repair	Improved	No Change
106	TGA	Mustard	Improved	Improved
	Tetralogy	Complete repair	Improved	Improved

Baseline measurement of patient's surviving anterior transmural myocardial infarction determined within 3 months of infarction. Peak CK levels at the time of infarction are also designated. The authors arbitrarily stratified patients based upon percent left ventricular asynergy documented during resting echocardiogram ($<$ versus $\geq$ 18% asynergy). Values are mean plus and minus 1 standard deviation with groups one and three being patients with asynergy $<$18% (17).

Abbreviations: AS = aortic stenosis, TGA = transposition of the great arteries, AVC = Atrioventricular canal, VO_{2max} = maximum oxygen consumption.

the improved treadmill performance was not associated with a change in $\dot{V}O_{2\,max}$. Bradley et al. demonstrated a significant improvement in both treadmill time and $\dot{V}O_{2\,max}$ in five patients who had undergone a Mustard procedure for TGA and in four patients posttetralogy repair (106). These findings are summarized in Table 5.

REFERENCES

1. Christiansen, J.L., and Strong, W.B., in *Heart Disease in Infants, Children and Adolescents* (F.H. Adams, G.C. Emmanouilldes, and T.A. Riemenschneider, eds.). Williams & Wilkins, Baltimore, pp. 93–106 (1989).
2. Braden, D.S., and Strong, W.B., in *Youth Exercise, and Sport* (C.V. Gisolfi and D.R. Lamb, eds.). Benchmark Press, Indianapolis, pp. 293–333 (1989).
3. Astrand, P.O., and Rodahl, K., *Textbook of Work Physiology: Physiological Basis of Exercise.* 3rd Ed. McGraw-Hill, New York (1986).
4. Nutter, D.O., Schlant, R.C., and Hurst, J.W., *Mod. Concepts Cardiovasc. Dis., 41*: 11–15 (1972).
5. MacDougall, J.D., Tuxen, D., Sale, D.G., et al., *J. Appl. Physiol., 58*: 785–790 (1985).
6. Bar-Or, O., *Pediatric Sports Medicine for the Practitioner: From Physiologic Principles to Clinical Applications.* Springer-Verlag, New York (1983).
7. Doyle, E.F., Arumugham, P., Lara, E., Rutkowski, M.R., and Kiely, B., *Pediatrics, 53*: 481–489 (1974).
8. Wagner, H.R., Weidman, W.H., Ellison, R.C., and Miettinen, D.S., *Circulation, 56*(Suppl. 1): 20–23 (1977).
9. Flamm, M.D., Braniff, B.A., Kimball, R., and Hancock, E.W., *Circulation, 35, 36*(Suppl. II): 109 (1967) (Abst.).
10. Mark, A.L., Dioschos, J.M., Abboud, F.M., et al., *Clin. Invest., 52*: 1138–1146 (1973).
11. Jokl, E., *Med. Sport, 5*: 148–149 (1971).
12. James, F.W., and Kaplan, S., *Primary Cardiol., 3*: 34 (1977).
13. James, F.W., Blomquist, C.G., Freed, M.D., Miller, W.W., Moller, J.H., Nugent, E.W., Riopel, D.A., Strong, W.B., and Wessel, H.U., *Circulation, 66*: 1377A–1397A (1982).
14. Alpert, B.S., Kartodihardjo, W., Harp, P., et al., *J. Pediatr., 98*: 763–765 (1981).
15. Cueto, L., and Moller, J.H., *Br. Heart J., 35*: 93–98 (1973).
16. Hossack, K.F., and Neilson, G.H., *Aust. NZ J. Med., 9*: 169–173 (1979).
17. Riopel, D.A., and Hohn, A.R., *Pediatr. Res., 11*: 163 (1977) (Abst.).
18. James, F.W., Schwartz, D.C., Kaplan, S., et al., *Am. J. Cardiol., 50*: 769–775 (1982).
19. Orsmond, G.S., Bessinger, F.B., Moller, J.H., *Am. Heart J., 99*: 76–86 (1980).

20. Taylor, M.R.H., The Response to Exercise of Children with Congenital Heart Disease. Ph.D. Thesis, University of London (1972).
21. Cumming, G.R., In *Frontier of Activity and Child Health* (H. Lavallee and R.J. Shephard, eds.). Pelican, Quebec, pp. 17–45 (1977).
22. Goldberg, S.J., Weiss, R., Kaplan, E., and Adams, F.H., *J. Pediatr.*, 69: 56–60 (1966).
23. Kveselis, D.A., Rocchini, A.P., Rosenthal, A., et al., *Am. J. Cardiol.*, 55: 1133–1139 (1985).
24. Lewis, A.B., Hymann, M.A., Stanger, P., et al., *Circulation*, 49: 978–984 (1974).
25. Chandramoule, B., Ehmke, D.A., and Lauer, R.M., *J. Pediatr.*, 87: 725 (1975).
26. Taylor, S.H., and Donald, K.W., *Br. Heart J.*, 22: 117–139 (1960).
27. James, F.W., and Kaplan, S., *Circulation*, 49, 50(Suppl. II): 27–34 (1974).
28. Cumming, G.R., and Mir, G.H., *Br. Heart J.*, 32: 365–369 (1970).
29. James, F.W., Kaplan, S., and Schwartz, D.C., *Am. J. Cardiol.*, 37: 145 (1976) (Abst.).
30. Maron, B.J., Redwood, D.R., Hirshfeld, J.W., et al., *Circulation*, 48: 864–874 (1973).
31. Cumming, G.R., and Mir, G.H., *Can. J. Physiol. Pharmacol.*, 47: 137–142 (1969).
32. Finnegan, P., Ihenacho, H.N., Singh, S.P., and Abrams, L.D., *Br. Heart J.*, 36: 913–918 (1974).
33. Truccone, N.J., Steeg, C.N., Dell, R., and Gersony, W.M., *Circulation*, 56: 79–82 (1977).
34. Moller, J.H., Rao, S., and Lucas, R.V., *Circulation*, 46: 1018–1026 (1972).
35. Neal, W.A., Lucas, R.V., Rao, S., and Moller, J.H., *Circulation*, 49: 948–951 (1974).
36. Stone, F.M., Bessinger, F.B., Lucas, R.V., and Moller, J.H., *Circulation*, 49: 1102–1106 (1974).
37. Howitt, G., *Br. Heart J.*, 28: 152–160 (1966).
38. Bastanier, C., Kaltwasser, B., and Mocellin, R., *Z. Kardiol.*, 66: 587–593 (1977).
39. Johnson, A.M., *Br. Heart J.*, 24: 375–388 (1962).
40. Cumming, G.R., *Am. J. Cardiol.*, 42: 613–619 (1978).
41. Goldberg, S.J., Mendes, F., and Hurwitz, R., *Am. J. Cardiol.*, 23: 349–353 (1969).
42. Hugenholtz, P.G., and Nadas, A.S., *Pediatrics*, 32: 769–775 (1963).
43. Mocellin, R., Friedman, J., Sebering, W., and Buhlmeyer, K., *Z. Kardiol.*, 64: 1036–1052 (1975).
44. Duffie, E.R., and Adams, F.H., *Pediatrics*, 32: 757–768 (1963).
45. Bay, G., Abrahamsen, A.M., and Muller, C., *Acta Med. Scand.*, 190: 205–209 (1971).
46. Ellestad, M.H., *Stress Testing: Principles and Practice*. 3rd Ed. Davis, Philadelphia (1986).

47. Driscoll, D.J., Mottram, C.D., and Danielson, G.K., *J. Am. Coll. Cardiol.*, *11*: 831–836 (1988).
48. Barber, G., Danielson, G.K., Puga, F.J., et al., *J. Am. Coll. Cardiol.*, *7*: 630–638 (1986).
49. Driscoll, D.J., Staats, B.A., Heise, C.T., et al., *J. Am. Coll. Cardiol.*, *4*: 337–342 (1984).
50. Driscoll, D.J., Danielson, G.K., Puga, F.J., et al., *J. Am. Coll. Cardiol.*, *7*: 1087–1094 (1986).
51. Ben Schachar, G., Fuhrman, B.P., Wang, Y., et al., *Circulation*, *65*: 1043–1048 (1982).
52. Grant, G.P., Mansell, A.L., and Garofano, R.P., *Pedatric. Res.*, *24*: 1–5 (1988).
53. Matthews, R.A., Fricker, F.J., Beerman, L.B., Stephenson, R.J., et al., *Am. J. Cardiol.*, *51*: 1526–1529 (1983).
54. Parrish, M.D., Graham, T.P., and Bender, H.W., *Circulation*, *67*: 178–183 (1983).
55. Benson, L.N., Banet, J., McLaughlin, P., et al., *Circulation*, *65*: 1052–1059 (1982).
56. Musewe, N.N., Reisman, J., Benson, L.N., et al., *Circulation*, *77*: 1055–1061 (1988).
57. Murphy, J.H., Barlai-Kovach, M.M., Matthews, R.A., et al., *Am. J. Cardiol.*, *51*: 1520–1525 (1983).
58. Reybrauck, T., Dumoulin, M., and VanDer Hauwaert, L.G., *Am. J. Cardiol.*, *61*: 861–865 (1988).
59. Taylor, M.R.H., *Clin. Sci. Molec. Med.*, *45*: 99–105 (1973).
60. Godfrey, S., *Exercise Testing in Children. Applications in Health and Disease.* Saunders, Philadelphia (1974).
61. Gold, W.M., Mattioli, L.F., and Price, A.C., *Pediatrics*, *43*: 781–793 (1969).
62. Cumming, G.R., *Br. Heart J.*, *41*: 683–691 (1979).
63. Delisle, G., and Olley, P.M., *Union Med. Can.*, *103*: 886–889 (1974).
64. Garson, A., Jr., Gillette, P.C., Gutgesell, H.P., and McNamara, D.G., *Am. J. Cardiol.*, *46*: 1006–1012 (1980).
65. Hirschfeld, S., Tuboku-Metzger, A.J., Borkat, G., et al., *J. Thorac. Cardiovasc. Surg.*, *75*: 446–451 (1978).
66. Lambert, J., Ferguson, R.J., Gervais, A., and Gilbert, G., *Cardiology*, *66*: 120–131 (1980).
67. Mocellin, R., Bastanier, C., Hofacker, W., and Buhlmeyer, K., *Eur. J. Cardiol.*, *4*: 367–374 (1976).
68. Strieder, D.J., Aziz, K., Zaver, A.G., and Fellows, K.E., *Ann. Thorac. Surg.*, *19*: 397–405 (1975).
69. James, F.W., Kaplan, S., and Chou, T.-C., *Circulation*, *52*: 691–695 (1975).
70. Schwartz, D.C., James, F.W., and Koplan, S., *Circulation*, *52*: 258 (1975) (Abst.).

71. Ikkos, D., and Hanson, J.S., *Circulation, 22*: 583–590 (1960).
72. Thoren, C., Herin, P., and Vavra, J., *Acta Paediatr. Belg., 28* (Suppl.): 132–143 (1974).
73. Mocellin, R., and Bastanier, C., *Z. Kardiol., 66*: 298–302 (1977).
74. Taylor, M.R.H., and Godfrey, S., *Br. Heart J., 34*: 930–935 (1972).
75. Watson, G., Freed, D., and Strieder, J., in *Frontiers of Activity and Child Health* (H. Lavallee and R.J. Shepard, eds.). Pelican, Quebec, pp. 393–400 (1977).
76. Chawla, K., Serratto, M., Cruz, J., et al., *Circulation, 56*(Suppl. III): 171 (1977) (Abst.).
77. Winkler, R.B., Freed, M.D., and Nadas, A.S., *Am. Heart J., 99*: 87–92 (1980).
78. Monarrez, C.N., Strong, W.B., and Rees, A.R., *Paediatrician, 7*: 116–125 (1978).
79. Deal, B.J., Miller, S.M., Scagliotti, D., et al., *Circulation, 73*: 1111–1118 (1986).
80. Bricker, J.T., Traweek, M.S., Smith, R.T., et al., *Am. Heart J., 112*: 186–188 (1986).
81. Bricker, J.T., Porter, C.J., Garson, A., et al., *Am. J. Cardiol., 55*: 1001–1004 (1985).
82. Ya'acov, D., Strasberg, B., Fleischman, P., et al., *Am. Heart J., 112*: 854–855 (1986).
83. Zipes, D.P., Cobb, L.A., Garson, A., et al., *J. Am. Coll. Cardiol., 1225–1232* (1985).
84. Mitchell, J.H., Maron, B.J., Epstein, S.E., et al., *J. Am. Coll. Cardiol., 6*: 1186–1232 (1985).
85. Barton, C.W., Katz, B., Schork, M.A., and Rosenthal, A., *Clin Cardiol., 6*: 473–477 (1983).
86. Jokl, E., and Mackintosh, R.H., *Med. Sport, 5*: 150–152 (1971).
87. Keith, J.D., in *Heart Disease in Infancy and in Childhood* (J.D. Keith, R.D. Rowe, and P. Vlad, eds.). Macmillan, New York, pp. 736–760 (1978).
88. Shearer, W.T., Rutman, J.Y., Weinberg, W.A., and Goldring, D., *J. Pediatr., 77*: 1004–1009 (1970).
89. Carpenter, M.A., Damman, J.F., Watson, D.D., and Beller, G.A., *Circulation, 68*: 111–258 (1983).
90. Connor, T.M., *Am. J. Cardiol., 43*: 74–78 (1978).
91. Szekares, L., and Papp, G., *Acta Physiol. Hung., 32*: 143–162 (1967).
92. Alpert, B.S., Moes, D., DuRant, R.H., and Strong, W.B., *Pediatr. Res., 18*: 117A (1984) (Abst.).
93. Bjaske, B., *Scand. J. Thorac. Cardiovasc. Surg., 16*(Suppl.): 9–26 (1974).
94. Barlow, J.B., Bosman, C.K., Pocock, W.A., and Marchand, P., *Br. Heart J., 30*: 203–218 (1968).
95. Jeresaty, R.M., *Am. J. Cardiol., 37*: 317–319 (1976).
96. Cobbs, B.W., and King, S.B., *Am. Heart J., 93*: 741–758 (1977).
97. Bharati, S., Bauernfeind, R., Miller, L.B., Strasberg, B., and Lev, M., *J.*

Am. Coll. Cardiol., 13: 879–886 (1983).

98. Chesler, E., King, R.A., and Edwards, J.E., *Circulation, 67*: 632–639 (1983).
99. Pocock, W.A., Bosman, C.K., Chesler, E., Barlow, J.B., and Edwards, J.E., *Am. Heart J., 107*: 378–382 (1983).
100. Campbell, M., *Br. Heart J., 5*: 15–18 (1943).
101. Campbell, M., and Emanuel, R., *Br. Heart J., 29*: 577–587 (1967).
102. Fisch, C., *N. Engl. J. Med., 238*: 589–592 (1948).
103. Goldberg, B., Fripp, R.R., Lister, G., et al., *Pediatrics, 68*: 691–699 (1981).
104. James, F.W., Kaplan, S., Schwartz, D.C., et al., *Circulation, 54*: 671–000 (1976).
105. Ruttenburg, H.D., Adams, T.D., Orsmand, G.S., et al., *Pediatr. Cardiol., 4*: 19–24 (1983).
106. Bradley, L.M., Galioto, F.M., Vaccaro, P., et al., *Am. J. Cardiol., 56*: 816–818 (1985).

14

Potential Impact of Cardioactive Drugs

Nanette Kass Wenger

Emory University School of Medicine
Atlanta, Georgia

INTRODUCTION

The spectrum of patients with cardiovascular disease currently considered eligible for exercise training as well as those undergoing exercise testing for diagnosis, for assessment of functional capacity, for evaluation of therapeutic interventions, and for exercise prescription has broadened considerably. Patients arbitrarily excluded from exercise rehabilitation in former years, i.e., elderly individuals, patients with angina or exercise-induced ischemia, those with serious ventricular arrhythmias, and patients with substantial cardiac enlargement, ventricular dysfunction, or compensated congestive heart failure, among others, now constitute an increasing proportion of individuals for whom exercise training is recommended. These medically complex cardiac patients typically receive multiple drugs, many of which have the potential to alter, favorably or adversely, the determinants of exercise performance and the capacity for physical work. The impact of cardioactive drugs on exercise capability as well as exercise-drug interactions have thus assumed compelling importance.

Adapted in part, with permission, from Wenger, N. K., Ischemic heart disease: Exercise training, selected aspects of pharmacologic therapy, and drug-exercise interactions. *Emory J. Med.*, 3: 253 (1989).

HIGHLIGHTS OF EXERCISE PHYSIOLOGY: PATHOPHYSIOLOGICAL ALTERATIONS WITH MYOCARDIAL ISCHEMIA AND VENTRICULAR DYSFUNCTION

Myocardial Oxygen Demand and Exercise

The major determinants of myocardial oxygen demand include ventricular systolic wall tension, the heart rate, and the contractile state of the myocardium. Left ventricular wall tension is determined by both left ventricular pressure and volume; elevation of the systemic arterial pressure (left ventricular pressure) or ventricular dilatation (increased ventricular volume) thus engenders an increase in left ventricular wall tension, and thereby increases myocardial oxygen demand.

Dynamic exercise results in an increase of all of the determinants of myocardial oxygen demand: the heart rate (generally proportional to the intensity of the exercise), myocardial contractility, and ventricular wall tension. In the normal heart, virtually the maximal amount of available oxygen is extracted by resting myocardium; thus, in contrast to skeletal muscle, myocardium cannot respond to an increase in oxygen demand by the extraction of additional oxygen from its perfusing blood. An increase in myocardial oxygen demand can be met only by an increase in coronary blood flow, rendering it the determining factor in increasing oxygen delivery to the myocardium. A decrease in coronary vascular resistance normally occurs in response to an increased myocardial oxygen demand. In young healthy subjects, this decrease in coronary vascular resistance enables an augmentation of coronary blood flow from 60 ml/100 g of left ventricular myocardium at rest to as much as 300 ml/100 g of myocardium at peak exercise.

Exercise-induced tachycardia not only augments myocardial oxygen demand (the cardiac work rate per minute increases with the increase in the heart rate), but it may also limit myocardial oxygen delivery. Rapid heart rates encroach on the percentage of the cardiac cycle allotted to diastole, the predominant period for coronary and myocardial perfusion. Thus, tachycardia concomitantly engenders a progressive increase in the myocardial oxygen demand and a lessened time for the delivery of blood and oxygen to myocardium.

In addition to its effects on the myocardial oxygen demand, exercise may also induce arrhythmias; with exercise there is a progressive lessening of vagal tone with an increase in circulating catecholamines and sympathetic nervous system activity. The latter two factors can enhance myocardial automaticity and late potentials, while shortening myocardial conduction time and refractory periods (1).

Response to Exercise in the Coronary Patient: Factors in the Genesis of Myocardial Ischemia

Atherosclerotic obstruction of the coronary arteries limits their ability to increase coronary blood flow in response to an increase of myocardial oxygen demand. Inadequate delivery of oxygen to the working myocardium results in a variety of pathophysiological responses that underlie the clinical presentations of coronary atherosclerotic heart disease.

As discussed above, the myocardial oxygen supply is determined primarily by the coronary blood flow, and, to a lesser extent, by the arteriovenous oxygen difference. In addition to the duration of diastole (a function of the heart rate), the coronary blood flow is affected by the coronary vascular resistance (whose determinants are a combination of fixed and dynamic coronary arterial obstructive lesions), and by the gradient between the aortic diastolic pressure and the left ventricular end-diastolic pressure (the latter increasing with ventricular dysfunction).

The increase of coronary blood flow is typically insufficient to meet the increased myocardial oxygen demands when atherosclerotic obstruction of the coronary arterial luminal diameter is in excess of 50%. When the blood flow and the resultant oxygen supply are inadequate to meet the increased myocardial oxygen demand, there are manifestations of myocardial ischemia: angina pectoris, ventricular dysfunction with a depressed ejection fraction and a compensatory increase in systolic ventricular volume, and abnormalities of cardiac rhythm.

The ischemic threshold in patients with chronic stable angina can vary with the type of exercise, particularly when dynamic changes in coronary vasomotor tone occur at the site of stenosis. Isometric handgrip can worsen the ischemia, which is reversed by intracoronary nitrates. In other patients, warm-up exercise can increase the ischemic threshold and abrupt onset of exercise can decrease it (1a).

In patients with atherosclerotic obstruction of the coronary arteries, a number of factors influence the balance between the myocardial oxygen supply and demand. Some of these variables have diagnostic value in that exercise-based procedures (exercise testing with and without radionuclide studies) accentuate the discrepancy between myocardial oxygen supply and demand, enabling confirmation of the likelihood of ischemic heart disease. Conversely, a variety of medical interventions used in the management of patients with symptomatic coronary atherosclerotic heart disease—pharmacotherapy and prescriptive exercise training—appear to alter the myocardial oxygen supply/

demand equation favorably by decreasing the myocardial oxygen demand; they limit or control one or more of the factors that increase the myocardial oxygen requirements: increased heart rate, increased blood pressure, and increased myocardial contractility. Alternatively, the blood supply to the myocardium can be increased and the myocardial oxygen supply improved by revascularization procedures that either reduce or bypass the obstructing lesions in the epicardial coronary arteries: coronary angioplasty (PTCA) or coronary bypass surgery (CABG). Both categories of intervention restore the coronary blood flow and improve the myocardial oxygen supply, limiting the difference between the myocardial oxygen supply and demand, and thereby decreasing or eliminating the resultant clinical ischemic syndromes. Improvement in contractile function characteristically occurs in areas of previously ischemic myocardium following revascularization. The degree of residual ventricular dysfunction is typically determined by the extent of prior myocardial infarction and scarring.

Manifestations of Myocardial Ischemia

The most common symptomatic manifestation of myocardial ischemia is the pain of angina pectoris or myocardial infarction. Symptoms and signs of ischemic ventricular dysfunction may also occur.

When an adequate blood supply is present, myocardial glucose and free fatty acids are metabolized by oxidative mechanisms to support the mechanical activity of the heart. If the oxygen supply is inadequate an anaerobic glycolytic pathway is used for energy production. Because of the lesser efficiency of anaerobic glycolysis, areas of ischemic myocardium may show inadequate mechanical activity (poor contractility). Finally, myocardial ischemia may result in electrical instability of the heart, with resultant electrocardiographic abnormalities and disturbances of cardiac rhythm.

The work load required to precipitate manifestations of myocardial ischemia is a reasonable predictor of future coronary events. Thus, exercise testing (with and without a radionuclide or echocardiographic procedure) is used to categorize high-risk patients following a coronary event. Evidence of myocardial ischemia at a low work load, even in asymptomatic patients recovered from myocardial infarction, defines a population with a high risk of recurrent myocardial infarction or sudden cardiac death. This subgroup requires urgent coronary arteriography and subsequent appropriate therapy (2–5). In recent years, risk stratification has assumed particular importance in myocardial infarction patients who have undergone successful thrombolysis. Patients with residual myocardial ischemia at exercise testing must be evaluated for prompt coronary angioplasty or coronary bypass surgery designed to salvage the ischemic myocardium (6,7).

Atherosclerosis of the coronary arteries may result in the loss of the endothelial-dependent vasodilatation with exercise, with exercise-induced vasoconstriction occurring at the site of coronary stenosis.

MECHANISMS BY WHICH ANTIANGINAL (ANTI-ISCHEMIC) DRUGS LIMIT MYOCARDIAL OXYGEN DEMAND: IMPLICATIONS FOR EXERCISE TESTING AND EXERCISE TRAINING

Nitrate Drugs

Nitrate drugs, the oldest class of antianginal drugs, uniformly improves exercise tolerance, so that an increased duration and/or intensity of exercise can be performed prior to the onset of symptoms or signs of myocardial ischemia. Based on these data, physicians traditionally recommend the prophylactic use of nitroglycerin; for example, advising a patient unable to walk a flight of steps without developing angina to use a sublingual nitroglycerin tablet before attempting to do so. The stairs are then typically negotiated without difficulty. Exercise testing confirms that the administration of sublingual nitroglycerin can improve treadmill exercise capacity by as much as 1 MET (metabolic equivalent) (8). Comparable benefit is provided by new formulations, such as chewable, swallowed, or sublingual long-acting nitrate tablets, nitroglycerin ointments, long-acting patch preparations, and oral sprays. However, a nitrate-free interval of several hours is required to prevent the development of nitrate tolerance when long-acting formulations are used (9). The action of nitrate drugs in improving exercise tolerance reflects not only an alleviation of the symptoms of myocardial ischemia, but also an improvement in activity-precipitated ischemic ventricular wall motion abnormalities; enhancement of the ventricular ejection fraction and thereby of cardiac output further increases the exercise capacity (10,11).

When nitrate drugs are administered a number of mechanisms operate concomitantly to limit the myocardial oxygen demand. Nitrate drugs relax vascular smooth muscle. The predominant effect is venodilatation, with a resultant decrease in left ventricular filling pressure and volume (a reduction of the myocardial oxygen demand by reduction of preload). By decreasing left ventricular end-diastolic volume and pressure, nitrate drugs favor coronary collateral flow; coronary collateral vessels are thin-walled conduits, located predominantly in the subendocardium and they are vulnerable to compression when intraventricular pressures are raised during diastole (the major interval for the coronary blood flow). Nitrate drugs limit the elevation of the left ventricular diastolic pressure that is associated with exercise-related angina and probably with spontaneous angina. Nitrate drugs are also arteriolar vasodilators; they decrease peripheral vascular resistance (with a resultant lowering of the systemic arterial pressure), and thereby reduce the left ventricular work load. They improve left ventricular function during isometric exercise in coronary patients with left ventricular dysfunction, presumably by reduction of both the ventricular preload and ventricular afterload (11).

Nitrate-related coronary vasodilatation can increase the myocardial oxygen supply. Although nitrate drugs, administered to normal subjects, result in vasodilatation of the epicardial coronary arteries, the role of vasodilatation in patients with coronary atherosclerotic obstruction is uncertain. Whereas coronary vasodilitation may contribute to an increase of exercise performance prior to the onset of signs or symptoms of myocardial ischemia, nitrates are unlikely to induce coronary vasodiliatation in already ischemic areas of myocardium; myocardial ischemia, per se, is such a potent stimulus to vasodilatation that maximal local vasodilatation may have already been induced by the ischemia. Because nitrate drugs have substantial peripheral effects, they remain beneficial for patients with severe coronary disease who cannot dilate their coronary vessels.

In patients with only a modest severity of angina and myocardial ischemia, administration of nitrates may be sufficient to reduce or eradicate both the symptomatic and the electrocardiographic manifestations of myocardial ischemia at exercise testing (10).

The typical instruction to patients to sit down when using sublingual nitroglycerin has particular importance during exercise training. The patient with substantial exercise-induced vasodilatation who takes several sublingual nitroglycerin tablets may experience nitrate-related hypotension and syncope if not seated. Additionally, the combination of drug and exercise-related vasodilatation may initiate baroreceptor-mediated reflex tachycardia; the resultant increase in the myocardial oxygen demand could increase the angina, despite some concomitant coronary vasodilatation. Further, a seated patient is immediately identifiable to the exercise supervisor(s) as a person requiring attention.

β-Adrenergic Blocking Drugs

β-Blocking drugs are frequently administered to patients who have recovered from myocardial infarction to decrease the risk of both reinfarction and cardiac death (12,13). Further, β-blockade has been shown to increase the chances of survival following thrombolysis (14).

Both cardioselective and noncardioselective β-blocking drugs improve exercise tolerance and decrease the signs and symptoms of myocardial ischemia by reducing the patient's response to catecholamine stimulation. The major effect is a decrease in the exercise-related increases of the heart rate and the systolic blood pessure; that is, a decrease of the exercise rate-pressure or double product, with a lesser diminution of the resting heart rate and systemic arterial blood pressure. Myocardial contractility decreases concomitantly because β-blocked myocardium is less responsive to catecholamine stimulation. Thus, this class of compounds enables patients to exercise to a greater intensity and for a longer duration before they reach the rate-pressure product that previously evoked myocardial ischemia.

The decrease in the heart rate seems a more important contributor to the decrease in the myocardial oxygen demand than the decreases of systemic arterial pressure and myocardial contractility. This is clinically evident as a more dramatic response to β-blockade among patients whose resting heart rates are initially high. The prolongation of diastolic time, attendant on a slowing of the heart rate, allows an improvement in myocardial perfusion, with a particular enhancement of subendocardial coronary collateral flow. If β-blockade leads to an excessive depression of myocardial contractility, as may occur with preexisting borderline ventricular function or ventricular dysfunction at rest, there may be a paradoxical worsening of activity tolerance and increased angina pectoris. Depression of myocardial contractility results in an increased left ventricular filling pressure and volume, with an increase in pulmonary capillary pressure. Because of compensatory cardiac dilatation, an increase in myocardial wall tension is required to initiate contraction; this increases the myocardial oxygen demand, with resultant activity-related myocardial ischemia. Noncardioselective β-blocking drugs may precipitate bronchoconstriction in patients with reactive airways disease, limiting the ability to exercise.

Because β-blockade so effectively reduces the myocardial oxygen demand in patients for whom its application is appropriate, patients who undergo exercise testing for risk stratification while they are receiving β-blocking drugs may not develop the myocardial ischemia that would occur at low intensities of exercise in the absence of such drug therapy. Therefore, the predictive accuracy of risk stratification by exercise testing is decreased in patients who are receiving β-blocking drugs; the early appearance of adverse features retains an unfavorable prognostic significance (15), but some patients may not show exercise intolerance and/or evidence of myocardial ischemia until moderate levels of exercise are reached (15,16). This pharmaco-therapy-modified exercise tolerance may preclude the recognition of some patients at increased risk of recurrent coronary events. Data from serial exercise tests performed for up to 36 months following myocardial infarction in patients with and without metoprolol therapy showed a significantly higher maximal heart rate in the placebo-treated group throughout the study. Termination of exercise due to angina pectoris or ST-segment depression on the ECG occurred more frequently in the placebo group (17).

Exercise training is both feasible and effective in patients of all ages who train while being treated with β-blocking drugs (18). Functional improvements of as much as 30% have been described with both cardioselective and noncardioselective β-adrenergic–blocking drugs in coronary patients as in healthy subjects (19,20). The presumed basis for the increased work load and increased duration of activity achieved prior to myocardial ischemia is that β-blockade does not alter the cardiac, peripheral vascular, or skeletal muscle adaptive responses to exercise training: an increase in oxidative enzymes, an increase in capillary supply, and a decrease in exercise-induced blood lactate levels (21,22) (see below). The lack of change in the anaerobic (lactate) threshold with both selective and nonselective β-blocking drugs suggests that the blood flow to exercising muscles is unaltered by these therapies. This suggests that peripheral vasoconstriction is not an important adverse effect.

Calcium Entry–blocking Drugs

Calcium entry–blocking drugs, the newest class of antianginal (anti-ischemic) drugs, selectively block calcium-dependent excitation-contraction coupling, both in the myocardium and in vascular smooth muscle; they inhibit calcium entry into the conduction system as well. The predominant anti-ischemic effect is due to potent peripheral arteriolar vasodilatation and a resultant decrease in the myocardial oxygen demand (23,24). The decrease in afterload substantially decreases cardiac work. Despite potent coronary vasodilatation, there is only a limited increase in the myocardial oxygen supply following the oral administration of diltiazem. Intracoronary administration of diltiazem decreases the exercise-induced vasoconstriction of stenotic coronary arteries. The vasodilator effect on stenotic vessel segments of diltiazem and nitroglycerin seem additive (25), although the precise mechanisms underlying the vasodilatation remain uncertain.

The three compounds currently available for clinical use in the United States—verapamil, nifedipine, and diltiazem—are characterized by different chemical formulations and differing negative inotropic and electrophysiological properties. Verapamil, which is also an effective agent to correct supraventricular tachyarrhythmias, is most likely to depress atrioventricular conduction; nifedipine characteristically induces considerable tachycardia, secondary to a profound vasodilatation; and diltiazem appears to cause fewer problems with these two aspects than do the other drugs. All may worsen preexisting ventricular dysfunction.

Because this class of compounds so effectively decreases myocardial oxygen demand, exercise test risk stratification has less predictive accuracy for patients thus treated (26). As with the β-blocked patient, calcium-blocking drug therapy may increase exercise tolerance and reduce or delay evidence of myocardial ischemia until moderate levels of exercise have been accomplished. Patients may thus not be recognized as being at high risk, although this would have been evidence prior to the institution of pharmacotherapy. It remains uncertain whether the deferring of an abnormal response to moderate levels of exercise suggests a more favorable outcome while receiving pharmacotherapy.

This class of drugs interacts with a number of aspects of exercise training. Because nifedipine administration often results in an increased heart rate, even at rest, the amount of exercise that can be performed prior to attainment of the prescribed training heart rate range may be limited. Conversely, when verapamil is given, the occurrence of atrioventricular conduction abnormalities may alter the heart rate and require assessment of the exercise prescription.

The profound peripheral vasodilatation resulting from the administration of calcium-antagonist drugs may cause ankle edema, at times sufficiently pronounced to limit the use of this class of agents. Such edema is due to local factors; it may be more prominent in elderly patients with poor tissue turgor, but should not be misconstrued as evidence of heart failure. If this error is made and diuretic drugs are administered, inappropriately, to reduce ankle edema, they will concomitantly reduce the circulating blood volume. When additional exercise-induced vasodilatation occurs, symptomatic hypotension and occasionally syncope may result. The use of support hose is recommended to limit ankle edema. If the dosage of a calcium entry-blocking drug has been increased or diuretic drug has been added to a calcium-blocking drug regimen, it is wise to check the patient's body mass prior to the initiation of exercise. Patients whose weight is less than usual should have their blood pressure assessed in the sitting and standing positions prior to exercise in order to be sure that hypovolemic postural hypotension is not present.

This emphasizes the importance of volume status as a determinant of hemodynamic competence in patients who are receiving drugs with major arteriolar vasodilator effects. Patients who are taking calcium-blocking drugs should be cautioned that any viral or other illness characterized by nausea, vomiting, and diarrhea may result in hypovolemia, with adverse effects upon the ability to exercise; in such circumstances, it is prudent to assess body weight and postural changes in blood pressure prior to the initiation of exercise.

MECHANISMS BY WHICH EXERCISE TRAINING FAVORABLY AFFECTS THE MYOCARDIAL OXYGEN SUPPLY:DEMAND RATIO

Individualized prescriptive exercise is the hallmark of rehabilitative physical activity for the coronary patient. Its major goal is the improvement of cardiorespiratory fitness, with resultant lessening of symptoms and enhancement of functional capacity.

Dynamic exercise training lessens the myocardial oxygen demand by decreasing the heart rate and systolic blood pressure responses to any given submaximal work load. There is a lessened myocardial work load and oxygen demand at any level of total body work and oxygen demand. The main mechanism for functional improvement and a lessening of ischemic symptoms after aerobic training appears to be regulatory changes in the peripheral circulation, adaptations that allow exercise to be performed more efficiently. These include an increase in overall arteriovenous oxygen extraction, a decrease in systemic vascular resistance, and an improved distribution of the cardiac output during exercise; all these responses decrease the demand for oxygen transport. Specific adaptive changes in skeletal muscle include an increased percentage of type I (slow twitch) fibers, an increase in mitochondrial oxidative enzymes, an increase in capillary density around muscle fibers, and an increase in the myoglobin content. The combination of increased oxygen extraction, increased vagal tone, lessened catecholamine release, and probably a number of other factors may decrease the rate-pressure product and other determinants of myocardial oxygen demand by as much as 18%. An added favorable effect of exercise training is an increase in maximal oxygen uptake of about 20%, with even more benefit in previously sedentary or physically unfit patients.

As a result, the symptoms and signs of myocardial ischemia in the exercise-trained coronary patient first appear at a greater work load and/or a long work duration than prior to training. Trained coronary patients function further from their ischemic threshold during usual daily activities; any submaximal task is perceived as requiring a lessened intensity of exertion because it is a lesser percentage of their now increased work capacity. The improvement in functional capacity after exercise training reflects a lessened myocardial oxygen demand for any submaximal task. The patient shows (a) an increase of the maximal oxygen consumption, (b) a lower heart rate and systolic blood pressure at rest, (c) a lesser increase in the heart rate and systolic blood pressure at any submaximal work load, (d) a more rapid return to normal of the heart rate following exercise, (e) lessened or absent angina at work loads that previously induced this symptom, and (f) decreased or absent ST-segment changes on the exercise ECG at work loads that previously precipitated these changes (27–29).

There is little evidence that the moderate-intensity, short-term exercise training typically undertaken by middle-aged or older adults following myocardial infarction or myocardial revascularization procedures improves either myocardial contractility or total ventricular systolic function. Prolonged, high-intensity exercise training has been reported to improve the cardiac function in coronary patients (29–31). The effects of exercise training on the ventricular diastolic function of coronary patients have been less well studied. Further, there is little or no evidence that the coronary collateral circulation or myocardial perfusion improves as a result of dynamic exercise training. Training favorably affects systemic vascular resistance; the increase in systemic vasodilatation that occurs with training is an important contributor to the improved stroke volume and cardiac output.

INTERACTIONS OF COMMONLY USED CARDIOVASCULAR
DRUGS WITH EXERCISE TESTING AND TRAINING

There has been a progressive increase in the use of exercise testing and training in the management of patients with coronary atherosclerotic heart disease, most of whom are likely to be prescribed a variety of cardiovascular drugs.

The exercise-related features of the antianginal (anti-ischemic) drugs—nitrate preparations, β-adrenergic–blocking drugs, and calcium entry–blocking drugs—have been discussed (see below). It appears appropriate to review the drug-exercise interactions of antihypertensive drugs, antiarrhythmic drugs, digitalis, and other preparations used to treat congestive heart failure.

Most evaluations of the functional capacity and of the coronary risk status that involve exercise testing address the heart rate and blood pressure responses to graded intensities of exercise and the resultant symptomatic, electrocardiographic, or other objective abnormalities (including those demonstrated by radionuclide imaging). Typically, both symptomatic and objective responses of the coronary patient relate prominently to changes in the rate-pressure product. Cardiovascular drugs that alter the balance between the myocardial oxygen supply and demand by influencing any of its determinants—but particularly the heart rate and systolic blood pressure—are likely to modify the results obtained at exercise testing and the ability to exercise.

Changes in the exercise electrocardiogram associated with pharmacotherapy may reflect hemodynamic changes, direct effects of the drug on the myocardium, or both. Because the exercise test response and the exercise capacity of many patients with coronary disease are substantially altered by a number of the commonly used cardiovascular drugs, alone or in combination, the effects of pharmacotherapy must be considered when evaluating the results of an exercise test (as discussed above) as well as when prescribing exercise training. In contradistinction to the drug-free state that is desirable for diagnostic and prognostic exercise testing, exercise testing that is undertaken to derive an exercise prescription should be performed with the patient on an optimal medical regimen.

Subsequently, any major change in pharmacotherapy requires repetition of the exercise test and revision of the exercise prescription; this is not only because of the specific consequences of the altered drug therapy, but also because alterations in drug treatment usually reflect an alteration in clinical status. Nonetheless, patients receiving virtually all cardiovascular drugs can undergo exercise testing and the treated individuals retain their capability and suitability for exercise training.

Diuretic Drugs

The potassium-wasting diuretics, predominantly thiazide preparations and loop diuretics, may factitiously suggest myocardial ischemia on the exercise electrocardiogram if hypokalemia has been induced. Hypokalemia-related abnormalities of the ST-segment and T-wave may appear both at rest and with exercise. Diuretic-induced hypomagnesemia may also contribute to an abnormal ECG. Even if serum potassium levels are normal, intracellular potassium levels may be inadequate with magnesium deficiency, since adequate magnesium levels are needed to transport potassium ions across the cellular membrane into the myocytes.

Further, hypokalemia may lead to skeletal muscle weakness and fatigue; the latter may be misinterpreted as a consequence of myocardial ischemia or other causes of cardiac dysfunction, particularly if fatigue limits exercise tolerance. In the patient who is receiving digitalis, hypokalemia may induce arrhythmias both at rest and with exercise. Serum potassium levels increase with vigorous exercise if total body potassium is not depleted, so that an excessive risk of arrhythmia with exercise should not be anticipated.

Excessive diuresis may reduce the circulating blood volume. When exercise-induced vasodilatation also occurs symptomatic hypotension may result from the hypovolemic state.

Antihypertensive Drugs

The ability of the previously hypertensive patient to exercise is improved by virtually all categories of antihypertensive drugs owing to a reducing in both the resting and the exercise-induced cardiac work load when the blood pressure is controlled (32). Antihypertensive drugs lessen the increase in blood pressure induced by both dynamic and isometric exercises.

For patients participating in an exercise regimen, the response to antihypertensive therapy should be checked both at rest and with exercise. Many antihypertensive drugs, including β-adrenergic-blocking drugs, calcium entry–blocking drugs, reserpine, guanethadine, and prazosin, among others, limit the heart rate, autonomic responses, or effect significant vasodilatation. If excessive, these changes may result in exercise-related symptomatic hypertension, dizziness, and even syncope. Alternatively, when there is inadequate control of the blood pressure during exercise, the increased myocardial oxygen demand of the exercise-related hypertension may limit the ability to exercise.

Vasodilator Drugs

Vasodilator drugs have been discussed as therapy for myocardial ischemia and hypertension, but they also figure prominently in the therapy of congestive cardiac failure. Although they produce prompt symptomatic and hemodynamic improvement in the patient with congestive heart failure, they effect little or no immediate objective improvement of exercise tolerance in such individuals. Exercise tolerance, as documented objectively by exercise testing, may improve later; this is postulated to be due in part to alterations in regional blood flow, and in part to a "spontaneous" training effect as the previously sedentary patients, now with an improved symptomatic status, undertake reasonable levels of physical activity.

Vasodilator therapy, administered to the patient with heart failure, is designed to overcome the excessive vasoconstriction that attempts to compensate for the limited cardiac output; "compensatory" vasoconstriction imposes an increased work load on the failing left ventricle. The improvement in exercise capacity attendant on vasodilator therapy, particularly in the patient with myocardial dysfunction and congestive cardiac failure, depends in part on the type of vasodilator agent that is used (33) because the various vasodilator drugs act on different vascular beds and involve different mechanisms of vasodilatation.

Vasodilator drugs such as hydralazine and the calcium entry-blocking drugs act directly on arteriolar smooth muscle, independently of the mechanism or mechanisms causing the vasoconstriction, but they may not improve exercise tolerance even when the symptoms and hemodynamic abnormalities of the heart failure are improved. With exercise, vasoconstriction normally occurs in the renal and splanchnic vascular beds to enhance delivery of blood to the exercising muscles. In patients treated with hydralazine or calcium entry-blocking drugs, these changes in regional blood flow cannot occur because of the direct vasodilator action of the drug upon smooth muscle. The most important mechanism effecting the redistribution of blood flow with exercise appears to be an α-adrenergic—mediated vasoconstriction. When α-adrenergic–blocking drugs such as prazosin are used to overcome the vasoconstriction of congestive cardiac failure, they result in substantial generalized vasodilatation without any diversion of blood flow to the exercising muscle, creating the need for an excessive increase in cardiac output. Energy output is "wasted" when the viscera are perfused during exercise; therefore, improvement of the exercise capacity is either absent or is substantially limited if the patient with heart failure is so treated.

Vasodilator drugs such as the angiotensin-converting enzyme inhibitors counteract the excessive vasoconstriction of congestive cardiac failure by decreasing angiotensin II, vasopressin, and norepinephrine, but they permit normal sympathetic regulation of the vascular tone during exercise; the resultant vasoconstriction of the renal and splanchnic vascular beds decrease the blood flow to the viscera and permits an increased blood flow to the exercising muscle. This in part explains the early improvement in exercise capacity when angiotensin-converting enzyme inhibitor preparations are administered to patients with congestive cardiac failure (34).

Milrinone, a selective phosphodiesterase inhibitor, effects substantial symptomatic improvement in some patients with severe heart failure; however, it remains controversial whether there has been an objective improvement in maximal exercise tolerance (35,36).

Digitalis Glycosides

There is a minimal increase in myocardial oxygen demand when digitalis is administered to normal individuals owing to the increase in myocardial contractility. In contrast, when digitalis is administered to patients with congestive cardiac failure the beneficial effect on the ventricular dimensions, heart rate, and wall tension decreases the net cardiac work load and myocardial oxygen demand despite the increase of myocardial contractility (37,38). The exercise-induced increase of left ventricular end-diastolic pressure seen in the patient with congestive cardiac failure is at least partially corrected after treatment with digitalis.

Digitalis typically accentuates any underlying repolarization abnormalities on the electrocardiogram, and it may produce repolarization abnormalities both at rest and with exercise. Although ST-segment and T-wave changes are dose dependent, repolarization abnormalities may be present even with subtherapeutic dosages of digitalis. Because of these repolarization abnormalities, the predictive accuracy of ST-segment changes with exercise is lessened in patients who are receiving digitalis glycosides. However, the amplitude of

digitalis-induced repolarization abnormalities is greatest at heart rates
between 110 and 130 beats/min, and does not progress with increasing
exercise intensity as is characteristic of the ST-segment abnormalities
of myocardial ischemia (39).

As previously noted, a combination of digitalis therapy and
diuretic-related hypokalemia increases the likelihood of exercise-
related arrhythmias.

Antiarrhythmic Agents

All patients who are receiving antiarrhythmic drugs must be considered at increased risk of arrhythmic complications because of the
characteristics of their underlying clinical problem. Ventricular ectopic
beats pose a greater risk of progression to ventricular tachycardia or
ventricular fibrillation when they are associated with myocardial
ischemia and/or myocardial dysfunction.

All type IA antiarrhythmic agents—quinidine, procainamide,
disopyramide—may, paradoxically, by arrhythmogenic by virtue of
their prolongation of the QT-interval of the electrocardiogram.

Quinidine depresses sinus node function, slowing the heart rate.
It also has a vagolytic effect that increases the heart rate, and an α-
receptor–blocking effect; the resultant vasodilatation and reflex
increase in sympathetic activity further increase the heart rate. The net
result is an increased heart rate at rest and at low levels of activity, but
quinidine has little effect on the heart rate or blood pressure with
moderate- to high-level exercise (40). Neither procainamide nor disopyramide produces significant alterations of the resting or exercise
heart rate and blood pressure (41). However, disopyramide substantially depresses myocardial contractility; patients who are receiving
this preparation require careful surveillance for exercise-induced ventricular dysfunction.

Mexilitine, tocainide, encainide, and flecainide do not appear to
have any adverse effect upon exercise tolerance; comparable peak
heart rates, blood pressures, exercise duration, and peak rate-pressure
products are described before and after drug administration (42).
Flecainide-induced QRS prolongation is increased by exercise.
Exercise-induced wide-complex tachycardias have been described with
flecainide therapy, and exercise testing has been suggested to evaluate
the possible proarrhythmic effects of this agent (43). This observation
is important, since the proarrthymic effects of encainide and flecainide
have recently been documented in coronary patients in a controlled

clinical trial (44). Exercise causes a rate-dependent augmentation of flecainide's effects on ventricular conduction, enhancing state-dependent sodium channel blockade, and potentially causing ventricular arrhythmias (45).

Psychotropic Drugs: Cardiovascular Effects and Interaction with Cardiovascular Drugs

Many patients with coronary disease have associated emotional problems, and they may thus be prescribed phenothiazine drugs or tricyclic antidepressant compounds. Many psychotropic drugs produce repolarization abnormalities during exercise testing and they may also cause orthostatic hypotension. Further, many tricyclic antidepressant drugs may be arrhythmogenic, as their effect on cardiac conduction resembles that of type IA antiarrthymic drugs; they may also depress myocardial contractility.

Tricyclic antidepressants (TCAs) block the synaptic reuptake of norepinephrine and they may also block the synaptic uptake of guanethidine or clonidine, interfering with blood pressure control; conversely, withdrawl of TCAs may cause serious hypertension because there is no longer antagonism to the guanethidine or clonidine. Tricyclic antidepressants also impair the hepatic metabolism of dicoumarol, causing excessive anticoagulation in patients receiving the drug. At least in early reports, a newer TCA, alprazolam, appears to have little or no cardiotoxicity or adverse drug-drug interactions.

Lithium carbonate is used to treat affective disorders. Although it does not interfere with exercise tolerance (46), abnormalities of sinus node and AV conduction have been described (47), as has potentiation of heart failure. Sodium restriction and/or administration of thiazide diuretics can precipitate lithium toxicity.

Phenothiazine tranquilizers may decrease myocardial contractility, induce heart failure and arrhythmias, produce cardiac conduction abnormalities, and cause a variety of ECG changes (predominantly QT prolongation and ST-T abnormalities) both at rest and with exercise (48).

ACKNOWLEDGMENT

With appreciation to Jeanette Zahler and Julia Wright for assistance in manuscript preparation and review.

REFERENCES

1. Podrid, P.J., Venditti, F.J., Levine, P.A., et al., *Am. J. Cardiol.*, *62*: 24H (1988).
1a. Pupita, G., Kaski, J.C., Galassi, A.R., et al., *Am. Heart J. 118*: 539 (1989).
2. DeBusk, R.F., Blomqvist, C.G., Kouchoukos, N.T., et al., *N. Engl. J. Med.*, *314*: 161 (1986).
3. Hamm, L.F., Stull, G.A., and Crow, R.S., *Prog. Cardiovasc. Dis.*, *28*: 463 (1986).
4. Stone, P.H., Titi, Z.G., Muller, J.E., et al., *J. Am. Coll. Cardiol.*, *8*: 1007 (1986).
5. Wenger, N.K., *Am. Coll. Cardiol.*, *1*: 14 (1986).
6. Melin, J.A., DeCoster, P.M., Renkin, J., et al., *Am. J. Cardiol.*, *56*: 705 (1985).
7. Schaer, D.H., Leiboff, R.H., Wasserman, A.G., et al., *Circulation*, 72(Suppl. III): III-462 (1985).
8. Markes, J.E., Gorlin, R., Mills, R.M., et al., *Am. J. Cardiol.*, *43*: 265 (1979).
9. Schaer, D.H., Buff, L.A., and Katz, R.J., *Am. J. Cardiol.*, *61*: 46 (1988).
10. Glancy, D.L., Richter, M.A., Ellis, E.V., et al., *Am. J. Med.*, *62*: 39 (1977).
11. Flessas, A.P., and Ryan, T.J., *Am. Heart J.*, *105*: 239 (1983).
12. Frishman, W.H., Furberg, C.D., and Friedewald, W.T., *Curr. Probl. Cardiol.*, *9*: 1 (1983).
13. Pederson, T.R., *N. Engl. J. Med.*, *313*: 1055 (1985).
14. The TIMI Study Group, *N. Engl. J. Med.*, *320*: 618 (1989).
15. Murray, D.P., Tan, L.B., Salih, M., et al., *Br. Heart J.*, *60*: 474 (1988).
16. Ho, S.W.-C., McComish, M.J., and Taylor, R.R., *Am. J. Cardiol.*, *55*: 258 (1985).
17. Olsson, G., Rehnqvist, N., Freyschuss, U., et al., *Am. J. Cardiol.*, *61*: 519 (1988).
18. Hare, T.W., Lowenthal, D.T., Hakki, H.H., et al., *Clin. Pharmacol. Ther.*, *33*: 206 (1983).
19. Pratt, C.M., Welton, D.E., Squires, W.G., Jr., et al., *Circulation*, *64*: 1125 (1981).
20. Sweeney, M.E., Fletcher, B.J., and Fletcher, G.F., *Am. Heart J.*, *118*: 941 (1989).
21. Wolfel, E.E., Hiatt, W.R., Brammell, H.L., et al., *Circulation*, *74*: 664 (1986).
22. Vanhees, L., Fagard, R., and Amery, A., *Am. Heart J.*, *108*: 270 (1984).
23. Moskowitz, R.M., Piccini, P.A., Nacarelli, G.V., et al., *Am. J. Cardiol.*, *44*: 811 (1979).
24. Bonow, R.O., Leon, M.B., Rosing, D., et al., *Circulation*, *65*: 1337 (1982).
25. Nonogi, H., Hess, O.M., Ritter, M., et al., *J. Am. Coll. Cardiol.*, *12*: 892 (1988).
26. Mukharji, J., Kremers, M., Lipscomb, K., et al., *Am. J. Cardiol.*, *55*: 267 (1985).

27. Saltin, B., *Ann. N.Y. Acad. Sci.*, *301*: 224 (1977).
28. Clausen, J.P., *Prog. Cardiovasc. Dis.*, *18*: 459 (1976).
29. Paterson, D.H., Shephard, R.J., Cunningham, D., et al., *J. Appl. Physiol.*, *47*: 482 (1979).
30. Hagberg, J.M., Ehsani, A.A., and Holloszy, J.O., *Circulation*, *67*: 1194 (1983).
31. Ehsani, A.A., Martin, W.W., III, Heath, G.W., et al., *Am. J. Cardiol.*, *50*: 246 (1982).
32. Virtanen, K., Janne, J., and Frick, M.H., *Eur. J. Clin. Pharmacol.*, *21*: 275 (1982).
33. Tan, L.B., *Cardiovasc. Res.*, *21*: 615 (1987).
34. Creager, M.A., Massie, B.M., Faxon, D.P., et al., *J. Am. Coll. Cardiol.*, *6*: 163 (1985).
35. LeJemtel, T.H., Gumbardo, D., Chadwick, B., et al., *Circulation*, *73*(Suppl. III): III–213 (1986).
36. Weber, K.T., Janicki, J.S., and Maskin, C.S., *Circulation*, *73*(Suppl. III): III–196 (1986).
37. Gross, G.J., Warltier, D.C., Hardman, H.F., et al., *Am. Heart J.*, *93*: 487 (1977).
38. Parker, J.O., West, R.O., Jr., Ledwich, J.R., et al., *Circulation*, *40*: 453 (1969).
39. Sundqvist, K., Atterhog, J.-H., and Jogestrand, T., *Am. J. Cardiol.*, *57*: 661 (1986).
40. Fenster, P.E., Dahl, C., Marcus, F.I., et al., *Am. Heart J.*, *104*: 1244 (1982).
41. Fenster, P.E., Comess, K.A., and Hanson, C.D., *Cardiology*, *69*: 366 (1982).
42. Lampert, S., and Lown, B., *Circulation*, *66*(Suppl. II): 186 (1982).
43. Anastasiou-Nana, M.I., Anderson, J.L., Stewart, J.R., et al., *Am. Heart J.*, *113*: 1071 (1987).
44. Special Report, *N. Engl. J. Med.*, *321*: 406 (1989).
45. Ranger, S., Talajic, M., Lemery, R., et al., *Circulation*, *79*: 1000 (1989).
46. Tilkian, A.G., Schroeder, J.S., and Kao, J., *Am. J. Cardiol.*, *38*: 701 (1976).
47. Hagman, A., Arnman, K., and Ryden, L., *Acta Med. Scand.*, *205*: 467 (1979).
48. Grant, D., Crawford, M.H., and O'Rourke, R.A., *Am. Heart J.*, *102*: 465 (1981).

15

Cardiovascular Problems of the Wheelchair Disabled

Roger M. Glaser

Wright State University School of Medicine
Dayton, Ohio

INTRODUCTION

In recent years, there has been an increased awareness of the problems and needs of individuals who depend upon wheelchairs for locomotion. Many of these individuals suffer from neuromuscular disorders (for example, stroke, multiple sclerosis, muscular dystrophy, cerebral palsy, and traumatic injury to the central nervous system) which have led to lower-limb paralysis, paresis, and/or spasticity. Others suffer from orthopedic problems or amputations of the lower limbs. Although wheelchairs help in rehabilitation by permitting more independence and greater participation in societal activities, insufficient or inappropriate amounts of daily exercise can give rise to secondary cardiovascular problems (19,45,54). Some of these cardiovascular problems can be avoided or alleviated by incorporating specialized fitness programs into one's lifestyle. In addition, the enhanced physical capability can improve the outcome of rehabilitation. This chapter focuses on the limitations of exercise capability among wheelchair users (in particular, the spinal cord injured); problems associated with wheelchair confinement and use; techniques for the assessment of physical fitness in this group; techniques for improving physical fitness; and the use of functional neuromuscular stimulation to exercise paralyzed lower limb muscles. Clinical applications of new technologies will be addressed, as will their potential to reduce the incidence of cardiovascular problems.

Although this chapter will use spinal cord injury (SCI) as a model of a wheelchair-dependent population, many of the principles presented can be applied to wheelchair users with other types of neuromuscular and orthopedic disorders. Spinal cord injury can result in complete paraplegia or quadriplegia (tetraplegia), with sudden and drastic changes in lifestyle. Major causes include motor vehicle accidents (over 38%), accidents during sports or physical activities, and trauma during violent crimes (10,103). There are currently more than 200,000 SCI individuals in the United States, and each year approximately 8000 new patients with SCI survive to join this population (103). Prior to World War II, 80% of SCI victims died within 3 years of injury (64), primarily due to kidney and pulmonary infections (90). With the advent of antibiotic drugs and advances in surgical techniques, paraplegics now have a near normal life expectancy, but quadriplegics still have a life expectancy that is about 10% shorter than that of the able-bodied (AB) (90). Generally, the greater the age at the time of SCI, the higher the level of SCI, and the more complete the SCI, the shorter is the life expectancy (21). Currently, common long-term causes of death in the SCI population (and lower limb amputees) are a variety of cardiac and vascular disorders (62,68,102,103).

Le and Price (68) reported a death rate 228% greater for their SCI group than that of an age- and gender-matched AB group. This was apparently due in part to adoption of a sedentary lifestyle with consequent degenerative changes in the cardiovascular system (20,57,67,102). The high risk of coronary heart disease among sedentary SCI individuals is indicated by low blood high-density lipoprotein-cholesterol (HDL-C) concentrations relative to SCI athletes, sedentary AB, and active AB individuals (20,57,67). Thus, arm exercise training may increase the health status and reduce the cardiovascular risks of SCI individuals just as leg exercise benefits AB individuals.

LIMITATIONS IN EXERCISE CAPABILITY OF SCI INDIVIDUALS

The higher the level and the more complete the SCI, the more widespread is the loss of somatic and autonomic nervous system function (Fig. 1) (45). With respect to somatic function, cervical lesions typically result in quadriplegia, whereas thoracic or lumbar lesions typi-

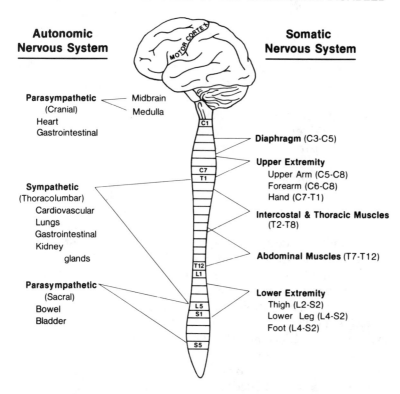

Figure 1 Schematic diagram of the central nervous system showing neural outflows from the somatic nervous system (providing skeletal muscle innervation) and autonomic nervous system (providing internal organ innervation). General innervations from each spinal cord level are indicated. (From Ref. 45; used with permission.)

cally result in paraplegia. The more skeletal muscles that are paralyzed, the lower is the voluntary exercise capability, and the lower is the aerobic fitness that may be achieved through exercise training. In higher-level SCI patients, paralysis of the intercostal muscles can severely limit pulmonary ventilation; this further reduces exercise capability and leads to secondary pulmonary problems. Furthermore, paralysis of the leg muscles usually results in marked atrophy of the affected muscles and osteoporosis of the bones. Immobilization of the lower limbs may also precipitate venous stasis, blood pooling, and edema due to loss of normal venous muscle pumping. This may lead to deep venous thrombosis (DVT) and subsequent pulmonary embolism. Prolonged pressure on supporting tissues and an inadequate local circulation frequently lead to decubitus ulcers.

The aerobic exercise capability of SCI individuals can also be limited by a diminished sympathetic outflow (see Fig. 1). Sympathetic reflexes normally augment blood flow to the metabolically active skeletal muscles by inducing vasoconstriction in relatively inactive tissues (such as the gut, kidneys, and skin); vasodilatation of skeletal muscles arterioles; venoconstriction (which facilitates venous return); and increases in the heart rate and myocardial contractility (which augment stroke volume and cardiac output) (45,54). These reflexes are absent to varying degrees in most SCI individuals; those with lesions above T1 have interruption of all sympathetic nerves that innervate the heart (from T4 to T1), markedly limiting cardioacceleration, myocardial contractility, and augmentation of stroke volume and cardiac output (32); any cardioacceleration in such individuals reflects a withdrawal of vagal parasympathetic tone at the S-A node. A reduced sympathetic outflow also impairs thermoregulatory capacity owing to an inappropriate blood flow distribution and an insufficient sweating response below the lesion level.

Thus, the loss of functional skeletal muscle mass and inactivity of the venous muscle pump in the lower extremities are compounded by diminished or nonexistent cardiovascular reflexes during exercise. The active arm muscles are fatigued quickly because of their relatively small mass, an inadequate blood flow secondary to the hypokinetic circulation, a limited aerobic energy supply, and a greater component of anaerobiosis with the accumulation of metabolites in the muscles (45,49,51,54). The early fatigue of the arm muscles during both wheelchair locomotion and exercise training discourages many wheelchair users from leading active lives. Unfortunately, a sedentary lifestyle leads to a further decrement of physical fitness and an even greater reduction of functional capability. Specific exercise training programs are needed to break this vicious cycle (45,54).

Special Exercise Precautions

Patients with SCI performing strenuous exercise are exposed to the usual risks known for AB individuals as well as additional risks due to their central nervous system (CNS) damage and the resulting motor, sensory, and autonomic dysfunction. Because of potential health risks, wheelchair users should have a thorough medical examination (including an ECG) prior to beginning a strenuous exercise program. Risks unique to SCI individuals include exercise hypotension, orthostatic hypotension, autonomic dysreflexia (sudden and inappropriate blood pressure responses), trunk instability, pressure sores, and muscle spasms (13,14,65,77). Thermoregulation is also a problem for some patients. Health care professionals involved with exercise for SCI individuals should be aware of these risks and take appropriate safety precautions.

The blood pressure responses of SCI patients during exercise are quite different and inconsistent relative to those shown by AB individuals. High-level SCI patients may exhibit a paradoxical drop in blood pressure as exercise progresses; this reflects a lowering of total peripheral resistance as blood vessels in active muscles dilate in response to hypoxia and increased concentrations of local metabolites, without a corresponding increase in cardiac output. Exercise in an upright posture also causes blood pooling in the lower extremities, with an inadequate venous return and a low cardiac output; this leads to orthostatic hypotension, with dizziness or possible loss of consciousness. The risk may be reduced by regular orthostatic training (for example, head-up tilt, assisted standing, brace ambulation), maintenance of proper hydration, use of compression stockings or an abdominal binder, and physical conditioning.

Occasionally, high-level SCI patients exhibit a sudden episode of extreme hypertension due to autonomic dysreflexia (hyperreflexia); this can be fatal if it is not corrected in a timely manner. Measures that help to avoid this condition include prevention of bowel impaction, bladder overdistension, and skin tissue trauma. The bladder should be emptied just prior to exercise and during prolonged exercise bouts, and the blood pressure should be monitored at regular intervals (at least during initial sessions) (65). Exercise must be discontinued immediately if there are adverse reactions. Appropriate action must be taken to alleviate the problem (tilting up for hypertension and reclining for hypotension or fainting).

A security belt should be fitted around the SCI individual's upper trunk during arm exercise to prevent falls due to trunk instability and poor sitting balance. In addition, it is essential that pressure on weight-bearing tissues be minimized to prevent decubitus ulcers. Cushions should be placed under the ischial tuberosities and other weight-bearing areas, and pressure should be relieved periodically by raising the body off the cushion for 30-60 s every 20-30 mins. Furthermore, many SCI individuals experience occasional spasms in the paralyzed lower limb muscles, ranging from mild to hazardous in their severity. So care must be taken to avoid damage to the lower limbs by strong spasms and rapid limb movements. Oral antispasmodic and muscle relaxant drugs help to control muscle spasms, but further limit exercise capability by reducing skeletal muscle excitability. Additional side effects include dizziness, ataxia, and depression (90).

Careful consideration also should be given to ambient temperature, relative humidity, and clothing worn as well as to exercise intensity and duration. Many SCI individuals have a limited thermoregulatory capacity due to inadequate sweat secretion and impaired cardiovascular system control, so that overheating occurs more easily in this population than in the AB. Exercise in cold environments may result in excessive heat loss. If there are symptoms of either hyperthermia or hypothermia, exercise should be discontinued, and clothing and environmental conditions should be appropriately adjusted.

PROBLEMS ASSOCIATED WITH WHEELCHAIR USE

Individuals who depend upon manual wheelchairs for locomotion use their relatively small and weak upper body musculature. This places them at a marked disadvantage on account of the limited peak oxygen intake ($\dot{V}O_2$) and maximal power output (PO) capability for arm exercise. This is approximately two-thirds of leg exercise values for AB individuals who are not arm exercise trained (2,7,91,104). Arm exercise capability may be further reduced by the disability (as indicated above) as well as by a diminished muscular and cardiopulmonary fitness resulting from a sedentary lifestyle. Arm exercise is mechanically inefficient, and it is stressful to both the skeletal muscles and the cardiovascular and pulmonary systems in comparison to the same intensities of leg exercise (8,44,91,95). Indeed, when comparing wheelchair propulsion with walking and leg cycling, greater physiological stresses generally have been reported for handrim stroking (35,42,43,93,101). The difference is more pronounced at the greater exercise intensities needed at high locomotive velocities and when negotiating architectural barriers such as carpeting and upward grades.

In studies comparing arm and leg exercise (for example, arm crank or wheelchair ergometry versus leg cycle ergometry for AB subjects at matched submaximal PO levels), arm exercise elicited greater metabolic stress, as indicated by higher $\dot{V}O_2$ and blood lactate values; a heavier cardiac load, with a higher heart rate (HR), peripheral vascular resistance, intra-arterial blood pressure, and stroke work; and a greater demand on the pulmonary system (with a larger respiratory minute volume, $\dot{V}E$). A given absolute intensity of arm exercise also tends to elicit a lower cardiac output ($\dot{Q}$) and ventricular stroke volume (SV) (3,6,8,35,36,87,91). The lower $\dot{Q}$ and SV may be due to a greater afterload on the heart (because of the higher peripheral vascular resistance) and a lower end-diastolic volume (due to an attenuated return of venous blood to the heart) associated with inactivity of the venous muscle pump in the paralyzed legs (45,54). Furthermore, the elevated intrathoracic pressure during handrim stroking might decrease the effectiveness of the thoracic pump. These factors together reduce the effective blood volume during wheelchair activity, limiting peak $\dot{V}O_2$ and PO_{max}. Therefore, wheelchair locomotion, even at a low PO, can represent a relatively high exercise load for the SCI individual, with rapid onset of fatigue. Excessive cardiovascular and pulmonary stresses can hinder rehabilitation, imposing risks upon certain patients, including the elderly and those with cardiovascular or pulmonary impairments (35,45,54).

TECHNIQUES OF PHYSICAL FITNESS ASSESSMENT

With AB individuals, leg exercise (treadmill walking, bench stepping, or cycle ergometry) is typically used for stress testing. Here, a large muscle mass is contracted rhythmically, stimulating optimal (maximal) metabolic, cardiovascular, and pulmonary responses for valid functional evaluation of these systems. The primary factor that limits maximal PO and $\dot{V}O_2$ during these tests is *central circulatory* in nature; the cardiovascular system is not able to deliver sufficient oxygen to the large exercising muscle mass (1,12,70,82). In contrast, arm exercise (wheelchair locomotion, arm crank, and wheelchair ergometry) activates a relatively small muscle mass; the primary limiting factors are thus *peripheral* in nature, and local fatigue of the heavily stressed arm musculature can occur despite the delivery of sufficient blood and oxygen (4,34,49,59). Another peripheral factor that may limit the performance of arm exercise is an inadequate venous return of blood to the heart owing to deficient skeletal muscle pump activity (49). This can in turn limit $\dot{Q}$ and the delivery of blood and oxygen to the arm muscles. Because of the lower PO capability and the early onset of fatigue, arm exercise may not provide sufficient stimulus to drive the metabolic, cardiovascular, and pulmonary systems to full output, making valid functional evaluation of these systems difficult. Since the highest level of $\dot{V}O_2$ reached during maximal arm exercise is somewhat lower than the true physiological maximum expected for leg exercise in AB individuals, the term peak $\dot{V}O_2$ rather than maximal $\dot{V}O_2$ is typically used.

Arm Exercise Modes

Clinical exercise stress testing as well as the training of wheelchair users typically involve arm crank ergometers (ACE), since they are commercially available and the exercise intensity can be accurately set to desired levels. Wheelchair ergometers (WERG), which closely simulate wheelchair locomotion (9,34,36,39,98,99), are custom designed and constructed, and are mostly located in research laboratories. Figure 2 illustrates a combination of WERG-ACE designed and constructed by Glaser et al. (38). A conventional Monark cycle ergometer serves as the basis of this device, so it is relatively easy to construct and calibrate. Additional wheelchair exercise modes include operating a wheelchair on a motor-driven treadmill (24,33,58,94), and actual wheelchair locomotion over a predetermined course at specific velocities (11,37,42,43). To establish repeatable testing and training protocols, it is important to quantify the exercise PO. To estimate the PO requirements for actual wheelchair locomotion, Glaser et al. (37) used a strain-gauge transducer to measure the average force needed to push a standard medical wheelchair and its occupant over various terrains at a constant velocity. Figure 3 provides the linear regression equations to calculate PO based on body mass, floor surface and grade, and velocity (37). The validity of this technique was established by demonstrating

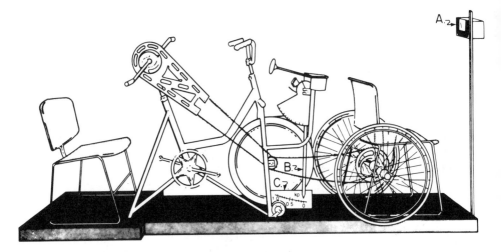

Figure 2 Diagram of the combination wheelchair–arm crank ergometer: A is electronic speedometer, B is lengthened pendular arm, and C is expanded braking force scale. (From Ref. 38; used with permission.)

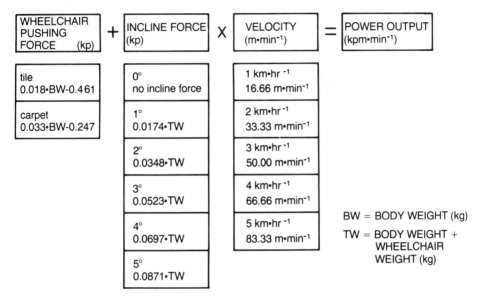

Figure 3 Composite summary of linear regression equations used to predict power output requirements (kpm min^{-1}) for wheelchair locomotion over given terrains (floor surface and incline) at various velocities. Units of kpm min^{-1} can be converted to units of watts (W) by dividing by 6.12. (From Ref. 37; used with permission.)

the similarity of metabolic and cardiopulmonary responses during actual wheelchair locomotion and exercise on a WERG set to the same PO levels (40).

Sawka et al. (84) compared WERG to ACE exercise at the same *submaximal* PO levels of 5, 15, 25, and 35 W. They found that WERG exercise generally elicited a higher oxygen intake, respiratory minute volume, cardiac output, stroke volume, systolic blood pressure, and heart rate (Fig. 4A,B,C). In another study, Glaser et al. (38) found that *maximal* effort WERG and ACE exercise elicited similar peak oxygen intake and respiratory minute volume. But, significantly lower maximal PO, peak heart rate, and blood lactate concentrations were elicited for WERG exercise (Table 1). It appears that both WERG and ACE can be used with similar results for exercise testing and training of wheelchair users. But lower submaximal and maximal PO levels would be employed for WERG exercise. Furthermore, the concept of ''exercise specificity'' suggests that WERG exercise may be more appropriate than ACE exercise for wheelchair-dependent populations because it

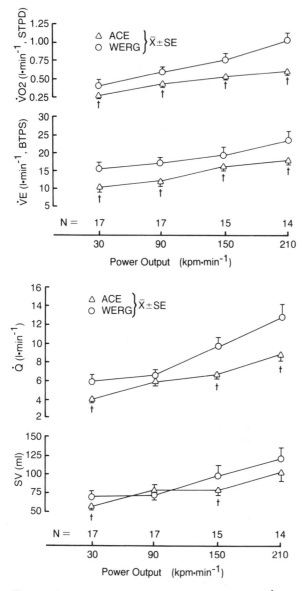

Figure 4 A, Comparison of oxygen intake ($\dot{V}O_2$) and respiratory minute volume ($\dot{V}E$); B, Comparison of cardiac output ($\dot{Q}$) and stroke volume (SV); and C, Comparison of heart rate (HR) and systolic blood pressure (SBP) data between wheelchair (WERG) and arm crank (ACE) ergometer exercise at equal power output levels. $*p < 0.05.$, $\dagger p < 0.01$. (Modified from Ref. 84; used with permission.)

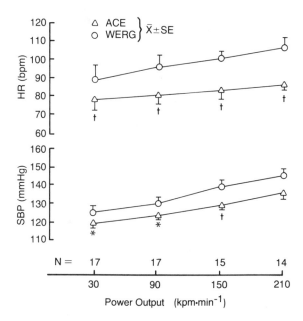

more closely resembles actual wheelchair locomotion (38,72). The lower metabolic rate and cardiopulmonary responses found for submaximal ACE exercise as well as the greater maximal PO achieved suggest that arm cranking may be superior to handrim stroking as a means of wheelchair locomotion. Smith et al. (89) found a lower oxygen intake (-32%), respiratory minute volume (-30%), and heart rate (-19%) when operating an arm crank propelled wheelchair relative to handrim propulsion under the same locomotive conditions.

Stress Testing Protocols

The fundamental principles followed for the lower limb stress testing of AB individuals are employed during upper limb stress testing of wheelchair-dependent individuals. Tests are usually progressive with respect to exercise intensity, and have well-defined submaximal or maximal effort endpoint criteria. Either a *continuous* or a *discontinuous* protocol may be used. Discontinuous, submaximal protocols on a WERG are preferable, since they are relatively safe and are task specific relative to stresses encountered during daily locomotive activity. Criteria for test termination include: (a) voluntary cessation, (b) symptoms of cardiovascular or pulmonary abnormalities (for example, chest discomfort, ECG changes, marked hypertension, dyspnea),

Table 1 Maximal Effort Wheelchair (WERG) and Arm Crank (ACE) Ergometer Exercise

| | PO_{max} (W) | | Peak $\dot{V}O_2$ (L min^{-1}) | | $\dot{V}E_{max}$ (L min^{-1}) | | HR_{max} (beats/min) | | LA_{max} (mmol L^{-1}) | |
	ACE	WERG	ACE	WERG	ACE	WERG	ACE	WERG	ACE	WERG
$\bar{X}$	93	59	1.77	1.73	71.8	71.5	169	158	8.4	6.2
±SE	7	5	0.14	0.14	5.7	6.5	4	4	0.6	0.5
p<	0.01		NS		NS		0.01		0.01	
%Δ	-36		-2		0		-7		-26	
r	0.86		0.92		0.78		0.72		0.52	

n = 16. p, probability level; NS, not significantly different; %Δ, percent difference between WERG and ACE exercise values; r, correlation coefficient between values for WERG and ACE exercise. PO_{max}, maximal power output; Peak $\dot{V}O_2$, peak oxygen intake, $\dot{V}E_{max}$, maximal respiratory minute volume; HR_{max}, maximal heart rate; LA_{max}, maximal blood lactate concentrations.
Source: Ref. 38; used with permission.

(c) achievement of the required maximal PO, and (d) attainment of a predetermined heart rate (for example, 75% of the age-adjusted HR reserve (34,45). However, the HR criterion may not be usable for high-level SCI patients owing to the interruption of sympathetic pathways to the heart and a limited HR response.

Basic exercise testing may be achieved by having the patient propel his or her own wheelchair over an established test course at paced or self-selected velocities (37,42,43). A suitable submaximal protocol would use locomotive tasks of 4–6 min in duration separated by 5–10 min of rest. Steady-rate physiological responses can be determined during the last minute of each exercise bout by using portable or radiotelemetry monitors. Wheelchair velocity increments of 0.5–1.0 $km \cdot h^{-1}$ are recommended.

For WERG and ACE tests, the propulsion velocity is typically held constant (for example, a wheel velocity of 3 km h^{-1} and a crank rate of 50 rpm, respectively) while the braking force is increased. With WERG, 5 W appears to be an appropriate initial PO, as it is frequently encountered during daily wheelchair locomotion (37). Increments of 5–10 W are appropriate for many patients, and the peak PO can be limited to 25–35 W for submaximal tests (34,35,84,85). For more fit patients, the PO increment and the maximal PO permitted can be greater. With ACE, the protocol is similar, but the PO increments are about two times those for WERG. Figure 5 illustrates the data of Glaser et al. (34) for a graded WERG test employing up to five 4-min exercise bouts, each followed by a 5-min rest. Since the subjects used were AB, the heart rate response was linear with respect to both PO and oxygen intake. Extrapolation of the submaximal data to the predicted maximal heart rate would only be appropriate with lower-level SCI patients whose cardioacceleration is not impaired. The maximal heart rate for arm exercise is 10–20 beats/min lower than for leg exercise. Thus, values obtained by using the formula 220 beats/min minus age should be reduced by 10–20 beats/min in order to predict the maximal heart rates for WERG and ACE exercises (83,91,99).

To determine maximal PO and peak oxygen intake, the discontinuous, submaximal test can be extended to maximal effort by increasing the number of exercise bouts. But much time would then be required to complete the test, and the multiple bouts of exercise could lead to fatigue and underestimation of maximal PO and peak oxygen intake. Therefore, if maximal testing is desired, and submaximal data are not needed, a continuous, maximal exercise protocol can be utilized. This shorter protocol begins at a low-to-moderate PO as a warm-up. The PO is then increased every 1–2 min until maximal effort is

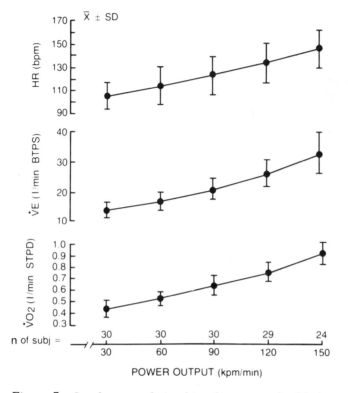

Figure 5 Steady-rate relationships between wheelchair ergometer power output and oxygen intake ($\dot{V}O_2$), respiratory minute volume ($\dot{V}E$), and heart rate (HR) for 30 able-bodied female subjects. (Modified from Ref. 34; used with permission.)

reached. By estimating fitness with previous submaximal testing, the initial PO and the magnitude of increments can be set so that the individual will complete the test in several minutes (4,15,23,63,66,75, 97,96).

Fitness criteria are based upon the metabolic and cardiopulmonary responses at given PO levels as well as the maximal PO achieved (34). During submaximal exercise, fit individuals have smaller responses. The lower oxygen intake indicates a lower aerobic energy expenditure and a higher mechanical efficiency, whereas the lower respiratory minute volume and heart rate imply a greater cardiopulmonary fitness with a lower relative stress. However, care must be taken not to interpret the low exercise HR of high-level SCI patients as an indication of superior cardiovascular fitness. With maximal exercise, the achieved PO, oxygen intake, respiratory minute volume, cardiac and stroke volume are greater in fit individuals. However, the maximal heart rate may not differ greatly between more and less fit individuals.

EXERCISE TRAINING TECHNIQUES

Normal daily wheelchair activity may not provide sufficient exercise to train the cardiopulmonary system. Supplemental arm exercise is necessary to improve fitness (58,65). Such training programs could increase the reserve capability and make the activities of daily living (such as wheelchair locomotion) less stressful, since they would be performed at lower percentages of maximal PO and peak oxygen intake. This could possibly contribute to an improved functional independence and rehabilitation outcome (41). Indeed, with wheelchair locomotion at 7 W, well-trained wheelchair athletes with an average age of 25 years utilize less than 7% of their maximal PO and 18% of peak oxygen intake. This is in contrast to the 9% of maximal PO and 29% of peak oxygen intake used by their sedentary cohorts. Older, sedentary wheelchair users have a more difficult plight, 50- to 60-year-old patients use 44% of maximal PO and 51% of peak oxygen intake, whereas those aged 80–90 use 100% of their maximal PO and peak oxygen intake for this routine locomotive task (43,85). Regular exercise training may thus reduce the stresses of wheelchair locomotion, and lower some of the risks associated with secondary cardiovascular disabilities.

Arm Exercise Protocols

To promote improved muscular and cardiopulmonary fitness as well as enhanced performance arm exercise, like leg exercise training, follows the fundamental principle of "overload" (45,54). Exercise is performed at intensities (and/or durations) beyond those encountered during normal daily activities. In addition, exercise intensity (and/or duration) is progressively increased as performance improves, until the desired fitness goals are reached. Maintenance of this fitness status involves periodic exercise at the final intensity/duration levels achieved. If exercise is discontinued, detraining occurs and fitness diminishes within several weeks (80,92).

Traditionally, ACE exercise has been used for the endurance training of wheelchair users. However, WERG exercise may be advantageous because a similar peak oxygen intake can be elicited, and it more closely resembles actual wheelchair activity so that it may better enhance locomotive performance (38,41). Training protocols may be either continuous or discontinuous. If enhanced cardiopulmonary fitness is the primary goal, PO should be adjusted to allow moderate levels of exercise of relatively long durations (15–60 min for continuous bouts and 3–5 min for each of the several discontinuous bouts) without excessive fatigue or respiratory distress. Exercise sessions should occur two to five times per week (31,71).

When prescribing aerobic leg exercise for AB individuals, marked anaerbiosis and metabolic acidosis should be avoided, since these can severely limit exercise duration. However, the heart rate may not be a usable indicator of exercise stress with SCI individuals, since cardioacceleration may not be proportional to the increases in the metabolic rate. To set the exercise intensity with this population, the direct determination of oxygen consumption, ventilation, and blood lactate concentration is desirable if instrumentation is available. Otherwise, the subjective feeling of stress and the actual exercise duration capability may be used. It is likely that several trials will be needed with each patient in order to set the training PO.

Physiological Adaptations to Arm Exercise Training

Studies on lower limb disabled individuals indicated that several weeks of endurance-type arm exercise training can significantly increase the PO capability, peak oxygen intake, and cardiopulmonary performance (22,65,73,75,79). Training with ACE of active wheelchair users increased their peak oxygen intake by 12–19% in 7–20 weeks (75,79). Even greater gains in cardiopulmonary fitness were obtained when quadriplegics who had relatively low initial fitness levels were trained for only 5 weeks (22). Using WERG exercise, Miles et al. (73) reported that over 6 weeks of interval training (three times per week) eight wheelchair athletes increased their maximal PO capability by 31%, peak oxygen intake by 26%, and peak respiratory minute volume by 32% (Table 2). These gains were sizable considering that the subjects had relatively high levels of fitness prior to training.

Although arm exercise training imposes a lower limit to the aerobic fitness that can be achieved, most participants can expect some cardiopulmonary benefits. The magnitudes of increments in aerobic fitness and exercise performance with training depend upon initial fitness and the size of the muscle mass available for exercise. Generally, gains in fitness are greater if individuals initiate training programs at relatively low fitness levels (depending upon their pathological limitations) (45,54). Many of the observed gains in arm exercise per-

Table 2 Individual and Mean ($\pm$SD) Values for Respiratory Minute Volume ($\dot{V}E$ L $\cdot$ min^{-1}), Tidal Volume (V_T, l), Respiratory Frequency (R_f, beats $\cdot$ min^{-1}), Power Output (W), and Peak Oxygen Intake ($\dot{V}O_2$ L $\cdot$ min^{-1}) Attained During Maximal Wheelchair Ergometer Exercise Before (B) and After (A) Six wk of Interval Training by Eight SCI Wheelchair Athletes

Subject	$\dot{V}_E$ B	$\dot{V}_E$ A	V_T B	V_T A	R_f B	R_f A	Power output B	Power output A	Peak $\dot{V}O_2$ B	Peak $\dot{V}O_2$ A
1	74.7	111.2	2.49	3.09	30	36	70	96	2.05	2.41
2	136.9	180.8	4.56	3.12	30	58	100	140	3.34	3.73
3	115.2	145.1	1.92	2.20	60	66	72	100	2.41	2.98
4	99.2	116.3	2.20	1.87	45	62	80	90	1.89	2.18
5	103.3	143.7	1.72	2.40	60	60	90	105	2.00	2.65
6	68.2	109.2	1.71	1.82	40	60	52	83	1.57	2.31
7	80.4	106.7	1.61	2.05	50	52	83	95	2.04	2.60
8	119.0	137.3	2.77	2.54	43	54	81	110	219	326
Mean	99.6	131.3	2.37	2.38	44.8	56.0	78.3	102.3	2.19	2.76
SD	22.4	23.8	0.91	0.47	10.9	8.6	14	16	0.49	0.49
	$P<0.05$		NS		$P<0.05$		$P<0.05$		$P<0.05$	

Source: From Ref. 73; used with permission

formance could be due to peripheral adaptations such as improved capillary density and/or metabolic capability within muscles (which would increase arteriovenous O_2 difference) rather than central circulatory adaptations (41,49,69,88). Nevertheless, regular arm exercise training appears to increase maximal PO capability and peak oxygen intake, and it may also decrease levels of physiological responses for given submaximal exercise tasks such as wheelchair locomotion (41).

Hooker and Wells (61) reported a significant increase in the HDL-C level (+20%) and a decrease in the total cholesterol (−8%) and low-density lipoprotein–cholesterol (LDL-C) levels (−15%) in SCI subjects following 8 weeks of moderate-intensity WERG training (60–70% peak $\dot{V}O_2$; 20 min/day, three times per week). These alterations in the blood lipid profile extrapolated to a mean decrease of 20% in the group's risk of future coronary artery disease. More research is necessary to develop appropriate exercise models and protocols, and to document their efficacy in reducing the risk of cardiovascular disease in this population.

Body Position and Arm Exercise Capability

In some individuals with lower limb paralysis, the etiology of upper body muscle fatigue may be a central factor secondary to a peripheral factor. Inactivity of the venous muscle pump can restrict the venous return of blood from the legs to the heart (a peripheral factor), thereby restricting the cardiac output capability during arm exercise (a central factor). Thus, pooling of blood in the leg veins can potentially lead to a hypokinetic circulation, reducing the availability of blood to the active upper body musculature, and limiting its exercise capability (45,49,54). Since SCI individuals typically perform arm exercise in an upright, sitting position, the hydrostatic pressure favors blood pooling in the leg veins. It seems plausible that the arm exercise capability would be enhanced by placing the individual in a supine position. This would minimize pooling, facilitate venous return, elevate cardiac output, increase arm muscle blood flow, and boost fatigue resistance.

Figoni et al. (27) had quadriplegic patients perform maximal effort ACE in a sitting and in a supine position on separate occasions. The maximal PO, peak oxygen intake, respiratory minute volume, stroke volume, and cardiac output were all greater when supine, suggesting that the cardiopulmonary training capability might be enhanced by using the supine position. Although these acute data are encouraging, research is needed to determine if prolonged exercise training in the supine position is superior for improving the aerobic fitness of lower limb paralyzed individuals.

USE OF FUNCTIONAL NEUROMUSCULAR STIMULATION-INDUCED EXERCISE OF THE PARALYZED LOWER LIMB MUSCULATURE

During the past 10 years, functional neuromuscular stimulation (FNS; sometimes referred to as functional electrical stimulation, FES) research has been conducted with the goal of inducing exercise in paralyzed lower limb muscles (5,16,47,74). Typically, electrical impulses from a stimulator are used in conjunction with skin surface electrodes placed over motor points in order to induce tetanic contractions of controlled intensity. This type of exercise of the paralyzed legs has the potential of utilizing a large muscle mass that otherwise would be dormant. In addition, FNS-induced exercise augments the circulation by activation of the venous muscle pump. Ultimately, FNS may bring SCI patients to higher fitness levels than can be attained with arm exercise alone. Quadriplegics will probably find such involuntary exercise particularly advantageous on account of the small muscle mass that is under voluntary control.

Special Considerations and Precautions

The foremost requirement for FNS use is that the muscles to be exercised are paralyzed due to upper motor neuron damage, and that the motor units (the lower motor neurons and the skeletal muscle fibers they innervate) are intact and functional. The existence of stretch reflex activity and spasticity indicate that the individual is a potential candidate for FNS exercise. However, if the patient retains some degree of sensate skin (which is common with incomplete SCI), FNS may cause discomfort or pain and the high stimulation current that is required to induce forceful contractions may not be tolerated. Although much of the instrumentation for FNS exercise was specially designed and constructed, the availability of commercial stimulators and exercise devices for clinical and home use is increasing.

Prior to initiating an FNS exercise program, a thorough medical examination is essential. This should include radiographs of the paralyzed limbs, range of motion testing, neurological examination, an ECG, and, preferably, evaluation of psychological status. The patient should be informed of the potential benefits and risks of FNS exercise, and clearly understand that FNS *will not* regenerate damaged neurons or cure paralysis. It should also be understood that, as with voluntary exercise training, any health and fitness benefits derived from FNS exercise training will be lost several weeks after this activity is discontinued.

Since the muscles, bones, and joints of the paralyzed lower limbs tend to be deteriorated, FNS-induced contractions should be kept as smooth as possible, and the contraction force generated should be limited to a safe level in order to prevent injury. Although FNS exercise training can improve the strength and endurance of the paralyzed muscles, there is currently no evidence that osteoporosis can be reversed by such activity (47). Therefore, it is conceivable that the muscles will ultimately generate more force than the bones can withstand. In addition, FNS may trigger severe spasms in some muscles, so it is important to observe the quality of the contractions to be certain that they are not hazardous (47,56). In some patients (especially quadriplegics), FNS exercise may provoke autonomic dysreflexia, with episodic dangerously high blood pressure (47,56). Therefore, it is essential that blood pressure be monitored periodically, especially during the initial FNS exercise sessions. Such exercise should be discontinued immediately if any response is observed that places the patient at risk.

Promoting Venous Return with FNS During Voluntary Arm Exercise

Arm exercise performance and the capability of developing high levels of cardiopulmonary fitness may both be limited by a hypokinetic circulation owing to an inadequate venous muscle pump. Although arm exercise in a supine position may help to alleviate this situation, FNS-based contractions of the paralyzed leg muscles is a promising alternative approach. Rhythmic contractions promote the venous return of blood, enhancing cardiac output and blood flow to the upper body musculature.

Glaser et al. (48) demonstrated that rhythmic patterns of FNS-induced isometric contractions (1.5–2.5 s on-off cycle) of the calf and thigh muscles increased the stroke volume and cardiac output (12–30% gain) in able-bodied and SCI individuals while resting in a sitting position. Davis et al. (17,18) and Figoni et al. (25) showed that this FNS technique augmented the stroke volume and cardiac output during both rest and ACE exercise a various gravitational loads (sitting, supine, and head-up tilt body positions). Thus, it appears that this technique can diminish venous pooling and alleviate the hypokinetic circulation in SCI patients. However, gains of maximal ACE PO and peak oxygen intake owing to the addition of FNS-induced leg muscle contractions and the impact upon long-term exercise training adaptations have yet to be determined. The FNS technique may have several other clinical applications, including deep venous thrombus prophylaxis, reducing excessive edema, and alleviating orthostatic hypotension (48). Again, research is needed to document the efficacy of FNS for these applications.

FNS-Induced Cycle Ergometry

In an effort to develop higher levels of cardiopulmonary fitness in SCI patients, a cycle ergometer propelled by the paralyzed legs was designed and constructed by Petrofsky et al. (76). Therapeutic Technologies Inc. (Tampa, Florida) began manufacturing sophisticated versions of this FNS cycle ergometer for clinical and home use in 1984. Computer-controlled FNS of the quadriceps, hamstrings, and gluteus maximus muscle groups is used to induce contractions at appropriate pedal positions (Fig. 6). When operating at the 50 rpm target, these

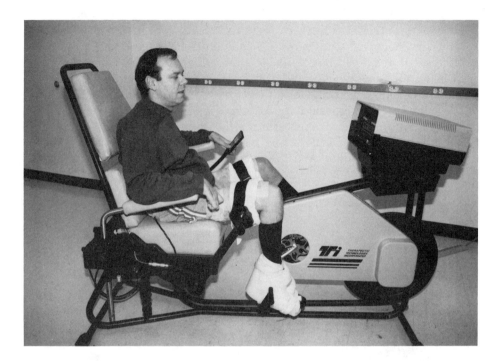

Figure 6   Functional neuromuscular stimulation (FNS) cycle ergometer exercise being performed by a spinal cord injured person on an ERGYS I device (Therapeutic Technologies, Inc.).

cycle ergometers induce 50 contractions of each contralateral muscle group per minute (a total of 300 muscle contractions per minute), the cyclic stimulation pattern and intensity being controlled by a microprocessor. When the pedal rate falls below 35 rpm, exercise is automatically terminated. The FNS cycle ergometry appears well suited for endurance training, as many SCI patients can pedal continuously for 30 min.

Training is typically scheduled three times per week. Initially, the patient pedals the FNS cycle ergometer at a PO of 0 W for up to 30 min. If fatigue occurs, three bouts are given in an attempt to achieve a total of 30 min of exercise. Each exercise bout is followed by 10 min of rest. When 30 min of continuous exercise can be achieved at 0 W, subsequent sessions are conducted at a PO of 6.1 W. When 30 min of continuous pedaling at this higher PO can be achieved, the PO is increased further by 6.1 W for subsequent sessions. As performance improves, intensity is further progressed to a limit of 42.7 W.

Physiological studies on SCI individuals indicate that FNS exercise elicits relatively large aerobic and cardiopulmonary responses as well as quite favorable central and peripheral hemodynamic responses (26,28,49,50,81). This suggests that it may provide more effective cardiopulmonary fitness training than arm exercise, especially for quadriplegics who have weakened arm musculature. Figure 7 provides data from Glaser et al. (50) depicting a steady-rate oxygen intake, respiratory minute volume, and heart rate of 12 SCI patients during

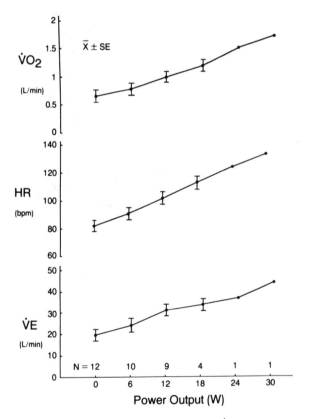

Figure 7 Steady-rate oxygen intake ($\dot{V}O_2$), respiratory minute volume ($\dot{V}E$), and heart rate (HR) responses of patients with spinal cord injury in relationship to power output for FNS cycle ergometry. (Modified from Ref. 50; used with permission.)

progressive-intensity FNS cycle ergometry. The relationships between PO and $\dot{V}O_2$, $\dot{V}E$, and HR seem quite linear. For this relatively untrained group of SCI patients, the PO ranged from 0 to 30 W. Only one patient could pedal at 30 W. He had a peak oxygen intake of 1.77 L/min, a respiratory minute volume of 45 L/min, and a heart rate of 135 beats/min. It is predicted from these data that a well-trained individual who could pedal at the PO limit of 42.7 W would have a peak oxygen intake of about 2 L/min with correspondingly high respiratory minute volume and heart rate responses. For comparison purposes, many able-bodied individuals jog at oxygen intakes of 1.5–2.0 L/min (50–60% of their maximal oxygen intake). Therefore, FNS cycling offers SCI patients a potential means of training at a similar aerobic metabolic rate to AB subjects. It is unlikely that arm exercise could elicit this magnitude of oxygen intake for a sufficient time (30 min) to stimulate marked cardiopulmonary adaptations. However, patients would need to be highly trained in order to achieve such high PO and oxygen intakes for long periods. Most SCI individuals perform FNS cycle ergometry at PO levels equivalent to walking (for example, an oxygen intake of about 1 L/min; 4 METs [metabolic equivalents]).

The PO levels used by SCI individuals for FNS cycle ergometry are quite low. For example, if a SCI patient can perform FNS cycling at 42.7 W, the oxygen intake is about 2 L/min. In contrast, an AB individual pedaling voluntarily at the same PO would have an oxygen intake of less than 0.9 L/min. Exercise utilizing FNS is mechanically *inefficient*, possibly owing to the nonphysiological activation of the paralyzed muscles, histochemical changes in these muscles, and inappropriate joint biomechanics (47,49,53). However, this inefficiency appears to be *desirable*, since greater metabolic and cardiopulmonary responses can be elicited by SCI patients for a given mechanical stress to their paralyzed muscles, bones, and joints.

Functional neuromuscular stimulation cycle ergometry may induce greater central hemodynamic responses than voluntary arm cranking in SCI patients. Figoni et al. (26) had six quadriplegic men perform FNS cycle ergometer exercise and, on another occasion, arm cranking exercise at POs that elicited an oxygen intake of approximately 1 L/min (11 and 38 W, respectively). The FNS cycling elicited a 59% greater stroke volume (92 versus 58 ml/beat) and a 20% greater cardiac output (8.01 versus 6.66 L/min). Figure 8 illustrates individual data of cardiac output against oxygen intake in 17 quadriplegics during voluntary ACE and FNS cycling exercise at an increasing PO (30). The likely mechanism for these responses is that FNS-induced contractions

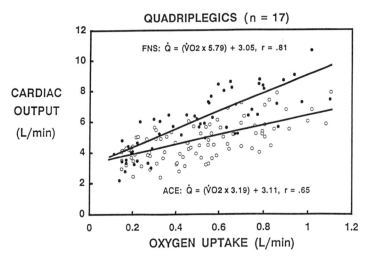

Figure 8 Individual data for cardiac output vs oxygen intake of 17 quadriplegics during voluntary ACE and FNS cycle ergometer exercise using progressive intensity power output levels. Linear regression equations and lines of best fit for ACE and FNS cycling are provided. (From Ref. 30; used with permission.)

of the paralyzed leg muscles activate the venous muscle pump and promote venous return, increasing cardiac preload. Figoni et al. (26) also found a 25% lower heart rate (87 versus 116 beats/min) and a 19% lower rate-pressure product during FNS cycling, suggesting that the higher cardiac volume load was achieved with lower myocardial O_2 demands. Therefore, FNS cycling is potentially more effective than arm cranking for cardiopulmonary training of quadriplegics, and also causes a lower cardiovascular risk.

Simultaneous FNS Cycling and Voluntary Arm Cranking Exercise

It appears likely that the cardiopulmonary fitness training capability of SCI patients could be further enhanced using a hybrid form of exercise (simultaneous FNS cycling and voluntary arm cranking) (Fig. 9). The physiological responses to this hybrid exercise (and other combination FNS–voluntary exercise modes) suggest that they provide superior cardiopulmonary training over either mode of exercise performed alone (17,46,55). This is to be anticipated because of the larger muscle mass

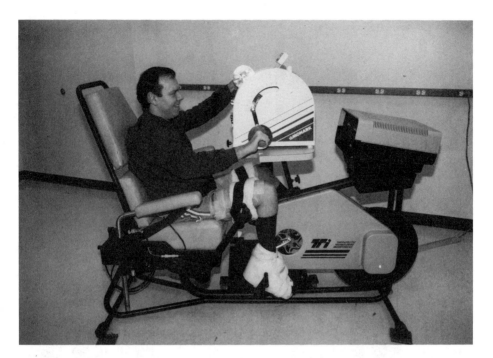

Figure 9 Hybrid (simultaneous FNS cycle ergometer and voluntary ACE) exercise being performed by a SCI person. The adjustable stand supporting the arm crank ergometer was specially designed and constructed.

utilized, the greater magnitudes of metabolic and cardiopulmonary responses elicited, and possible improvements in the circulation of blood to both the upper and lower body muscles.

Glaser (52) reported additive effects upon aerobic metabolism when combining the ACE and FNS leg cycling exercise. The oxygen intake of a T8 male paraplegic was 0.25 L/min at rest; 0.75 L/min during FNS cycling alone at 6.1 W; 0.75 L/min during voluntary arm cranking alone at 25 W; and 1.25 L/min during hybrid exercise at a total of 31.1 W. Hooker et al. (60) studied eight quadriplegics while performing this hybrid exercise, finding a significantly higher peak oxygen intake, respiratory minute volume, and cardiac output and a lower total peripheral resistance than when performing either arm cranking or FNS cycling alone. The similar stroke volumes obtained for FNS cycling and hybrid exercise were higher than for ACE (Fig. 10). Figoni et al. (29) combined 0-W (unloaded) FNS cycling with *maximal*

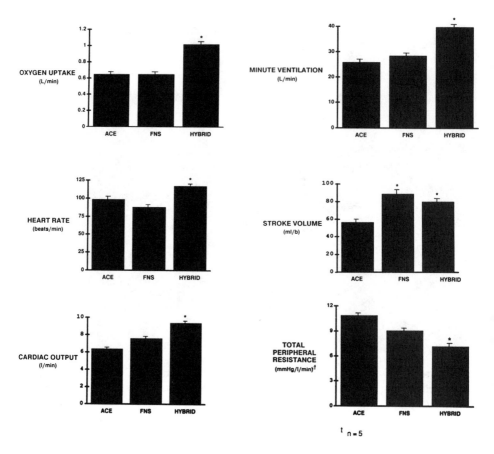

Figure 10 Oxygen intake, respiratory minute volume, heart rate, stroke volume, cardiac output, and total peripheral resistance of eight quadriplegics during voluntary ACE ($\bar{x}$ PO = 19.4 W), FNS cycling alone ($\bar{x}$ PO = 3.0 W), and hybrid exercise ($\bar{x}$ PO = 22.4 W). Values are $\bar{x} \pm$ SE. *Significant difference from ACE ($p < 0.05$). (Data to construct graphs from Ref. 60.)

effort arm cranking for nine quadriplegic subjects and found significant increases in peak oxygen intake (+0.3 L/min, +35%), stroke volume (+11 ml/beat, +26%), cardiac output (+2.7 L/min, +46%) and heart rate (+11 beats/min, +18%). The greater responses during hybrid exercise indicated that maximal effort arm cranking by itself is not a sufficient stimulus to drive the central circulation to full output. This apparently can be accomplished with the hybrid exercise owing to the substantially larger muscle mass utilized and the enhanced venous return and cardiac output that occurs with lower limb FNS.

Special attention needs to be given to the setting of arm and leg PO in order to attain the best compromise between a high oxygen intake and an extended exercise duration (30 min). In administering this hybrid exercise to a number of SCI paraplegics and quadriplegics, we noted an interaction between arm and leg exercises. That is, if the arm exercise intensity was increased beyond a certain level, it decreased the exercise capacity of the legs (shortening the exercise time at a given leg PO) and vice versa. This may be due to competition between the arms and legs for the available blood supply. It is thus probable that *central* circulatory factors rather than *peripheral* factors limit the capacity for this hybrid exercise. Therefore, hybrid exercise appears to provide optimal metabolic and cardiopulmonary responses for the aerobic conditioning of SCI individuals, whereas providing training benefits to both the upper and lower body musculature.

We find that hybrid exercise frequently results in peak oxygen intakes of over 1.5 and 2.0 L/min from nonathletic quadriplegic and paraplegic persons, respectively. Considering that maximal effort arm exercise for aerobically trained wheelchair athletes elicits peak oxygen intake values in the 2–3 L/min range (45), hybrid exercise appears to be superior, since similar peak oxygen intakes can then be obtained from the general population of SCI paraplegics.

Additionally, it is unlikely that arm exercise by itself can improve the lower limb circulation or integrity of the leg musculature. More research is needed to establish optimal protocols for hybrid exercise training, and to document the extent that cardiopulmonary fitness can be improved with long-term training by this technique.

CONCLUSIONS

During the past 20 years, much research has been dedicated to developing exercise techniques that can be used to evaluate and to improve the cardiopulmonary fitness of SCI patients. Traditionally, arm exercise modes (particularly ACE and WERG) have been used for these purposes. However, recent innovations in FNS techniques appear to be opening new avenues to more effective training. By using FNS to exercise paralyzed leg muscles, a greater muscle mass can be utilized and peripheral and central hemodynamic responses may be improved. The use of FNS-induced cycle ergometer exercise can elicit aerobic metabolic and cardiopulmonary responses of sufficient magnitudes and durations to stimulate cardiopulmonary training. These responses seem superior to those elicited by voluntary ACE exercise, especially for quadriplegics. Functional neuromuscular stimulation leg exercise is best used in conjunction with arm exercise (separately and combined) to optimize upper body, lower body, and cardiopulmonary fitness. Hybrid-type exercise is the most promising exercise technique for promoting the effective and efficient development of aerobic fitness in paraplegic and quadriplegic individuals. Ultimately, FNS exercise may contribute to improved health, physical fitness, and the rehabilitative potential of SCI individuals. However, more research is needed to develop safe and effective FNS exercise techniques and protocols, and to document the physiological responses, training benefits, and any reductions in cardiovascular problems.

ACKNOWLEDGMENTS

The author wishes to thank the Dayton Veterans Affairs Medical Center and the Rehabilitation Institute of Ohio at Miami Valley Hospital for enabling implementation of his research projects on wheelchair users. Most of the research projects from the author's laboratory were supported by the Rehabilitation Research and Development Service of the U.S. Department of Veterans Affairs.

REFERENCES

1. American College of Sports Medicine, *Guidelines for Graded Exercise Testing and Exercise Prescription*. Lee & Febiger, Philadelphia (1980).
2. Åstrand, P.-O., and Saltin, B., *J. Appl. Physiol.*, *16*: 977–981 (1961).
3. Åstrand, P.-O., Ekblom, B., Messin, R., Saltin, B., and Sternberg, J., *J. Appl. Physiol.*, *20*: 253–256 (1965).
4. Bar-Or, O., and Zwiren, L.D., *J. Appl. Physiol.*, *38*: 424–426 (1975).
5. Benton, L.A., Baker, L.L., Bowman, B.R., and Waters, R.L., *Functional Electrical Stimulation: A Practical Clinical Guide*. Professional Staff Association of the Rancho Los Amigos, Hospital, Downey, California (1981).
6. Bevegård, S., Freyschuss, U., and Strandell, T., *J. Appl. Physiol.*, *23*: 37–46 (1966).
7. Bergh, U., Kanstrup, I.-L., and Ekblom, B., *J. Appl. Physiol.*, *41*: 191–196 (1976).
8. Bobbert, A.C., *J. Appl. Physiol.*, *15*: 1007–1014 (1960).
9. Brattgard, S.-O., Grimby, G., and Höök, O., *Scand. J. Rehabil. Med.*, *2*: 143–148 (1970).
10. Bruce, D.A., Schut, L., and Sutton, L.N., *Primary Care, 11*: 175–194 (1984).
11. Clarke, K.S., *Arch. Phys. Med. Rehabil.*, *47*: 427–435 (1966).
12. Clausen, J.P., Klausen, K., Rasmussen, B., and Trap-Jensen, J., *Am. J. Physiol.*, *225*: 675–682 (1973).

13. Cole, T.M., Kottke, F.J., Olson, M., Stradal, L., and Niederloh, J., *Arch. Phys. Med. Rehabil.*, *14*:359–368 (1967).
14. Corbett, J.L., Frankel, H.L., and Harris, P.J., *Paraplegia*, *9*: 113–119 (1971).
15. Coutts, K.D., Rhodes, E.C., and McKenzie, D.C., *J. Appl. Physiol.: Respir. Environ. Exerc. Physiol.*, *55*:479–482 (1983).
16. Cybulski, G.R., Penn, R.D., and Jaeger, R.J., *Neurosurgery*, *15*: 132–146 (1984).
17. Davis, G.M., Servedio, F.J., Glaser, R.M., Collins, S.R., Gupta, S.C., and Suryaprasad, S.G., "Hemodynamic Responses During Electrically-Induced Leg Exercise and Arm Crank Ergometry in Lower-Limb Disabled Males." *Proc. 10th Ann. RESNA Conf. Rehabil. Tech.*, pp. 591–593.
18. Davis, G.M., Figoni, S.F., Glaser, R.M., Servedio, F.J., Gupta, S.C., and Suryaprasad, A.G., "Cardiovascular Responses in FNS-Induced Isometric Leg Exercise During Orthostatic Stress in Paraplegics." *Proc. Int. Conf. Assoc. Adv. Rehabil. Tech.*, pp. 326–327.
19. Davis, G.M., and Glaser, R.M., *Physiotherapy: Foundations for Practice Series* (L. Ada and C. Canning, eds.). Neurology Volume. Heinemann, London (in press).
20. Dearwater, S.P., LaPorte, R.E., Robertson, R.J., Brenes, G., Adams, L.L., and Becker, D., *Med. Sci. Sports Exerc.*, *18*: 541–544 (1986).
21. DeVivo, M.J., Fine, P.R., Maetz, H. M., and Stover, S.L., *Arch. Neurol.*, *37*: 707–708 (1980).
22. DiCarlo, S.E., Supp, M. D., and Taylor, H.C., *Phys. Ther.*, *63*: 1104–1107 (1983).
23. Emes, C., *Res. Q. Am. Assoc. Health Phys. Ed. Recreat.*, *48*: 209–212 (1977).
24. Engle, P., and Hildebrandt, G., *Paraplegia*, *11*:105–110 (1973).
25. Figoni, S.F., Davis, G.M., Glaser, R.M., Servedio, F.J., Gupta, S.C., Suryaprasad, A.G., Rodgers, M.M., and Ezenwa, B.N., "FNS-Assisted Venous Return in Exercising SCI Men." *Proc. Int. Conf. Assoc. Adv. Rehabil. Tech.*, pp. 328–329 (1988A).
26. Figoni, S.F., Glaser, R.M., Hendershot, D.M., Gupta, S.C., Suryaprasad, A.G., Rodgers, M.M., and Ezenwa, B.N., "Hemodynamic Responses of Quadriplegics to Maximal Arm-Cranking and FES Leg Cycling Exercise." *Proc. 10th Ann. IEEE Conf. Eng. Med. Biol.*, pp. 1636–1637 (1988).
27. Figoni, S.F., Gupta, S.C., Glaser, R.M., et al., *Rehabil. RD Prog. Rep.*, *25*: 108 (1988).
28. Figoni, S.F., Glaser, R.M., Hooker, S.P., Rodgers, M.M., Ezenwa, B.N., Faghri, P.D., Suryaprasad, A.G., Gupta, S.C., and Matthews, T., "Peak Hemodynamic Responses of SCI Subjects During FNS Leg Cycle Ergometry." *Proc. 12th Ann. RESNA Conf. Rehab. Tech.*, pp. 97–98 (1989).
29. Figoni, S.F., Glaser, R.M., Rodgers, M.M., Ezenwa, B.N., Hooker, S.P., Faghri, P.D., and Gupta, S.C., *Med. Sci. Sports Exerc.*, *21*: S96 (1989).
30. Figoni, S.F., Hooker, S.P., Glaser, R.M., Rodgers, M.M., Faghri, P.D.,

Ezenwa, B.N., Mathews, T., Suryaprasad, A.G., and Gupta, S.C., *Med. Sci. Sports Exerc.*, (Abst.) (in press).

31. Fox, E.L., and Mathews, D.K., *Interval Training: Conditioning for Sports and General Fitness.* Saunders, Philadelphia (1974).
32. Freyschuss, U., and Knuttson, E., *Life Sci.*, 8:421–424 (1969).
33. Gass, G.C., and Camp, E.M., *Med. Sci. Sports*, 11:256–259 (1979).
34. Glaser, R.M., Foley, D.M., Laubach, L.L., Sawka, M.N., and Suryaprasad, A.G., *Paraplegia, 16:* 341–349 (1978–79).
35. Glaser, R.M., Laubach, L.L., Sawka, M.N., and Suryaprasad, A.G., "Proceedings—International Conference on Lifestyle and Health, 1978: Optimal Health and Fitness for People with Physical Disabilities" (A.S. Leon and G.J. Amundson, eds.). University of Minnesota Press, Minneapolis, pp. 167–194 (1979).
36. Glaser, R.M., Sawka, M.N., Laubach, L.L., and Suryaprasad, A.G., *J. Appl. Physiol.: Respir. Environ. Exerc. Physiol., 46:* 1066–1070 (1979).
37. Glaser, R.M., Collins, S.R., and Wilde, S.W., "Power Output Requirements for Manual Wheelchair Locomotion." *Proc. IEEE Natl. Aerospace Elect. Conf., 2:* 502–509.
38. Glaser, R.M., Sawka, M.N., Brune, M.F., and Wilde, S.W., *J. Appl. Physiol.: Respir. Environ. Exerc. Physiol., 48:* 1060–1064 (1980).
39. Glaser, R.M., Sawka, M.N., Young, R.E., and Suryaprasad, A.G., *J. Appl. Physiol.: Respir. Environ. Exerc. Physiol., 48:* 41–44 (1980).
40. Glaser, R.M., and Collins, S.R., *Am. J. Phys. Med., 60:* 180–189 (1981).
41. Glaser, R.M., Sawka, M.N., Durbin, R.J., Foley, D.M., and Suryaprasad, A.G., *Am. J. Phys. Med., 60:* 67–75 (1981).
42. Glaser, R.M., Sawka, M.N., Wilde, S.W., Woodrow, B.K., and Suryaprasad, A.G., *Paraplegia, 19:* 220–226 (1981).
43. Glaser, R.M., Simsen-Harold, C.A., Petrofsky, J.S., Kahn, S.E., and Suryaprasad, A.G., *Ergonomics, 26:* 687–697 (1983).
44. Glaser, R.M., Sawka, M.N., and Miles, D.S., "Efficiency of Wheelchair and Low Power Bicycle Ergometry." *Proc. IEEE Natl. Aerospace Elect. Conf., 2:* 946–953 (1984).
45. Glaser, R.M., *Exercise and Sports Sciences Reviews, Vol. 13* (R.L. Terjung, ed.). Macmillan, New York, pp. 263–303 (1985).
46. Glaser, R.M., Strayer, J.R., and May, K.P., "Combined FES Leg and Voluntary Arm Exercise of SCI Patients." *Proc. 7th Ann. IEEE Conf. Eng. Med. Biol. Soc.*, pp. 308–313 (1985).
47. Glaser, R. M., *Cen. Nerv. Syst. Trauma, 3:* 49–62 (1986).
48. Glaser, R.M., Rattan, S.N., Davis, G.M., Servedio, F.J., Figoni, S.F., Gupta, S.C., and Suryaprasad, A.G., "Central Hemodynamic Responses to Lower-Limb FNS." *Proc. 9th Ann. IEE Conf. Eng. Med. Biol. Soc.*, pp. 615–617 (1987).
49. Glaser, R.M., *1988 American Association EMG Electrodiagnostic Didactic Progress*, pp. 21–26 (1988).
50. Glaser, R.M., Figoni, S.F., Collins, S.R., Rodgers, M.M., Suryaprasad, A.G., Gupta, S.C., and Mathews, T., "Physiologic Responses of SCI

Subjects to Electrically Induced Leg Cycle Ergometry." *Proc. 10th Ann. IEEE Conf. Eng. Med. Biol. Soc.*, pp. 1638–1640 (1988).

51. Glaser, R.M., *Med. Sci. Sports Exerc.*, 21: S149–S157 (1989).
52. Glaser, R.M., in *Current Therapy in Sports Medicine—2* (J.S. Torg, R.P. Welsh, and R.J. Shephard, eds.). B.C. Decker, Toronto, pp. 166–170 (1989).
53. Glaser, R.M., Figoni, S.F., Hooker, S.P., Rodgers, M.M., Ezenwa, B.N., Suryaprasad, A.G., Gupta, S.C., and Mathews, T., "Efficiency of FNS Leg Cycle Ergometry." *Proc. 11th Ann. IEEE Intl. Conf. Eng. Med. Biol. Soc.*, pp. 961–963 (1989).
54. Glaser, R.M., and Davis, G.m., in *Exercise in Modern Medicine: Testing and Prescription in Health and Disease* (B.A. Franklin, S. Gordon, and G.C. Timmis, eds.). Williams & Wilkins, Baltimore, pp. 237–267 (1989).
55. Glaser, R.M., in *Fitness for Aged, Disabled and Industrial Workers* (M. Kanecko, ed.). Human Kinetics, Champaign, Illinois, pp. 127–134 (1990).
56. Gruner, J.A., Glaser, R.M., Feinberg, S.D., Collins, S.R., and Nussbaum, N.S., *J. Rehabil. R D*, 20: 21–30 (1983).
57. Heldenberg, D., Rubinstein, A., Levtov, D., Werbin, B., and Tamir, I., *Atherosclerosis*, 39: 163–167 (1981).
58. Hildebrandt, G., Voigt, E.-D., Bahn, D., Berendes, B., and Kroger, J., *Arch. Phys. Med. Rehabil.*, 51: 131–136 (1970).
59. Hjeltnes, N., *Scand. J. Rehabil. Med.*, 9: 107–113 (1977).
60. Hooker, S.P., Glaser, R.M., Figoni, S.F., Rodgers, M.M., Ezenwa, B.N., Faghri, P.D., Mathews, T., Gupta, S.C., and Suryaprasad, A.G., "Physiologic Responses to Simultaneous Voluntary Arm Crank and Electrically-Stimulated Leg Exercise in Quadraplegics." *Proc. 12th Ann. RESNA Conf. Rehabil. Tech.*, pp. 99–100 (1989).
61. Hooker, S.P., and Wells, C.L., *Med. Sci. Sports Exerc.*, 21: 18–22 (1989).
62. Hrubec, Z., and Ryder, R.A., *J. Chron. Dis.*, 33:239–250 (1980).
63. Huang, C.-T., McEachran, A.B., Kuhlemeier, K.V., DeVivo, M.J., and Fine, P.R., *Arch. Phys. Med. Rehabil.*, 64:578–582 (1983).
64. Jackson, R.W., and Fredrickson, A., *Am. J. Sports Med.*, 7: 293–296 (1979).
65. Knutsson, E., Lewenhaupt-Olsson, E., and Thorsen, M., *Paraplegia, 11*: 205–216 (1973).
66. Kofsky, P.R., Davis, G.M., Shephard, R.J., Jackson, R.W., and Keene, G.C.R., *Eur. J. Appl. Physiol.*, 51: 109–120 (1983).
67. LaPorte, R.E., Adams, L.L., Savage, D.D., Brenes, G., Dearwater, S., and Cook, T., *J. Epidemiol.*, 120: 507–517 (1984).
68. Le, C.T., and Price, M., *J. Chron. Dis.*, 35: 487–492 (1982).
69. Magel, J.R., McArdle, W.D., Toner, M., and Delio, D.J., *J. Appl. Physiol.: Respir. Environ. Exerc. Physiol.*, 45: 75–79 (1978).
70. McArdle, W.D., Glaser, R.M., and Magel, J.R., *J. Appl. Physiol.*, 30: 733–738 (1971).
71. McArdle, W.D., Katch, F., and Katch, V., *Exercise Physiology: Energy, Nutrition, and Human Performance*. Lea & Febiger, Philadelphia (1986).

72. McCafferty, W.F., and Horvath, S.M., *Res. Q. Am. Assoc. Health Phys. Educ. Recreat., 48*: 358–371 (1977).

73. Miles, D.S., Sawka, M.N., Wilde, S.W., Durbin, R.J., Gotshall, R.W., and Glaser, R.M., *Ergonomics, 25*: 239–246 (1982).

74. Mortimer, J.T., in *Handbook of Physiology. The Nervous System II* (J.M. Brookhart, V.B. Mountcastle, V.B. Brooks, and S.R. Geiger, eds.). American Physiological Society, Bethesda, Maryland, pp. 155–187 (1981).

75. Nilsson, S., Staff, P.H., and Pruett, E.D.R., *Scand. J. Rehabil. Med., 7*: 51–56 (1975).

76. Petrofsky, J.S., Phillips, C.A., Heaton, H.H., III, and Glaser, R.M., *J. Clin. Eng., 9*: 13–19 (1984).

77. Pierce, D.S., and Nickel, V.H., *The Total Care of Spinal Cord Injuries.* Little, Brown, Boston (1977).

78. Pollack, S.F., Axen, K., Spielholz, N., Levin, N., Haas, F., and Ragnarsson, K.T., *Arch. Phys. Med. Rehabil., 70*:214–219 (1989).

79. Pollock, M.L., Miller, H.S., Linnerud, A.C., Laughridge, E., Coleman, E., and Alexander, E., *Arch. Phys. Med. Rehabil., 55*: 418–424 (1974).

80. Pollock, M.L., Wilmore, J.H., and Fox, S.M., *Exercise in Health and Disease: Evaluation and Prescription for Prevention and Rehabilitation.* Saunders, Philadelphia (1984).

81. Ragnarsson, K.T., O'Daniel, W., Edgar, R., Pollack, S., Jr., Petrofsky, J., and Nash, M.S., *Arch. Phys. Med. Rehabil., 69*: 672–677 (1988).

82. Reybrouck, T., Heigenhauser, G.F., and Faulkner, J.A., *J. Appl. Physiol., 38*: 774–779 (1975).

83. Sawka, M.N., Glaser, R.M., Wilde, S.W., Miles, D.S., and Suryaprasad, A.G., *Fed. Proc., 39*: 287 (1980) (Abst.).

84. Sawka, M.N., Glaser, R.M., Wilde, S.W., and von Luhrte, T.C., *J. Appl. Physiol.: Respir. Environ. Exerc. Physiol., 49*: 784–788 (1980).

85. Sawka, M.N., Glaser, R.M., Laubach, L.L., Al-Samkari, O., and Suryaprasad, A.G., *J. Appl. Physiol.: Respir. Environ. Exerc. Physiol., 50*: 824–828 (1981).

86. Sawka, M. N., in *Exercise and Sport Sciences Review.* Vol. 14 (K.B. Pandoff, ed.). Macmillan, New York: pp. 175–210 (1986).

87. Schwade, J., Blomqvist, C.G., and Shapiro, W., *Am. Heart J., 94*: 203–208 (1977).

88. Simmons, R., and Shephard, R. J., *Int. Z. Angew. Physiol., 30*: 73–84 (1971).

89. Smith, P.A., Glaser, R.M., Petrofsky, J.S., Underwood, P.D., Smith, G.B., and Richards, J.J., *Arch. Phys. Med. Rehabil., 64*: 249–254 (1983).

90. Stauffer, E.S., in *The Total Care of Spinal Cord Injuries* (D.S. Pierce and V.H. Nickel, eds.). Little, Brown, Boston, pp. 81–102 (1978).

91. Stenberg, J., Åstrand, P.-O., Ekblom, B., Royce, J., and Saltin, B., *J. Appl. Physiol., 22*: 61–70 (1967).

92. Thorstensson, A., *Acta Physiol., Scand., 100*: 491–493 (1977).

93. Traugh, G.H., Corcoran, P.J., and Reyes, R.L., *Arch. Phys. Med. Rehabil.*, *56*: 67–71 (1975).
94. Voight, E.-D., and Bahn, D., *Scand. J. Rehabil. Med.*, *1*: 101–106 (1969).
95. Vokac, Z., Bell, H., Bautz-Holter, E., and Rodahl, K., *J. Appl. Physiol.*, *39*: 54–59 (1975).
96. Whiting, R.B., Dreisinger, T.E., and Abbott, C., *South. Med. J.*, *76*: 1225–1227 (1983).
97. Wicks, J.R., Lymburner, K., Dinsdale, S.M., and Jones, N.L., *Paraplegia*, *15*: 252–261 (1977–78).
98. Wicks, J.R., Oldridge, N.B., Cameron, B.J., and Jones, N.L., *Med. Sci. Sports Exerc.*, *15*: 224–231 (1983).
99. Wilde, S.W., Glaser, R.M., Sawka, M.N., Miles, D.S., and Fox, E.L., *Fed. Proc.*, *39*: 289 (Abst.) (1980).
100. Wilde, S.W., Miles, D.S., Durbin, R.J., Sawka, M.N., Suryaprasad, A.G., Gotshall, R.W., and Glaser, R. M., *Am. J. Phys. Med.*, *60*: 277–291 (1981).
101. Wolfe, G.A., Waters, R., and Hislop, H.J., *Phys. Ther.*, *57*: 1022–1027 (1977).
102. Yekutiel, M., Brooks, M.E., Ohry, A., Yarom, J., and Carel, R., *Paraplegia*, *27*: 58–62 (1989).
103. Young, J.S., Burns, P.E., Bowen, A.M., and McCutcheon, R., *Spinal Cord Injury Statistics: Experience of the Regional Spinal Cord Injury Systems*. Good Samaritan Medical Center, Phoenix (1982).
104. Zwiren, L.D., and Bar-Or, O., *Med. Sci. Sports*, *7*:94–98 (1975).

16

The Costs and Benefits of Exercise Programs in Secondary and Tertiary Prevention

Roy J. Shephard

University of Toronto
Toronto, Ontario, Canada

INTRODUCTION

It is now widely considered that physical inactivity is a costly luxury, in large part because it increases the risk of chronic conditions such as ischemic heart disease. However, the extent of the resultant economic loss remains uncertain for several reasons (42,43,48):

1. There is no clear agreement as to the value of various types of exercise program in the secondary and tertiary prevention of chronic disease.*

2. Some estimates of the costs of chronic disease have "lumped" expenses for a major element in the accounts (chronic cardiovascular disease) as a single composite item, whereas the periods of hospitalization and thus the costs of treating the different cardiovascular diseases, such as hypertension, ischemic heart disease, and congestive failure, vary substantially from one disorder to another (38).

3. Many of the imputed costs of chronic disease are indirect, attributable to losses in productivity, the biggest expense being premature death. If a person survives and continues working through to the

---

*Secondary prevention is used here in its epidemiological sense—the prevention of clinical manifestations in a person who already has subclinical disease. Tertiary prevention refers to exercise prescribed after the onset of clinical symptoms.

normal age of retirement, there is no agreement as to whether one should calculate the economic gain *as the full additional salary that is earned* (20), or merely as the added value of the individual's contribution to society, perhaps 25% of the annual income (38).

4. The rate of participation in the labor force is currently changing quite rapidly; because of automation there will in the future be progressively less societal need for people to continue working through 65 or 70 years of age (48).

5. Some allowance must be made for losses of production that arise from caring for the sick and from the grief of bereavement; however, in the absence of better information, most authors merely ascribe an arbitrary percentage of total costs to this term (19).

6. Chronic disease, by definition, has a long and uncertain lag period before disabling clinical manifestations appear. The predicted benefits from secondary and tertiary prevention lie some years distant, and are highly susceptible to the investigator's assumptions regarding the discount rate (this rate is a device that economists use to assess the willingness of society to sacrifice now for future good). Different authors have applied values, ranging widely from 0 to 10% per annum; if benefit is not anticipated for 10–20 years, variations of discount rate have a major impact upon estimated savings from preventive programs (39).

Despite these problems and other difficulties to be discussed below, there is agreement that the costs of chronic disease are very large, possibly approaching $8000 per worker per year, measured in 1990 U.S. dollars (20). Moreover, a substantial part of the expense is related to conditions associated with a poor lifestyle (including a lack of physical activity).

In this final chapter, we will attempt to relate potential savings from a planned increase of physical activity to the costs of the necessary programs, looking at the issues of both secondary and tertiary prevention.

COST/BENEFIT AND COST/EFFECTIVENESS ANALYSES

The principles governing cost/benefit and cost/effectiveness analyses of exercise programs in particular have been discussed in several recent monographs (39,42,43).

A cost/benefit analysis suffers from certain important limitations. While the minimization of medical costs is an important, and sometimes a highly ethical function, the optimizing of a simple cost/benefit equation cannot be the only concern of a health professional. Particular problems arise from the inclusion of lost production in such calculations. A rigid cost/benefit analysis makes it easier to justify the provision of an exercise program for a highly paid senior executive than for a lower-level production-line worker. By a further extension of such logic, little economic justification can be found for attempts at rehabilitating a severely disabled patient who is unlikely to return to work. Moreover, once the age of retirement has been reached, no patient has any apparent economic value, and a cost/benefit approach would argue against allocation of resources to an improvement of health in the senior citizen. Such a totalitarian view of society is ethically unacceptable, and ignores the real contribution that many old people, paralegics, and permanently disabled patients bring to a community.

Cost/effecitveness and cost/utility analyses avoid some of these pitfalls. The costs of various forms of treatment, such as the prolonged use of β-blockers, angioplasty, bypass surgery, and cardiac transplant operations can be compared with the costs of preventive and rehabilitative programs in terms of a specific outcome—a unit cost per added year of productive work, or per added year of quality-adjusted lifespan (10,16,23,56). The costs of many traditionally recommended medical treatments are quite high. For example, a main coronary artery bypass operation costs a health insurer about $5500 per year of quality-adjusted life in North American (53) or $2750 in the United Kingdom (56,57), but (because the prognosis without surgery is better than for main-vessel disease) a bypass operation for single-vessel disease costs about $55,000 to add a year of quality-adjusted life (QALY) (Table 1). In general, any treatment can be regarded as "effective" if the cost per QALY is less than $25,000, "ineffective" at a cost of over $125,000, and debatable between $25,000 and $125,000. However, the conclusion which is reached depends very much upon the completeness of costing. For example, account should be taken of the time that must be invested in hospital visits or participation in exercise programs. Such a time investment is of more concern to the time-conscious ("type A") personality than to a relaxed ("type B") individual; the type A individual will be anxious to ensure that a large part of the nominal class time is devoted to conditioning rather than to ancillary goals of the program such as social interaction between participants, and a time-oriented patient may also be tempted to exceed the prescribed intensity or duration of an exercise prescription in an attempt to hasten the training process.

Drastic surgical treatment such as a cardiac transplant operation may extend life by a couple of years, but it may also be necessary to spend a substantial part of the added lifespan in special investigative

Table 1   Concept of Quality Adjusted Lifespan

Mobility	Physical activity	Social activity
Drove car and used bus or train without help (5)	Walked without physical problems (4)	Did work, school, or housework and other activities (5)
Did not drive or had help to use bus or train (4)	Walked with physical limitations (3)	Did work, school, or housework but other activities limited (4)
In house (3)	Moved own wheelchair without help (2)	Limited in amount or kind of work, school, or housework (3)
In hospital (2)		
In special care unit (1)	In bed or chair (1)	Performed self-care but did no work, school, or housework (2)
		Had help with self-care (1)

Each year of survival is multiplied by a time-specific quality of wellness score which is integrated (in terms of utility, relative desirability, and social preference). Typical items considered in reaching an appropriate multiplier are listed.
Source: From Ref. 16; used with permission.

and treatment facilities, so that the apparent extension of lifespan must be heavily discounted in terms of QALY (16). Likewise, the exercising patient may invest much of any added survival time either in the prescribed exercise program itself or in traveling to and from an exercise facility. Accepting Paffenbarger's (31) estimate that an optimum exercise program extends the lifespan of a middle-aged adult by 2 years (Table 2), the corresponding physical activity (perhaps 5 h/week, continued over 50 years of adult life) requires more than 2 years of 16-h waking days to undertake (even ignoring related travel time). If the exercise (plus the associated travel to the chosen recreational site) is enjoyed (as in most rural recreation), this may be seen as a good investment of time, which need not necessarily be included in the final balance sheet. But if the program involves tedious urban driving to the recreational facility, and the prescribed physical activity is itself perceived as burdensome, then the time that is used or the "opportunity foregone" should probably be costed. Likewise, involvement in a community exercise program can make a very positive contribution to the

Table 2   The Influence of an Active Lifestyle[a] upon the Years of Added Life to an Age of 80 Years, as Estimated from Mortality Data on Harvard Alumni, 1962–1978

Starting age (years)	Years gained[b]
35–39	2.51
40–44	2.34
45–49	2.10
50–54	2.11
55–59	2.02
60–64	1.75
65–69	1.35
70–74	0.72
75–79	0.42
35–79[c]	2.15

[a] An active lifestyle is here defined as expending an average of 8.4 MJ/week (2000 kcal/week) or more in walking, stair climbing, and sports play, with gains expressed relative to all subjects with a lower energy expenditure.

[b] Data adjusted for cigarette smoking, hypertension, low gain of body mass since university, and early potential mortality.

[c] Weighted average for period specified.

Source: From Ref. 31; used with permission.

life of some families, but for others, a worksite, rehabilitation center, or even a community-based program is disruptive, to the point that a cost should be assessed, probably at an average industrial wage ($12 or even $15/h). If time is indeed costed in this way, then an interval program may appear to be less cost-effective than a continuous training plan, and the patient may be attracted to short bouts of intensive exercise in the hope that these will achieve results comparable to what could have been achieved by a longer period of more moderate activity.

A further variable is compliance. Surgery is a once-only event. However, most types of medical treatment require sustained patient compliance, and close enquiry reveals a major attenuation of the presumed effectiveness of treatment because the prescribed medication is no longer taken. Likewise, the number of patients persisting with an exercise prescription declines exponentially with time (21,41). The impact of any program thus depends upon the product of therapeutic effectiveness and anticipated compliance with the prescribed therapy.

JUSTIFICATION OF CARDIAC FOCUS

Exercise has a potential benefit in many areas of secondary and tertiary prevention. However, it is easiest to illustrate the issues of cost/effectiveness with reference to the secondary and tertiary prevention of ischemic heart disease for several reasons:

1. There have already been serious attempts to estimate the enormous direct and indirect costs attributable to cardiac disease (Table 3) (20,37,38).
2. Exercise is a very safe form of treatment even for the patient with advanced cardiac disease; Noakes (27) has estimated that a year of supervised exercise is six times less risky than the immediate chances of dying from coronary by-pass surgery. There is thus little danger that the adverse effects of exercise will outweigh the potential health benefits.
3. The costs of even a tertiary preventive program seem quite low relative to some surgical alternatives (for example, Noakes [27] has equated the cost of coronary vascular by-pass surgery with that of 74 years of participation in a supervised phase III tertiary exercise program).

Table 3   Annual Costs to U.S. Economy of Ischemic Heart Disease

	Annual cost (billion dollars)
Direct cost:	
Personal services and supplies (hospital care, services of physicians and nurses, provision of drugs)	2.6
Nonpersonal items (research, training, public health services, capital construction, and insurance schemes)	0.5
Indirect costs:	
premature death	19.4
loss of output from illness	3.0
intangible effects upon productivity (pain, suffering, orphanhood, etc.).	5.2
Total	30.7

All costs expressed in 1962 U.S. dollars; 1990 costs would be more than three times larger.
Source: From Ref. 19; used with permission.

4. Regular physical exercise has substantial therapeutic value in both the secondary (32,41,44) and the tertiary (29,47) prevention of ischemic heart disease.
5. An exercise prescription is pleasant and positive advice relative to the dour medical prohibitions that are a part of the advice needed by some cardiac patients; given effective leadership, the long-term compliance with an exercise program may be better than for other types of prolonged medical treatment (41).
6. Nevertheless, a need to practice "defensive medicine" has led to a substantial escalation of exercise program costs, particularly in the United States, to the point that some medical insurance schemes are now refusing reimbursement of the costs of exercise therapy for all except a few categories of patient (15).

The time thus seems particularly appropriate to make a critical analysis of the cost/effectiveness of exercise, with specific reference to chronic cardiovascular disease.

SOME PROBLEMS IN THE ANALYSIS OF ECONOMIC BENEFITS

We have already noted some major difficulties in assessing the costs of chronic disease. There are substantial problems when examining other elements in the cost/effectiveness calculation, including potential variations in the proposed treatment program and its social setting, disagreements about appropriate discount rates, uncertainties about the economic value of prolonged survival, and a need to reach decisions regarding the attribution of any fiscal benefits.

Variations of Treatment and Social Setting

It is important to emphasize at the outset of this section that the costs of an exercise program vary widely depending upon the type of regimen that is recommended and its social setting. Exercise, either for the secondary or for the tertiary prevention of chronic disease, can range from a simple home program with a minimum of supervision and equipment to a carefully monitored prescription pursued in a purpose-built facility (Table 3). In some instances, exercise is the sole direct form of intervention, but more commonly the patient receives associated lifestyle counseling, and (in the case of tertiary prevention) there is likely to be some monitoring of the medical condition and adjustment of drug prescriptions where needed.

The social setting ranges from the highly technological free-enterprise system of North America through social democracies and centralized state economies to developing societies with very limited resources. The social environment has a major impact upon the costs of both exercise and alternative forms of treatment. In North America, most adults expect an exercise program to be associated with a professionally supervised center that uses expensive testing and exercise equipment, but in Dunedin, New Zealand, moderate hill walking is an accepted low-cost alternative source of physical activity for the "postcoronary" patient, and in developing societies, the demands of daily occupation may still provide a sufficient source of energy expenditure. Likewise, the costs of medical and surgical treatment differ two- or threefold even between Canada and the United States, whereas in developing societies, both the available therapeutic options and their costs will be very different from the North American expectation.

The present calculations refer mainly to North American society, but where possible figures from other cultures are included for purposes of comparison. In general, a high-intensity program reduces the costs of exercise because its duration is shorter. However, if the increase of intensity is such as to demand more professional supervision, more sophisticated monitoring, or more elaborate exercise equipment, a low-intensity program may remain the most cost-effective type of treatment.

Discounting of Benefits

We have already noted that much of the benefit imputed to an exercise program develops after an extended and uncertain lag period, and is thus highly susceptible to assumptions about the discount rate. Some investigators have assumed a figure equal to the average inflation-adjusted return on government bonds or industrial investments. Others have applied an artificially high discount rate to compensate for what they regard as excessive claims for the benefits of exercise. Others, again, have based a sensitivity analysis upon several potential discount rates, ranging from 0 to 10% (39,48).

In comparing the benefits from various exercise programs it may be necessary to consider whether gains are likely to appear after a short or a long lag period, although in the steady state, uncertainties arising from differences of discount rate should disappear, since program costs are incurred by one cohort of patients as benefit is reaped by an earlier cohort, and the discount rate then effectively drops to zero.

Extended Survival

Assessments of the economic value of survival assume that the individual concerned is able and willing to work, and has the opportunity to do so. However, willingness to work in such groups as cardiac and wheelchair patients depends more upon social and psychological factors than upon any exercise-generated increase of physical working capacity (41,49). For example, the Toronto Rehabilitation Centre is an outpatient facility servicing a predominantly white-collar population. In this setting, the physical demands of work are low, motivation is high, and 86% of patients have returned to work within 6 months of sustaining a myocardial infarction. However, in a rural area of southeastern Sweden, where the main occupation is lumber cutting, the climate is cold, and government social benefits are easily obtained, only 50–55% of patients choose to return to work following myocardial infarction (35). A further imponderable is the *need* for work in a postindustrial society. Many economic analysts have assumed as a norm a 95% employment rate continuing through to an age of 65 or even 70 years, but a displacement of labor-intensive industries from North America to the Third World and the automation of factories are together steadily decreasing employment opportunities for older individuals in developed countries. An increasing proportion of patients are thus choosing not to return to work following myocardial infarction or spinal injury, while the retirement of employees is encouraged at an ever-earlier age.

Some actuaries have also expressed a concern that far from saving costs, a lengthening of lifespan will actually increase the load upon overburdened pension funds (39,46). In fact, both the economic and the personal impact of longer survival depend very much upon the quality of any added years of life. Is this likely to be a period of good health, or will there be gross incapacitation from angina and heart failure? Recent Canadian studies suggest that the average senior citizen spends 8–9 years with some degree of disability, and a final year of total dependency (3,45). The enormous societal costs of supporting a growing elderly population reflect the need for institutional care rather than the expense of feeding and clothing the fit elderly (42). Paffenbarger has stressed that the years added by an exercise program are quality living rather than a period of costly dependency, and available data suggest that the survival curves for active and sedentary individuals come together in extreme old age (32,34) (Fig. 1), in what Fries (9) has termed a "squaring" of mortality curves. The actuarial fears thus appear largely unwarranted.

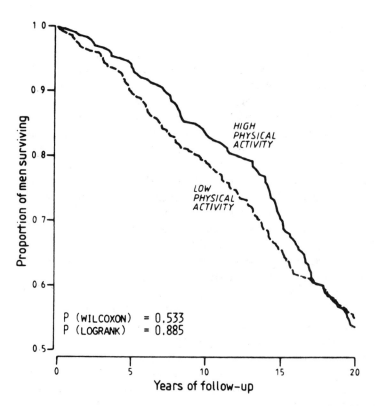

Figure 1 Cumulative mortality curves for inactive and active populations living in Finland. Note that survival curves for the two groups come together in old age. (From Ref. 34; used with permission.)

Attribution of Costs and Benefits

Most economic analyses ignore any transfer payments between one sector of the economy and another (39,48). Nevertheless, in worksite exercise programs, the attribution of any economic benefits between the employee and the worker becomes an issue of hot debate. Ideally, decisions should be based upon the implications of a given policy for society as a whole. However, if a company is being asked to sponsor a program of secondary exercise therapy, or an insuring agency is considering a scale of reimbursement for tertiary preventive programs (13,15,18), the tendency is to focus upon costs and benefits within a single sector of the economy. Thus, an insuring agency would be quite interested in a potential reduction of future cardiac incidents and resultant disability payments, but would take much less account of the opportunity costs that a patient might incur through the time committed to participation in a specific type of preventive program.

DIRECT COSTS OF AN EXERCISE PROGRAM

The direct costs of an exercise program include expenditures for personal services and supplies (for instance, the services of a physician and an exercise professional who are prescribing and supervising the activity, plus the patient's travel costs and the charges for any special clothing and equipment that are regarded as necessary for a particular pursuit), together with less readily measured nonpersonal items (research in the exercise sciences, investment in the training of sports physicians and exercise supervisors, the promotion of regular physical activity by government agencies, the capital construction of exercise facilities by municipalities and private enterprise, and the insurance of program operators against exercise-related accidents).

Secondary Exercise Therapy

The direct cost of secondary exercise therapy for the middle-aged, coronary-prone individual depends greatly upon the scale of intervention that is contemplated. Possible options include an increase of normal daily physical activity, the development of specific worksite programs, and the use of existing community resources.

In middle-aged and older people, substantial endurance training and thus the prevention of various "diseases of inactivity" can result from encouraging an increase of normal daily physical activities, particularly vigorous walking (25,32). In surveys of Harvard alumni, Paffenbarger and associates found that much of the protection against heart disease was attributable to deliberate walking; likewise Morris and associates found that British civil servants were protected against fatal heart attacks by what they termed "vigorous getting about" (apparently, rapid walking). The societal costs of activities such as walking are quite limited—certainly, there is no call for the patient to seek an extensive preliminary medical clearance, day-by-day supervision of the exercise is unnecessary, and costly facilities are not required. National governments may spend some money in promoting this type of activity through various forms of advertising, and municipalities may face a call for the paving (and in Canada and northern U.S. states snow ploughing) of sidewalks. However, if walking is seen as a means of transportation within the community, there may also be some economic savings because of a reduced demand for parking spaces and/or feeder bus lines. The individual will need to purchase additional shoes, socks, and food (a total expenditure of perhaps $300/year), but if the required walking is built into the daily schedule, the opportunity cost may be surprisingly small. It is interesting to contrast jogging with walking. Because the legs are subjected to a greater impact stress, the jogger finds a need to purchase special and often costly shoes. Body temperature rises to a much greater extent, so that the jogger is reluctant to wear normal clothing; instead, a special jogging suit is purchased (indeed, if the climate is extreme, the patient may buy several uniforms appropriate to different weather conditions). There is a need to shower after jogging, and except in the rare instances when such facilities are available at the place of work, jogging cannot be used as a method of daily transportation; it thus has a substantially higher opportunity cost than walking. Finally, because of the greater average intensity of activity, many middle-aged joggers find it prudent to have periodic medical evaluations and specific prescription of a suitable personal jogging pace.

It has been argued that worksite classes offer the most cost-effective type of organized exercise program (43). Many of the fixed overhead costs of an exercise program are lower at the worksite. Publicity channels and peer-support networks are already established, and easy access to the facility eliminates most of the opportunity cost of related travel (42). On the other hand, the quality of the recreational experience in a renovated office basement or a corner of the shop floor tends to be less than could have been found in the alternative setting of a rural resort; the hour devoted to exercise may thus be seen as a time-consuming duty rather than a pleasure. The accounting for some industrial programs takes little notice of the costs of serviced space, arguing that the area which has been allocated to the exercise class was previously underused or unused. However, the construction of a specially designed exercise facility is very expensive, particularly if it is located in a downtown office tower, and unless the hours of work are flexible, there is a danger that a worksite facility may lie empty for a large part of the day and most of the night. Typical program costs for a combination of staff, equipment, and serviced space range from $100 to $400 per worker (Table 4), or with 20% participation in the exercise class, $500–$2000 per participant per year. Unfortunately, such facilities currently attract only the keen 20% of employees (21). The marginal cost of attracting lazier employees would probably be much greater, and the usual worksite exercise/lifestyle program totally fails to reach such important target groups as the elderly, women with young children, the disabled, and the unemployed.

Table 4   Costs of Alternative Tactics for the Delivery of a Secondary Preventive Exercise Program Within the Context of Corporations of Varying Size

Expected number of participants	Recommended facility	Cost per participant-year
<400	Campus-wide facility with full-time supervisor	$300–500
5–50	Minimal facility, testing and exercise prescription only (? visiting team)	$150–500
75–250	150–300 m^2 facility with part- or full-time supervisor	$365–500
400–850	600–1,200 m^2 facility[a] with full-time supervisor	$300–500

All costs expressed in 1983 dollars.

[a] If participation rate is 20%, 600 m^2 for 400 participants provides a space standard of 0.3 m^2 per worker.

Note. Based in part on a concept of R.S. Wanzel, 1979, "Rationale for Employee Fitness Programs." In: *Employee Fitness, the How To.* Ed.: R.S. Wanzel (pp. 1–16), Toronto: Ontario Ministry of Culture and Recreation.

Land costs are much lower in the suburbs than in the center of a city, although the necessary acreage for the physical facility, parking, and access roads still represents a large fraction of total program costs (43). The per participant expense depends largely upon the degree of success in ensuring usage of the facility over a large part of the day throughout much of the year. For instance, swimming lakes and cross-country ski trails have great aesthetic appeal, reducing their opportunity cost; on the other hand, such facilities are relatively ineffective as a means of promoting greater physical activity within a community because their use is limited to a few weeks in each season. The cost of heavily used urban recreational facilities such as skating rinks lies in the range $38–$220 per citizen per year, or with $20 utilization, $190–$1100 per participant-year (43).

Tertiary Exercise Programs

Insurance companies are scrutinizing the direct costs of tertiary exercise programs ever more closely (15). For example, exercise treatment during the first 3 months after myocardial infarction (phase I and phase II programs) can be very expensive—particularly if the physician insists upon continuous electrocardiographic monitoring of exercise responses over this period (4,7,8,24,52). In the United States, costs for this early phase of treatment may amount to $4500–$5500, and because of a limited reimbursement by insurers, there are strong financial incentives to patient noncompliance. While debate continues on the merits of close electrocardiographic and medical surveillance of postcoronary patients (11,40,52), the optimal solution will probably lie in a careful gradation of risk and a corresponding stratification of monitoring procedures (11,33).

The costs during the third phase of postcoronary rehabilitation are more typical of clinical exercise programs for other conditions such as chronic chest disease. Figures still vary widely with the extent of medical supervision, counseling, and exercise testing that is made available. The most economical arrangement is a home program, with visits to a supervising clinic every 1–2 months (or sooner if untoward symptoms appear); some training is possible with such an arrangement, but both the intensity of effort and the conditioning response are less than can be obtained by more closely supervising activity (17); on the other hand, the risks of sudden death (although still less than 1 in 100,000 h of physical activity), appear to be several times higher when exercising alone than when exercising in a clinic (51). A typical small hospital program in Sweden involves a salaried physician, two physiotherapists, and one trainee physiotherapist to supervise a group of sixteen postcoronary patients; a total of 27 rehabilitation sessions are provided over a period of 2 years, and after adding an arbitrary 10% allowance for materials and equipment, a cost of $156, or about $6 per patient-session, is estimated (12,35). In the United States, the postcoronary patient often undertakes a phase III program at a community institution such as a YMCA. The main expense is then for medically supervised stress testing; with two stress tests per patient ($450 each) and a thrice-weekly program ($450, or about $2 per patient-session), the cost of a 21-month program would be about $1350. With such an arrangement, the weekly exercise sessions are lightly supervised by paramedical health professionals, but otherwise seem of good value; given the variability in such signs as ST segmental depression from one day to another (1), it is more debatable whether the stress tests are cost effective. In Australia, a typical combination of two exercise tests and a thrice-weekly conditioning program costs a total of about $825 per patient (37). At the Toronto Rehabilitation Centre, a medically supervised exercise program is provided throughout the treatment period; this involves one salaried physician, one physiotherapist, and three student assistants per class of 50 patients. The personal costs of a single 1-hr class per week then amount to about $3 per participant; figures of this order have also been cited for medically supervised programs in the United States (36,58). The main advantage of having a physician present at testing sessions is not the occasional cardiac resuscitation (paramedical professionals could undertake this just as effectively as a medically qualified doctor); rather, the physician has an opportunity to examine the reactions of the patient to exercise, to evaluate any symptoms that have been reported, and to match the objective conditioning response against the extent of training that has been noted in the patient's diary records. Many economic analyses of clinical exercise programs ignore the use of space; if a gymnasium is occupied by a single class of cardiac patients, meeting one to three times per week, the annual cost of this serviced space may easily amount to $400–$500 per patient. In Toronto, Johanna Kennedy (administrator of the Toronto Rehabilitation Centre), has estimated the total cost of a 4-year tapered phase III program at $1720 per participant; this figure includes five routine exercise tests per patient, medically supervised exercise sessions held once weekly for the first year, and monthly for a further 6 months, telemetry during exercise sessions, and a 24-h ambulatory monitoring of the ECG when required, further exercise tests if required, telephone or personal access to their exercise supervisor, and psychological screening. Although the cost of the program is quite high, it nevertheless compares very favorably with that of a briefer U.S. program that provides only paramedical supervision of exercise classes. The high costs in the United States reflect a combination of extensive patient surveillance by nonsalaried medical staff, attempts to recoup rapidly the costs of expensive test equipment, and a major allowance for insurance against contingency litigation.

In a large city such as Toronto, the opportunity costs associated with participation in a medically supervised exercise class are perhaps the heaviest expense faced by the patient. Program participants can easily invest 2 h in travel to and from the rehabilitation center, bringing the total opportunity cost to 3 h, or $36–$45 per session. Two years of thrice weekly attendance would thus demand a total investment of $10,800–$13,500, and even the simplified Toronto plan generates an opportunity cost of $2160–$2700 over 4 years, more than the direct costs of the program.

CALCULATING THE ECONOMIC BENEFITS OF EXERCISE

Although there are ethical objectives to basing treatment decisions upon a rigid cost/benefit analysis, it is nevertheless of interest to calculate the likely savings from participation in a secondary or tertiary program of preventive exercise.

Economic Benefits of Secondary Prevention

The potential economic benefits from a program of secondary preventive exercise include both acute and chronic gains. In the short term, the individual feels better. He or she is thus more productive at work and makes fewer demands for the medical treatment of minor complaints. In a longer-term perspective, there is a probable decrease in the direct personal and nonpersonal costs of illness, together with indirect savings related to lost production, premature death, and the associated intangible costs of pain, suffering, and invalid care imposed upon relatives.

In the North American economy, acute gains accrue mainly to the employer, providing an economic incentive for the development of employee fitness and lifestyle programs (42,43,48). Possible benefits include an improvement of corporate image, the recruitment of premium employees, a lesser rate of employee turnover, greater productivity, reduced absenteeism, and fewer industrial injuries (48). Depending upon the employee participation rate, the cumulative benefit to the company may be as large as $500/worker/year; however, the largest item in the balance sheet is a reduction in the costs due to employee turnover (Table 5). It is plainly arguable that if all companies developed similar worksite exercise programs, then a specific company program would provide little or no incentive to remain with a particular corporation, effectively removing this item from the benefit side of the ledger. Program participation is rapidly associated with a lesser

Table 5   Estimate of the Financial Benefits Accruing from an Employee Fitness Program

Benefit	Fiscal saving
Employment in fitness services	Labor-intensive
Worker satisfaction	Higher quality production—less warranty work
Productivity	$116/worker-year
Absenteeism	$ 30/worker-year
Turnover	$324/worker-year
Industrial injury	$ 43/worker-year
Health insurance premiums	Reduced (?32%)
Company image	Enhanced by in-house program
Total	$513/worker-year

All data expressed in 1982 U.S. dollars.
Source: From Ref. 42; used with permission.

demand for medical services, presumably because of an enhanced per-ceived health rather than an early reduction in organic illness (14). In Canada, the associated fiscal savings accrue to government health insurance programs, and only indirectly to the corporation or the indi-vidual (through a possible reduction in provincial taxation); however, in the United States, some companies have found reductions in medi-cal claims of up to $500/worker/year, and in consequence they have been able to negotiate more favorable contracts with medical insurance agencies (48). A final dividend, which is very difficult to cost, is the sense of personal health experienced by the exercise participant. In practical terms, this is perhaps one of the most important reasons why many people engage in regular physical activity.

In a long-term perspective, the most important anticipated saving is the avoidance of premature death, with resultant gains in produc-tion. Allowing 100% of the additional salary that the individual should earn through to the age of normal retirement, Klarman (19) set the total indirect costs of cardiac disease at $27.6B in the U.S. economy of 1962, or in 1990 dollars, more than $100B dollars, almost $1000/worker/year. Australian estimates (37,38) are only about a quarter of this figure, partly because the global term "cardiac disease" has been broken down into such elements as myocardial infarction, hyperten-sion, and congestive failure, but largely because the allowance for lost production has been set at 25% of the anticipated income through to normal retirement (43).

To what extent might participation in an exercise program curb these enormous costs? Studies of both worksite and community sug-gest that regular vigorous physical activity can decrease the "coronary" death rate by 25–50% (25,30,32,41,44). There is less evi-dence that the physical activity will reduce the incidence of non-fatal attacks; however, the proportion of fatal attacks becomes smaller, and a previously active person tends to develop a less severe infarct, so that the costs of convalescence are less than for a sedentary and obese patient. The imputed economic benefit depends greatly upon the vari-ous assumptions that are made, including the societal impact of a pro-longed loss of production (25% or 100% of the salary that is no longer earned?), the decrease in the incidence of "cardiac" deaths (25% or 50%?), and (since the benefit from exercise depends upon continuing participation) the anticipated long-term compliance with a fitness pro-gram (10 or 20%?). On the most optimistic set of assumptions, the sav-ing would be ($1000 × 100% × 50% × 20%) or $100/worker-year, but on the most conservative assumptions it would drop as low as ($1000 × 25% × 25% × 10%) or about $6.25/worker-year. Whichever figure is correct, the reduction of premature deaths would not in itself provide economic justification for more than the simplest of exercise programs. However, we can add to these figures more substantial savings arising from a short-term improvement of perceived health; the resultant decreases in medical consultations and usage of hospital beds have led to economies ranging from $142 to $500/worker-year (48). As already noted, the improvement of mood state also has a positive effect upon work performance (48) which would amount to $500/worker-year.

While an exercise program often cannot be justified in terms of its impact upon the costs of cardiac disease, it becomes an economically attractive option if the balance sheet also reflects the short-term benefits of an improved mood state.

Tertiary Prevention

Economic justification for exercise as a form of tertiary prevention might be sought in a prolongation of life, a decrease in the recurrence rate of events such as myocardial infarction, and an earlier return to work following an initial illness.

As with secondary prevention, most of the available information relates to the postcoronary patient. Current evidence suggests that there is a 20–30% reduction in the incidence of fatal reinfarctions in response to a program of endurance exercise (Table 6) (2,29,47), with no significant change in the number of nonfatal recurrences. The potential economic impact can be estimated as follows. The typical postcoronary mortality rate with standard treatment is about 4% a year (41). Given also an average age of 45 years, as in the Toronto Rehabilitation Centre population, and an annual income of $22,000, the cost in the first year would amount to $880 per patient. On the most optimistic assumptions (societal contribution 100% of salary, 30% reduction in fatal recurrence rate with exercise, 50% of patients sustain an appropriate dose of training) the estimated saving for 1 year would be (880 × 100% × 30% ×50%) or $132/patient. If the patients who have been spared the fatal heart attack continue to work and to exercise for an average of 10 years, the cumulative impact would amount to $1320/ patient-year. On less optimistic assumptions (average age of the patient 55 years, 25% societal contribution of salary, 20% reduction in fatal recurrence rate, 25% of patients sustain an appropriate dose of training, period of renewed work 5 years), the estimated saving would drop to (880 × 25% × 20% × 25%), $11 over the first year, with a cumulative impact of $55/patient-year. To such savings may be added a variable benefit from earlier return to work and a lesser likelihood of subsequent retirement. Differences in the number of patients working both 6 months and 5 years after myocardial infarction have favored exercise by a margin of 5–10% (5), 14% (19), 17% (26), 27% (55), or 30% (6). On an optimistic assumption (50% of patients participate effectively in the exercise program, with a resultant 30% difference in overall workforce participation), the economic impact might be ($22,000 × 50% × 30%), or $3300/patient-year, whereas on a more conservative assumption (25% effective exercise participation, 10% increase of workforce participation), the benefit would drop to ($22,000 × 25% × 10%), or $550/patient-year.

Detailed observation of blue-collar workers in a rural area of southeastern Sweden support the order of benefit indicated by these calculations, the rehabilitated group earning an average of $2552 per year more than controls over a 5-year period (35). Likewise, a Russian study (26) noted that over the first year of operation, an exercise rehabilitation program yielded dividends of 805 roubles per patient, about U.S. $1459 at official exchange rates, based mainly upon gains in productivity. A benefit of $4.30 per $1.00 invested was suggested, putting the cost of the Russian exercise program at $339/patient-year. Other analyses from Lithuania (6) have reported that standard patterns of treatment were associated with an economic loss that was 94% greater than that observed with exercise rehabilitation (this would correspond, for instance, with a return to work of 61 and 80% in the two groups of patients).

Variables modifying the above estimates plainly include the average age of the person when disability is first incurred, the success in sustaining enthusiasm for the exercise class, the extent of available social benefits and thus the personal incentives to seek employment after rehabilitation, opportunities for employment of the older worker, and (in heavy industry) the potential to modify the individual's job description to allow lighter work. Over the first year following myocardial infarction, it may be quite difficult to justify exercise therapy simply in terms of greater productivity, although in a 5- to 10-year perspective, the cumulative economic impact of a greater return to work and continuing production could well match the cost of a phase III exercise program. A further probable long-term benefit is an improvement of perceived health—particularly a lightening of depression. Mood state is important as a determinant of both productivity and demands for medical care even in the person without overt disease. It is likely to be of paramount importance after the establishment of a clinical illness.

Table 6 Results of Major Randomized Trials of Exercise in the Tertiary Prevention of Myocardial Infarction

Author	Sample size	Entry	Follow-up	Treatment	Exercise group			Control group			Therapeutic benefit
					N	deaths	annual%	N	deaths	annual%	ex/control
Kentala (1972)	298 (165)[a]	6–8 weeks	1 year	Individual supervised, 2–3/weeks	152 77[c]	26 11	17.1 7.2	146 81[c]	32 11	21.9 6.9	0.81 1.04
Kallio (1981)	375 (74F, 301M)	Hospital discharge (2 weeks)	3 year	Exercise + health education	188	41	7.3	187	56	9.9	0.73
Kallio et al. (1988)	375 (74F, 301M)	Hospital discharge (2 weeks)	10 year (3-year progress)	Exercise + health education	188[c]	82	8.2	187[c]	97	9.7	0.85
Hamalainen et al. (1988)	456	Hospital discharge (2 weeks)	6 years (3/12 program)	Exercise + health education (controls received community-based program)	228	45[d]	7.5	228	55[d]	9.2	0.82
Palatsi (1976)	380	2–3/12	29 months (1-year program)	Daily home program (nonrandomized allocation based on time of recruitment)	180	18	4.1	200	28	5.8	0.64
Wilhelmsen et al. (1975)	315 (35F, 280M)	3 months	4 years	Individually supervised 3/week (hospital-based)	158	28	4.4	157	35	5.6	0.80
Shaw (1981)	651	2–36 months	3 years	Individually supervised 3/week	323	15	1.3	328	24	2.1	0.63

Study	n		Duration of exercise	Duration of follow-up	Program	N	Deaths	%	N	Deaths	%	Ratio
Rechnitzer et al. (1983)	751	733 retained	2–12 months	3–4 years	Partially supervised (2–4/week); (controls received homeopathic exercise)	379	15[d]	0.98	354	13[d]	0.91	1.08
Vermuelen et al. (1983)	98	—	—	5 years	—	47	2	0.85	51	5	1.90	0.45
Marra et al. (1985)	161		2 months	4.5 years	Individually supervised, increasing to 4/week (controls received homeopathic exercise)	81	6	1.35	80	5	1.90	0.45
Roman (1985)	193		2 months	Up to 9 years	Individually supervised, 2–4/week	93	16	3.6	100	27	5.8	0.59
Carson et al. (1982)	303		6 weeks	25 months	Individually supervised	151	12	3.9	152	21	7.9	0.57
Lamm et al.[b] (1982)	1360		4–12 weeks	3 years (6-week/3-year program)	Individually supervised 3/week	705	105	5.0	655	105	5.3	0.93
Total	5325					(370)			(447)			(0.83)

[a] Numbers suitable for long-term follow-up.

[b] Excluding (1) data of Kallio, (2) centers with low-level of follow-up, and (3) centers with significant baseline differences (see Ref. 29 for details).

[c] Same subjects as previous sample.

[d] Coronary deaths + assuming 4-year follow-up of all subjects.

CONCLUSIONS

If conservative assumptions are made about the likely fiscal benefits from an increase of physical activity, it becomes quite difficult to justify the costs of either secondary or tertiary exercise programs simply in terms of a reduction in economic losses from continuing illness and premature death. However, regular exercise also has a marked effect upon mood state and perceived health. In the symptom-free adult, a secondary preventive program may thus lead to a substantial enhancement of industrial performance and a substantially reduced demand for incidental medical services. After myocardial infarction, such benefits are likely to be even more important, and in a 5- to 10-year perspective such items can more than repay the costs of a comprehensive phase III cardiac rehabilitation program. Exercise is indeed a cost-effective method of treatment.

Nevertheless, the primary reason for advocating exercise is not to save money. Rather, it is a pleasant, readily accepted form of therapy which is better received than most medical or surgical alternatives. It is on such grounds that we should commend it to our patients, both those who are ostensibly healthy and those who already have developed clinical disability.

REFERENCES

1. Bailey, D.A., Shephard, R.J., and Mirwald, R.L., *Can. J. Appl. Sport Sci.*, 1: 67–78.
2. Bobbio, M., "Does Post-myocardial Infarction Rehabilitation Prolong Survival? A Meta-analytic Survey." Proceedings of the Fourth World Congress of Cardiac Rehabilitation, Brisbane, p. 92 (1988) (Abst.).
3. Canada Health Survey, Ottawa: Health & Welfare Canada (1982).
3a. Carson, P., Phillips, R., Lloyd, M. *et al.* Exercise after a myocardial infarction: A controlled trial. *J. Roy. Coll. Phys. Surg.* 16: 141–147 (1982).
4. Dolatowski, R.P., Squires, R.W., Pollock, M.L., Foster, C.R., and Schmidt, D.H., *Med. Sci. Sports Exerc.*, 15;281–286 (1983).
5. Dwyer, T., and Rutherford, R., "Cost and Benefit in Cardiac Rehabilitation—Tertiary Rehabilitation." Proceedings of the Fourth World Congress of Cardiac Rehabilitation, Brisbane, p. 87 (1988) (Abst.).
6. Estany, E.R., de Leon, O.P., Chesa, C.S., Duenas, A., and Canero, A.H., "Influence of Comprehensive Cardiac Rehabilitation on Return to Work After Myocardial Infarction." Proceedings of the Fourth World Congress of Cardiac Rehabilitation, Brisbane, p. 145 (1988) (Abst.).
7. Fardy, P.S., Doll, N., Taylor, J., and Williams, M., Monitoring cardiac patients: How much is enough. *Physician. Sportsmed.*, 10(6): 145–154 (1982).

8. Fletcher, G.F., and Cantwell, J.D., *Chest, 71*: 27–32 (1977).
9. Fries, J.F., *N. Engl. J. Med., 303*: 130–135 (1980).
10. Gudex, C., *QALYs and Their Use by the Health Service*. Centre for Health Economics, University of York, England (cited in Ref. 24) (1986).
10a. Hamalainen, H., Kallio, V., and Arstila, M. Late mortality after first myocardial infarction: Effect on rehabilitation. Proceedings of IVth World Congress of Cardiac Rehabilitation, Brisbane, October, p. 93 (1988).
11. Haskell, W.L., in *Clin. Sports Med.—Symp. Cardiac Rehabil., 3*(2): 455–469 (1984).
12. Hedback, B., Perk, J., and Engvall, J., "Cardiac Rehabilitation After Coronary By-pass Grafting—Socio-economic Results." Proceedings of the Fourth World Congress of Cardiac Rehabilitation, Brisbane, p. 110 (1988) (Abst.).
13. Herbert, D.L., *Exerc. Stand. Malpract. Reporter, 2*(1): 1–6 (1988).
14. Herzlich, C., *Health and Illness*. Academic Press, London (1973).
15. Humphrey, R., *J. Cardiopulmon. Rehabil., 8*: 276–278 (1988).
15a. Kallio, V., Evaluation of earlier studies: Europe. In: L.S. Cohen, M.B. Mock, and I. Ringqvist (eds), *Physical Conditioning and Cardiovascular Rehabilitation*. New York: Wiley, pp. 257–270 (1981).
15b. Kallio, V., Hamalainen, H., Hakkila, J., Luurila, O., Knuts, L.-R., and Arstila, M. Multifactorial intervention programme after acute myocardial infarction; 10 years follow-up. Proceedings, IVth World Congress of Cardiac Rehabilitation, Brisbane, p. 67 (1988).
16. Kaplan, R.M., in *Behavioral Epidemology and Disease Prevention* (R.M. Kaplan and M.H. Criqui, eds.). Plenum Press, New York, pp. 31–56 (1985).
17. Kavanagh, T., and Shephard, R.J., *Arch. Phys. Med. Rehabil., 61*: 114–118 (1980).
18. Kelly, J.J., *Cardiac Rehabilitation Guidelines*. Blue Cross and Blue Shield of Virginia, Richmond (1986).
18a. Kentala, E. Physical fitness and feasibility of physical rehabilitation after myocardial infarction in men of working age. *Annals of Clinical Research 4* (Suppl. 9):1–84 (1972).
19. Klarman, H.E., in *The Heart and Circulation. Second National Conference on Cardiovascular Disease. Vol. 2, Community Services and Education* (E.C. Andrus, ed.). U.S. Public Health Service, Washington, D.C. (1964).
20. Klarman, H.E., in *Preventive and Community Medicine* 2nd Ed. (D.W. Clark and B. MacMahon, eds.). Little, Brown, Boston, pp. 603–615 (1981).
20a. Lamm, G., Denolin, H., and Dorossiev, D. Rehabilitation and secondary prevention of patients after acute myocardial infarction: WHO collaborative study. *Advances in Cardiology* 31:107–111 (1982).
21. Leatt, P., Hattin, H., West, C., and Shephard, R.J., *Can. J. Publ. Health, 79*: 20–25 (1988).
22. Luce, B.R., "Principles of Cost/Benefit Analysis." Proceedings of the Fourth World Congress of Cardiac Rehabilitation. Brisbane, p. 86 (1988) (Abst.).

22a. Marra, S., Paolillo, V., Spadaccini, E., and Angelino, P.F. Long-term follow-up after a controlled randomized post-myocardial infarction rehabilitation programme: Effects of morbidity and mortality. *European Heart Journal* 6:656–663 (1985).

23. Maynard, A., *Br. Med. J., 295*: 1537–1541 (1987).

24. Mitchell, M., Franklin, B., Johnson, S. and Rubenfire, M. *Arch. Phys. Med. Rehabil., 65*: 463–466 (1984).

25. Morris, J.N., Everitt, M.G., Pollard, R.L., Chave, S.P.W., and Semmence, A.M., *Lancet, 2*: 1207–1210 (1980).

26. Nikolaeva, L.F., Karpova, G.D., Rubanovich, A., Evdakov, V.A., Aronov, D.M., Aleshin, O.I., Modorova, A.A., Zhydko, N.I., and Deev, A.D. "Medical, Social and Economic Effectiveness of the USSR National Staged MI Patients Rehabilitation Programme." *Proceedings of the Fourth World Congress of Cardiac Rehabilitation.* Brisbane, p. 118 (1988) (Abst.).

27. Noakes, T.D., *S. Afr. Med. J., 62*: 238–240 (1982).

28. Office of Technology Assessment, *A Review of Selected Federal Vaccine and Immunization Policies.* United States Congress (1979).

29. Oldridge, N.B., Guyatt, G.H., Fischer, M.E., and Rimm, A.A., *J.A.M.A., 260*: 945–950 (1988).

30. Paffenbarger, R., in *Exercise in Cardiovascular Health and Disease* (E.A. Amsterdam, J.H. Wilmore, and A.N. deMaria, eds.). Yorke Medical Books, New York, pp. 35–49 (1977).

31. Paffenbarger, R., *Med. Sci. Sports Exerc., 20*: 426–438 (1988).

32. Paffenbarger, R., Hyde, R.T., Wing, A.L., and Hsieh, C.C., *N. Engl. J. Med., 314*: 605–613.

32a. Palatsi, I. Feasibility of physical training after myocardial infarction and its effects on return to work, morbidity and mortality. *Acta Medica Scandinavica 599* (Suppl):7–84 (1976).

33. Parmley, W.W., *Cardiology, 15*(3): 4–5 (1986).

34. Pekkanen, J., Marti, B., Nissinen, A., Tuomilehto, J., Punsar, S., and Karvonen, M.J., *Lancet,* 1(8548): 1473–1477 (1987).

35. Perk, J., and Hedback, B., "Cost Effectiveness of Cardiac Rehabilitation." Proceedings of the Fourth World Congress of Cardiac Rehabilitation. Brisbane, p. 110 (1988) (Abst.).

36. Pyfer, H.R., and Doane, B.L., in *Exercise Testing and Exercise Training in Coronary Heart Disease* (J.P. Naughton, H.R. Hellerstein, and I.C. Mohler, eds.). Academic Press, New York, pp. 365–369 (1973). 7–84.

36a. Rechnitzer, P.A., Cunningham, D.A., Andrew, G.M. Buck, C.W., Jones, N.L., Kavanagh, T., Oldridge, N.B., Parker, J.O., Shephard, R.J., Sutton, J.R., and Donner, A. Relation of exercise to the recurrence rate of myocardial infarction in men. Ontario Exercise-Heart Collaborative Study. *American Journal of Cardiology* 51:65–69 (1983).

37. Reznik, R., "The Cost of Cardiac Disease." Proceedings of the Fourth World Congress of Cardiac Rehabilitation. Brisbane, p. 86 (1988) (Abst.).

38. Roberts, A.D., *The Economic Benefits of Participation in Regular Physical Activity.* Recreation Ministers' Council of Australia, Canberra, Australia, pp. 1–32 (1982).

38a. Roman, O. Do randomized trials support the use of cardiac rehabilitation? *Journal of Cardiac Rehabilitation* 5:93–96 (1985).

39. Russell, L.B., *Is Prevention Better Than Cure?* Brookings Institute, Washington, D.C., pp. 1–129 (1986).
40. Sennett, S.M., Pollock, M.L., Pels, A.E., Foster, C., Dolatowski, R., Laughlin, J., Patel, S., and Schmidt, D.H., *J. Cardiopulmon. Rehabil.*, 7: 458–465 (1987).
40a. Shaw, L.W. Effects of a prescribed supervised exercise program on mortality and cardiovascular morbidity in patients after myocardial infarction. The National Exercise and Heart Disease Project. *American Journal of Cardiology* 48:39–46 (1981).
41. Shephard, R.J., *Ischemic Heart Disease and Exercise.* Croom Helm, London, pp. 1–428 (1981).
42. Shephard, R.J., *Economic Benefit of Enhanced Fitness.* Human Kinetics, Champaign, Illinois, pp. 1–210 (1986).
43. Shephard, R.J., *Fitness and Health in Industry.* Karger, Basel, pp. 1–316 (1986).
44. Shephard, R.J., *Sports Med.*, 3: 26–49 (1986).
45. Shephard, R.J., in *International Perspectives on Adapted Physical Activity* (M.E. Berridge and G.R. Wards, eds.). Human Kinetics, Champaign, Illinois, pp. 235–242 (1987).
46. Shephard, R.J., *Physical Activity and Aging.* 2nd Ed. Croom Helm, London, pp. 1–354 (1987).
47. Shephard, R.J., *Physician Sportsmed.*, 16(6): 116–127 (1988).
48. Shephard, R.J., *Sports Med.*, 7: 286–309 (1989).
49. Shephard, R.J., *Fitness Assessment and Programming for Disabled Populations—Research and Practice.* Human Kinetics, Champaign, Illinois (1990).
50. Shephard, R.J., Corey, P., and Kavanagh, T., *Med. Sci. Sports Exerc.*, 13: 1–5 (1981).
51. Shephard, R.J., Kavanagh, T., Tuck, J., and Kennedy, J., *J. Cardiac. Rehabil.*, 3: 321–329 (1983).
52. Simoons, M., Lap, C., and Pool, J., *Am. Heart J.*, 100: 9–14 (1988).
53. Torrance, G.W., *J. Health Economics*, 5: 1–30 (1986).
54. Van Camp, S.P., and Peterson, R.A., *J.A.M.A.*, 256: 1160–1163 (1986).
55. Vasilauskas, D., Krisciunasx, A., and Lazaravicius, A., "Rehabilitation of Post-Infarctional Patients: Socio-Economic Effectiveness." *Proceedings of the Fourth World Congress of Cardiac Rehabilitation.* Brisbane, p. 144 (1988) (Abst.).
55a. Vermeulen, A., Lie, K.I., and Durrer, D. Effects of cardiac rehabilitation after myocardial infarction: Changes in coronary risk factors and long-term prognosis. *American Heart Journal* 105:798–801 (1983).
55b. Wilhelmsen, L., Sanne, H., Elmfeldt, D., Grimby, G., Tibblin, G., and Wedel, H. Controlled trial of physical training after myocardial infarction. *Preventive Medicine* 4:491–508 (1975).
56. Williams, A., *Br. Med. J.*, 291: 326–329 (1985).
57. Williams, A., *Screening for Risk of Coronary Heart Disease* (M. Oliver, M. Ashley-Miller, and D. Wood, eds.). Wiley, London (1986).
58. Zohman, L.R., in *Exercise Testing and Exercise Training in Coronary Heart Disease* (J.P. Naughton, H.R. Hellerstein, and I.C. Mohler, eds.). Academic Press, New York, pp. 329–336 (1973).

Index

Acetohexamide, 329
Acute cardiac failure, 399–400
Acute responses to exercise, 2–5
  duration, 2–4
  psychological reactions, 4–5
β-Adrenergic blocking drugs,
  452–454
Aerobic exercise:
  intensity of, 90–93
  sustained, 4
Aerobic power (VO_{2max}), 55–57
  in the cardiac population,
    237–238
  changes in patients following
    CABGS/PTCA, 285–287
  in children with congenital
    heart disease, 414–416
  classification of, 71–72
  criteria used to establish
    attainment of, 70
  direct measurement of, 65–66
  effect of children's physical
    activity on, 114–119

(Aerobic power *continued*)
  in the elderly, 190–195
    benefits from endurance
      training program, 218
  in healthy children, 413–414
  improved, in DM patients,
    340–341
  measures of, 59–65
  prediction of, 57
  walking or jogging speed
    based on, 100
  the wheelchair disabled and,
    472–473
Aging:
  distinguishing disease from,
    189–190
  functional classification of, 188
  gradations of, 188
Air pollution effects on training
  program, 35–37
Ambulatory monitoring for the
  detection of myocardial
  ischemia, 383–384

527

About the Editors

ROY J. SHEPHARD is Professor of Applied Physiology, School of Physical and Health Education, and Department of Preventive Medicine and Biostatistics, Faculty of Medicine, University of Toronto, Ontario, Canada, and Consultant to the Toronto Rehabilitation Centre. The author of or coauthor of over 700 journal articles, book chapters, and abstracts, and author or coauthor of approximately 20 books, he is a former president of the American College of Sports Medicine and the Canadian Association of Sports Sciences, an Honorary Fellow and Vice-President of the British Association of Sport and Medicine, Honorary Fellow of the Belgian Society of Sports Medicine, and Fellow of the American Academy of Physical Education. Dr. Shephard received the B.Sc. degree (1949) in physiology, M.B.B.S. degree (1952) with distinction in forensic medicine and public health, Ph.D. degree (1954) in science, and M.D. degree (1959) from the University of London, England.

HENRY S. MILLER, Jr. is Professor of Internal Medicine/ Cardiology and Medical Director, Cardiac Rehabilitation Program, Section of Cardiology, Department of Medicine, Bowman Gray School of Medicine, Wake Forest University, Winston-Salem, North Carolina. The author or coauthor of nearly 70 journal articles, book chapters, and abstracts, he is a former president of the American College of Sports Medicine and a Fellow of the American College of Physicians,

American College of Cardiology, Council on Clinical Cardiology, American College of Sports Medicine, Council on Epidemiology, and American Association of Cardiovascular and Pulmonary Rehabilitation. Dr. Miller received the B.S. degree (1950) in medical science and M.D. degree (1954) from Wake Forest University, Winston-Salem, North Carolina.